Bayesian Analysis of Infectious Diseases

Chapman & Hall/CRC Biostatistics Series

Series Editors
Shein-Chung Chow, Duke University School of Medicine, USA
Byron Jones, Novartis Pharma AG, Switzerland
Jen-pei Liu, National Taiwan University, Taiwan
Karl E. Peace, Georgia Southern University, USA
Bruce W. Turnbull, Cornell University, USA

Recently Published Titles

Biomarker Analysis in Clinical Trials with R
Nusrat Rabbee

Interface between Regulation and Statistics in Drug Development
Demissie Alemayehu, Birol Emir, Michael Gaffney

Innovative Methods for Rare Disease Drug Development
Shein-Chung Chow

Medical Risk Prediction Models: With Ties to Machine Learning
Thomas A Gerds, Michael W. Kattan

Real-World Evidence in Drug Development and Evaluation
Harry Yang, Binbing Yu

Cure Models: Methods, Applications, and Implementation
Yingwei Peng, Binbing Yu

Bayesian Analysis of Infectious Diseases
COVID-19 and Beyond
Lyle D. Broemeling

Statistical Meta-Analysis using R and Stata, Second Edition
Ding-Geng (Din) Chen and Karl E. Peace

Advanced Survival Models
Catherine Legrand

Structural Equation Modeling for Health and Medicine
Douglas Gunzler, Adam Perzynski and Adam C. Carle

For more information about this series, please visit: https://www.routledge.com/Chapman--Hall-CRC-Biostatistics-Series/book-series/CHBIOSTATIS

Bayesian Analysis of Infectious Diseases

COVID-19 and Beyond

Lyle D. Broemeling

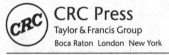

CRC Press
Taylor & Francis Group
Boca Raton London New York

CRC Press is an imprint of the
Taylor & Francis Group, an **informa** business

A CHAPMAN & HALL BOOK

First edition published 2021
by CRC Press
6000 Broken Sound Parkway NW, Suite 300, Boca Raton, FL 33487-2742

and by CRC Press
2 Park Square, Milton Park, Abingdon, Oxon, OX14 4RN

© 2021 Lyle D. Broemeling

CRC Press is an imprint of Taylor & Francis Group, LLC

ISBN: 978-0-367-63386-8 (hbk)
ISBN: 978-1-003-12598-3 (ebk)

Typeset in Palatino
by SPi Global, India

Contents

Author

Lyle D. Broemeling, Ph.D., is Director of Broemeling and Associates Inc., and is a consulting biostatistician. He has been involved with academic health science centers for about 20 years and has taught and been a consultant at the University of Texas Medical Branch in Galveston, The University of Texas MD Anderson Cancer Center and the University of Texas School of Public Health. His main interest is in developing Bayesian methods for use in medical and biological problems and in authoring textbooks in statistics. His previous books are *Bayesian Biostatistics and Diagnostic Medicine,* and *Bayesian Methods for Agreement.*

1

Introduction to Bayesian Inferences for Infectious Diseases

1.1 Introduction

This book will introduce the reader to the latest Bayesian techniques that analyze the behavior of infectious diseases. A preview of the book is presented, followed by a list of references, and ending with online resources that provide information about emerging infectious diseases and allied subjects.

1.2 A Preview of the Book

Chapter 2 describes the foundation of Bayesian statistics. First, Bayesian theorem is given for both discrete and continuous measurements. This necessitates an explanation of the components of Bayes theorem, namely prior information, the posterior distribution of the unknown parameters, and the predictive distribution of future observations. Also provided in this chapter are many examples that illustrate Bayes theorem, among then the standard populations, such as the binomial, the normal, the Poisson, the multivariate normal, and the multinomial, and the Dirichlet.

Chapter 3 explicates the biology and evolutionary behavior of infectious diseases, including viral and bacterial manifestations of the contagion. Next to be explained is that of the immune response via antibodies that attack the invading pathogens. The immune response involves various blood cells (white, red, and platelets) that defend against the disease. Next to be described are drugs that attempt to destroy the components of the disease. A good example of this is quinine and related drugs that control the malaria virus, and drugs that can nearly eradicate the HIV virus of AIDS patients. Although drugs have been very successful in controlling diseases, drug resistance can become a serious issue. This was the case for streptomycin, the breakthrough drug that controlled tuberculosis, but later developed a resistance. Of course, vaccines were a giant advance in medical theory, and one first thinks of the smallpox vaccine against polio. Of course, there are many examples of vaccines, such as those against measles, mumps, and diphtheria. It should be noted that for some viruses, a vaccine is yet to be developed. AIDS and Ebola do not have vaccines, but a very successful treatment for AIDS is successful, but not for Ebola. Of course, transmission of the disease from animals to humans plays an important role in the biology of emerging diseases. It is thought that the coronavirus first appeared in animals (birds, pigs, etc.) in China and was later transmitted to humans in the latter months in 2019. Ebola is believed to have been transmitted by nonhuman African primates to human.

Chapter 4 lays the foundation for Bayesian inference of discrete time Markov chain. The concepts of limiting distributions, transient and recurrent states, ergodic chains, and the period of a chain are defined and explained.

Chapter 5 presents biological examples of discrete time Markov chains including (1) birth and death processes, (2) logistic growth processes, (3) epidemic processes, (4) deterministic version of epidemics, (5) the stochastic version of epidemics, (6) chain binomial epidemic models, (7) the Greenwood Model, (8) The Reed-Frost Model, and (9) the duration and size of an epidemic. Lastly, the chapter consists of the explanation of statistical concepts necessary to understand epidemics.

Chapter 6 is about the Bayesian analysis of continuous time Markov chains, such as the Poisson process. Of primary importance is the estimation of the parameter of the Poisson process via its posterior distribution. Associated subjects of the Poisson process are thinning and superposition, the spatial Poisson process, and concomitant Poisson processes. Also discussed are nonhomogeneous Poisson processes and its intensity function. The chapter ends with an explanation of the important question about the coronavirus: Why are more tests needed than was originally thought to be necessary?

Chapter 7 begins with an explanation of Bayesian inferences for continuous time Markov processes. The fundamentals consist of the Markov property of the transition function, transition rates, the holding transition function with R, understanding the concepts of limiting and stationary distributions, the basic limit theorem, the mean time to absorption, and time reversibility. These ideas are illustrated with DNA evolution. Different interpretations of DNA are based on several modes, including the Kimura, the Jukes-Cantor, the Felsenstein, and the Churchill representation. Examples of these are the birth and death process, random walk, the Yule process, the birth and death process with immigration, the deterministic SI (susceptible infection) model, the stochastic SI model, and finally the SIS (Susceptible, infected, susceptible) version.

Chapter 8 begins with contagious diseases, a preview of data analysis models, the epidemic threshold theorem, and basic properties of the infection process.

Also described are the chain binomial representation, the size of the epidemic, and the chain binomial model for the evolution of epidemics. Examples given are those for the chain model for the common cold, generalized linear models for the analysis of binomial chains, examples for the common cold in households of size two and three. Of utmost importance is the measles epidemic. Next, the exponential growth of epidemics is explained mathematically where the growth rate of the epidemic is estimated by Bayesian techniques, that is to say, the posterior distribution of the growth rate is determined. This is illustrated by the coronavirus where the growth rate, mortality rate, and recovery rate are examined via Bayesian methods. Other examples of estimating the growth, mortality, and recovery rates are shown with the AIDS epidemic in HIV patients, where the CD4 count is the main response. Further examples are with smallpox and respiratory disease data.

1.3 Some Key References for Infectious Diseases and their Analysis

The following books are very relevant to the subject of infectious diseases.

1. Barry, J.M. (2004). *The Great Influenza: The Story of the Deadliest Pandemic in History*. Penguin Books, New York.
2. Blangiardo, M. and Cameletti, M. (2015). *Spatial and Spatio-temporal Bayesian Models with R-INLA*. John Wiley & Sons Ltd., Chichester, West Sussex, UK.
3. Becker, N.G. (1989). *Analysis of Infectious Disease Data*, Chapman and Hall, London, UK.
4. Broemeling, L.D. (2007). *Bayesian Biostatistics and Diagnostic Medicine*. Chapman & Hall/CRC, Taylor & Francis, Boca Raton, FL.
5. Broemeling, L.D. (2012). *Advanced Bayesian Methods for Medical Test Accuracy*, Chapman & Hall/CRC, Taylor & Francis, Boca Raton, FL.
6. Broemeling, L.D. *Bayesian Methods in Epidemiology*, Chapman & Hall/CRC, Taylor & Francis, Boca Raton, FL.
7. Desowitz, R.S. (1991). *The Malaria Capers, Tales of Parasites and People*, W.W Norton & Company, New York.
8. Drexler, M. (2002). *Secret Agents*, The Penguin Group, New York.
9. Glynn, I. and Glynn, J. (2004). *The Life and Death of Smallpox*, Profile Books Ltd. London, UK.
10. Held, L., Hens, N., O'Neil, P., and Wallinga, J. (2020). *Handbook of Infectious Disease Data Analysis*, Taylor & Francis Group, Boca Raton, FL.
11. Lee, P.M. (1989). *Bayesian Statistics: An Introduction*, Second edition, John Wiley & Sons Inc., New York.
12. Li, M.Y. (2018). *An Introduction to Modeling of Infectious Diseases*. Springer International Publishing, Cham, Switzerland.

13. Ryan, F. (1992). *The Forgotten Plague: How the Battle Against Tuberculosis Was Won and Lost*, Little Brown and Company, Boston, MA.

The Following Articles are Quite Appropriate for the Coronavirus Pandemic

1. Brian, T. (2020). The Covid-19 pandemic, *Significance*, 17(3), 12.
2. Ball, P. (2020). How do epidemiologists know how many people will get Covid-19?, *Significance*, 17(3), 12-14.
3. Bilder, R.C., Iwen, P.C., Abdalhamid, B., Tebbs, J.M., and McMahan, C.S. (2020). Tests in short supply? Try Group Testing, *Significance*, 17(3), 15.
4. Cochran, J.J. (2020). Why we need more coronavirus tests than we think we need, *Significance*, 17(3), 14-15.
5. Finazzi, F. and Fazo, A. (2020). The impact of the Covid-19 pandemic on Italian mobiity, *Significance*, 17(3), 17-18.
6. Frasier, S.L. (2002). False positive alarm, *Scientific American*, 323(1), 12-14.
7. Fischetti, M. (July 2002). Inside the coronavirus. What scientists know about the inner workings of the pathogen that has infected the world, *Scientific American*, 323(1), 32–37.
8. Nirala, V. (2002). ASA members show leadership during crisis, *AMSTATNEWS*, 515, 10-13.

Links to Infectious Disease Sources

The CDC is a Federal Agency Responsible for Gathering Information About Disease In the U.S.

https://www.cdc.gov/coronavirus/2019-ncov/cases-updates
https://www.cdc.gov/coronavirus/2019-ncov/whats-new-all.htm

Comments

The chapters to follow will show the reader how the Bayesian approach analyzes the evolutionary behavior of infectious diseases, including the coronavirus pandemic.

2

Bayesian Analysis

2.1 Introduction

Bayesian methods will be employed to make Bayesian inferences for time series, and this chapter will introduce the theory that is necessary in order to describe those Bayesian procedures. Bayes theorem, the foundation of the subject, is first introduced, followed by an explanation of the various components of Bayes theorem: prior information, information from the sample given by the likelihood function, the posterior distribution which is the basis of all inferential techniques, and lastly the Bayesian predictive distribution. A description of the main three elements of inference follows, namely estimation, tests of hypotheses, and forecasting future observations.

The remaining sections refer to the important standard distributions for Bayesian inference, namely the Bernoulli, the Beta, the multinomial, Dirichlet, normal, gamma, and normal-gamma, multivariate normal, Wishart, normal-Wishart, and the multivariate t-distributions. As will be seen, the relevance of these standard distributions to inferential techniques is essential for understanding the analysis of time series.

As will be seen, the multinomial and Dirichlet are the foundation for the Bayesian analysis of Markov chains and Markov jump processes. For normal stochastic processes such as Wiener and Brownian motion, the multivariate normal and the normal-Wishart play a key role in determining Bayesian inferences.

Posterior inferences by direct sampling methods are easily done if the relevant random number generators are available. On the other hand, if the posterior distribution is quite complicated and not recognized as a standard distribution, other techniques are needed. To solve this problem, Monte Carlo Markov Chain (MCMC) techniques have been developed and have been a major success in providing Bayesian inferences for quite complicated problems. This has been a great achievement in the field and will be described in later sections.

WinBUGS and R are packages that provide random number generators for direct sampling from the posterior distribution for many standard distributions, such as binomial, gamma, Beta, and t-distributions. On occasion these will be used; however, my preferences are WinBUGS and R, because they have been adopted by other Bayesians. This is also true for indirect sampling, where WinBugs and R are excellent packages and are adopted for this book. Many institutions provide special purpose software for specific Bayesian routines. For example, at MD Anderson Cancer Center, where Bayesian applications are routine, several special purpose programs are available for designing (including sample size justification) and analyzing clinical trials, and will be described. The theoretical foundation for MCMC is introduced in the following sections.

Inferences for time series consist of testing hypotheses about unknown population parameters, estimation of those parameters, and forecasting future observations. When a sharp null hypothesis is involved, special care is taken in specifying the prior distribution for the parameters. A formula for the posterior probability of the null hypothesis is derived, via Bayes theorem, and illustrated for Bernoulli, Poisson, and normal populations. If the main focus is estimation of parameters, the posterior distribution is determined, and the mean, median, standard deviation, and credible intervals are found, either analytically or by computation with WinBUGS or R. For example, when sampling from a normal population with unknown parameters and using a conjugate prior density, the posterior distribution of the mean is a t and will be derived algebraically. On the other hand, for making Bayesian inferences for time series such as autoregressive are univariate t for the individual coefficients are gamma for the precision of the error process of the time series. These posterior inferences are provided both analytically and numerically with WinBUGS or R. Of course, all analyses should be preceded by checking to determine whether the model is appropriate, and this is where the predictive distribution comes into play. By comparing the observed results of the experiment with those predicted, the model assumptions are tested. The most frequent use of the Bayesian predictive distribution is for forecasting future observation of time series.

2.2 Bayes Theorem

Bayes theorem is based on the conditional probability law:

$$P[A \mid B] = P[B \mid A]P[A] / P[B] \tag{2.1}$$

where P[A] is the probability of A before one knows the outcome of the event B, P[B | A] is the probability of B assuming what one knows about the event A, and P[A | B] is the probability of A knowing that event B has occurred.

P[A] is called the prior probability of A, while P[A | B] is called the posterior probability of A.

Another version of Bayes theorem is to suppose X is a continuous observable random vector and $\theta \in \Omega \subset R^m$ is an unknown parameter vector, and suppose the conditional density of X given θ is denoted by $f(x \mid \theta)$. If $x = (x_1, x_2, ..., x_n)$ represents a random sample of size n from a population with density f(x $\mid \theta$), and $\xi(\theta)$ is the prior density of θ, then Bayes theorem expresses the posterior density as

$$\xi(\theta|x) = c \prod_{i=1}^{i=} f(x_i | \theta) \xi(\theta), x_i \in R \quad \text{and} \quad \theta \in \Omega \tag{2.2}$$

where the proportionality constant is c, and the term $\prod_{i=1}^{i=n} f(x_i | \theta)$ is called the likelihood function. The density $\xi(\theta)$ is the prior density of θ and represents the knowledge one possesses about the parameter before one observes X. Such prior information is most likely available to the experimenter from other previous related experiments. Note that θ is considered a random variable and that Bayes theorem transforms one's prior knowledge of θ, represented by its prior density, to the posterior density, and that the transformation is the combining of the prior information about θ with the sample information represented by the likelihood function.

"An essay toward solving a problem in the doctrine of chances" by the Reverend Thomas Bayes [1] is the beginning of our subject. He considered a binomial experiment with n trials and assumed the probability θ of success was uniformly distributed (by constructing a billiard table) and presented a way to calculate $\Pr(a \leq \theta \leq b \mid x = p)$, where x is the number of successes in n-independent trials. This was a first in the sense that Bayes was making inferences via $\xi(\theta \mid x)$, the conditional density of θ given x. Also, by assuming the parameter as uniformly distributed, he was assuming vague prior information for θ. The type of prior information, where very little is known about the parameter, is called noninformative or vague information.

It can well be argued that Laplace [2] is the greatest Bayesian because he made many significant contributions to inverse probability (he did not know of Bayes), beginning in 1774 with "Mémoire sur la probabilite des causes par les événements," with his own version of Bayes theorem, and over a period of some 40 years culminating in "Théorie analytique des probabilités." See Stigler [3] and Chapters 9–20 of Hald [4] for the history of Laplace's contributions to inverse probability.

It was in modern times that Bayesian statistics began its resurgence with Lhoste [5], Jeffreys [6], Savage [7], and Lindley [8]. According to Broemeling and Broemeling [9], Lhoste was the first to justify noninformative priors by invariance principals, a tradition carried on by Jeffreys. Savage's book was a major contribution in that Bayesian inference, and decision theory was put on a sound theoretical footing as a consequence of certain axioms of probability and utility, while Lindley's two volumes showed the relevance of Bayesian inference to everyday statistical problems and was quite influential and set the tone and style for the later books such as Box and Tiao [10], Zellner [11], and Broemeling [12]. Box and Tiao and Broemeling were essentially works that presented Bayesian methods for the usual statistical problems of the analysis of variance and regression, while Zellner focused Bayesian methods primarily on certain regression problems in econometrics. During this period, inferential problems were solved either analytically or by numerical integration. Models with many parameters (such as hierarchical models with many levels) were difficult to use because at that time numerical integration methods had limited capability in higher dimensions. For a good history of inverse probability, see Chapter 3 of Stigler [3], and Hald [4], who present a comprehensive history and are invaluable as a reference.

The last 20 years is characterized by the rediscovery and development of resampling techniques, where samples, such as Gibbs sampling, are generated from the posterior distribution via MCMC methods. Large samples generated from the posterior make it possible to make statistical inferences and to employ multi-level hierarchical models to solve complex, but practical problems. See Leonard and Hsu [13], Gelman et al. [14], Congdon [15–17], Carlin and Louis [18], Gilks, Richardson, and Spiegelhalter [19], who demonstrate the utility of MCMC techniques in Bayesian statistics.

2.3 Prior Information

2.3.1 The Binomial Distribution

Where do we begin with prior information, a crucial component of Bayes theorem rule? Bayes assumed the prior distribution of the parameter is uniform, namely

$$\xi(\theta) = 1, 0 \le \theta \le 1$$

where, θ is the common probability of success in n-independent trials and

$$f(x|\theta) = \binom{n}{x}\theta^x (1-\theta)^{n-x},\qquad(2.3)$$

where x is the number of successes = 0, 1, 2, ..., n. The distribution of X, and the number of successes are binomial and denoted by $X \sim$ Binomial (θ, n).

The uniform prior was used for many years; however, Lhoste [5] proposed a different prior, namely

$$\xi(\theta) = \theta^{-1}(1-\theta)^{-1}, \quad 0 \le \theta \le 1, \tag{2.4}$$

to represent information which is noninformative and is an improper density function. Lhoste based the prior on certain invariance principals, quite similar to Jeffreys [6]. Lhoste also derived a noninformative prior for the standard deviation σ of a normal population with density

$$f(x \mid \mu, \sigma) = \left(1/\sqrt{2\pi}\sigma\right)\exp-(1/2\sigma)(x-\mu)^2, \; \mu \in R \; \text{ and } \; \sigma > 0. \tag{2.5}$$

He used invariance as follows: he reasoned that the prior density of σ and the prior density of $1/\sigma$ should be the same, which leads to

$$\xi(\sigma) = 1/\sigma \tag{2.6}$$

Jeffreys' approach is similar in that in developing noninformative priors for binomial and normal populations, but he also developed noninformative priors for multi-parameter models, including the mean and standard deviation for the normal density as

$$\xi(\mu, \sigma) = 1/\sigma, \quad \mu \in R \; \text{ and } \; \sigma > 0 \tag{2.7}$$

Noninformative priors were ubiquitous from 1920s to 1980s and were included in all the textbooks of that period. For example, see Box and Tiao [10], Zellner [11], and Broemeling [12]. Looking back, it is somewhat ironic that noninformative priors were almost always used, even though informative prior information was almost always available. This limited the utility of the Bayesian approach, and people saw very little advantage over the conventional way of doing business. The major strength of the Bayesian way is that it a convenient, practical, and logical method of utilizing informative prior information. Surely the investigator knows informative prior information from previous related studies.

How does one express informative information with a prior density? For example, suppose one has informative prior information for the binomial population. Consider

$$\xi(\theta) = [\Gamma(\alpha+\beta)/\Gamma(\alpha)\Gamma(\beta)]\theta^{\alpha-1}(1-\theta)^{\beta-1}, \quad 0 \le \theta \le 1, \tag{2.8}$$

as the prior density for θ. The Beta density with parameters α and β has mean $[\alpha/(\alpha+\beta)]$ and variance $[\alpha\beta/(\alpha+\beta)^2(\alpha+\beta+1)]$ and can express informative prior information in many ways.

As for prior information for the binomial, consider the analysis of Markov processes, namely in estimating the transition probability matrix of a stationary finite-state Markov chain. Consider the five–by–five transition matrix P with components

$$P = (p_{ij}),$$

where

$$P = \begin{pmatrix} .2,.2,.2,.2,.2 \\ .2,.2,.2,.2,.2 \\ .2,.2,.2,.2,.2 \\ .2,.2,.2,.2,.2 \\ .2,.2,.2,.2,.2 \end{pmatrix} \qquad (2.9)$$

Note that

$$p_{ij} = \Pr\left[X_{n+1} = j \mid X_n = i \right] \qquad (2.10)$$

where $n = 0, 1, 2, \ldots$ that is to say X_n is a discrete time Markov with state space

$$S = \{1,2,3,4,5\}$$

Note that p_{ij} are the one-step transition probabilities of the Markov chain X_n, where the first row is the conditional distribution (given $X_0 = 1$) of a discrete random variable with mass points 1, 2, 3, 4, and 5, with probabilities .2, .2, .2, .2, .2. The second row is the conditional distribution (given $X_0 = 2$) of a discrete random variable with mass points 1, 2, 3, 4, and 5 with probabilities .2, .2, .2, .2, .2, etc. This is an example of a Markov chain where each state is recurrent, that is, it is possible to reach any state from any other state.

Using a multinomial distribution with probability mass function

$$\prod_{i,j=1}^{i,j=5} p_{ij}^{n_{ij}}, \qquad (2.11)$$

where $\sum_{i,j=1}^{i,j=5} p_{ij} = 1$ and $\sum_{i,j=1}^{i,j=5} n_{ij} = n$.

98 n_{ij} values are generated from the chain with the result

1 2 5 1 4 1 5 3 3 2 4 4 2 5 5 5 3 2 2 2 3 2 1 4 5 3 2 1 2 3 4 3 3 4 2 4 5 1 5 1 1 4 5 1 4
1 3 4 4 2 5 1 5 1 3 1 2 4 1 3 1 3 5 5 4 1 4 1 2 1 2 5 4 4 4 2 4 2 5 5 4 5 2 4 3 2 2 3 2 1
2 1 2 4 2 3 1 4 4 2.

The R code below is used to simulate the 98 observations from the Markov chain with transition matrix P

RC 2.1

```
MC.sim<-function(n,P,x1){
sim<-as.numeric(n)
m<-ncol(P)
if (missing(x1)){
sim[1]<-sample(1:m,1)# random start
} else {sim[1]<-x1}
for ( i in 2:n){
newstate<-sample(1:m,1,prob=P[sim[i-1],])
sim[i]<-newstate
}
sim
}
P<-matrix(c(.2,.2,.2,.2,.2,.2,.2,.2,.2,.2,.2,.2,.2,.2,.
2,.2,.2,.2,.2,.2,.2,.2,.2,.2,.2),nrow=5,ncol=5,byrow=TRUE)
MC.sim(100,P,1)
```

These cell frequencies can be displayed as five-by-five matrix

$$N = \begin{pmatrix} 1,7,4,6,2 \\ 5,3,4,6,5 \\ 3,6,2,3,1 \\ 5,7,2,5,4 \\ 6,1,3,3,4 \end{pmatrix} \qquad (2.12)$$

Thus, there is one one-step transition from 1 to 1, 7 transitions from 1 to 2, and lastly two one-step transitions from 1 to 5. Since the simulation was based on the multinomial distribution, it is known that the marginal distribution of the cell frequency n_{ij} is binomial with parameters p_{ij} and $n = 98$. In order to perform a Bayesian analysis, a prior distribution is assigned to the unknown cell frequencies: The conjugate distribution to the multinomial is the Dirichlet, which induces a beta prior to the individual cell frequencies. This results in a Dirichlet for the posterior distribution of the transition probabilities p_{ij}, and consequently a beta for the individual transition probabilities. For the Dirichlet, the density is

$$f\left(p_{11},p_{12},\ldots p_{55}\right) \propto \prod_{i,j=1}^{i,j=5} p_{ij}^{\alpha_{ij}-1} \qquad (2.13)$$

where $\sum_{i,j=1}^{i,j=5} p_{ij} = 1$ and the α_{ij} are positive.

Later in this chapter, a posterior analysis for estimating the transition probabilities will be presented.

2.3.2 The Normal Distribution

Of course, the normal density plays an important role as a model for time series. For example, as will be seen in future chapters, the normal distribution will model the observations of certain time series, such as autoregressive and moving average series. How is informative prior information expressed for the parameters μ and σ (the mean and standard deviation)? Suppose a previous study has m observations $x = (x_1 x_2, ..., x_m)$, then the density of X given μ and σ is

$$f(x \mid \mu, \sigma) \propto \left[\sqrt{m} / \sqrt{2\pi\sigma^2} \right] \exp - \left(m/2\sigma^2 \right) \left(\bar{x} - \mu \right)^2$$

$$\left[(2\pi)^{-(n-1)/2} \sigma^{-(n-1)} \right] \exp - \left(1/2\sigma^2 \right) \sum_{i-1}^{i=m} \left(x_i - \bar{x} \right)^2 \tag{2.14}$$

This is a conjugate density for the two-parameter normal family and is called the normal-gamma density. Note it is the product of two functions, where the first, as a function of μ and σ, is the conditional density of μ given σ, with mean $\bar{x}$ and variance σ^2/m, while the second is a function of σ only and is an inverse gamma density. Or equivalently, if the normal is parameterized with μ and the precision $\tau = 1/\sigma^2$, the conjugate distribution is as follows: (a) the conditional distribution of μ given τ is normal with mean $\bar{x}$ and precision $m\tau$, and (b) the marginal distribution of τ is gamma with parameters $(m + 1)/2$ and $\sum_{i=1}^{i=m} (x_i - \bar{x})^2/2 = (m-1)S^2/2$, where S^2 is the sample variance. Thus, if one knows the results of a previous experiment, the likelihood function for μ and τ provides informative prior information for the normal population.

For example, the normal serves as the distribution of the observations of a first order autoregressive process

$$Y(t) = \theta Y(t-1) + W(t), t = 1, 2, ... \tag{2.15}$$

where

$$W(t), t = 1, 2, ... \tag{2.16}$$

is a sequence of independent normal random variables with mean zero and precision τ, and $\tau > 0$. It is easy to show that the joint distribution of the n observations from the AR(1) process is multivariate normal with mean vector 0 and variance covariance matrix with diagonal entries $1/\tau(1 - \theta^2)$ and k-th order covariance $Cov[Y(t), Y(t + k)] = \theta^k/\tau(1 - \theta^2)$, $|\theta| < 1$, $k = 1, 2, \ldots$

Note that it is assumed the process is stationary, namely $|\theta| < 1$. Of course, the goal of the Bayesian analysis is to estimate the processes autoregressive parameter θ and the precision $\tau > 0$. For the Bayesian analysis, a prior distribution must be assigned to θ and τ, which in the conjugate prior case is a normal-gamma. The posterior analysis for the autoregressive time series results in a univariate t-distribution for the distribution of θ as will be shown in Chapter 5.

2.4 Posterior Information

2.4.1 The Binomial Distribution

The preceding section explains how prior information is expressed in an informative or in a noninformative way. Several examples are given and will be revisited as illustrations for the determination of the posterior distribution of the parameters. Suppose a uniform prior distribution for the transition probability (of the five-state Markov chain) p_{ij} is used. What is the posterior distribution of p_{ij}?

By Bayes theorem,

$$f\left(p_{ij}|N\right) \propto \binom{n}{n_{ij}} p_{ij}^{n_{ij}} \left(1-p_{ij}\right)^{n-n_{ij}} \tag{2.17}$$

where n_{ij} is the observed transitions from state i to state j, and n is the total cell counts for the five-by-five cell frequency matrix N. Of course, this is recognized as a Beta $(n_{ij} + 1, n - n_{ij} + 1)$ distribution, and the posterior mean is $(n_{ij} + 1/n + 2)$. On the other hand, if the Lhoste [5] prior density (2.4) is used, the posterior distribution of p_{ij} is Beta $(n_{ij}, n - n_{ij})$ with mean n_{ij}/n, which is the usual estimator of p_{ij}.

2.4.2 The Normal Distribution

Consider a random sample $x = (x_1, x_2, \ldots, x_n)$ of size n from a normal $(\mu, 1/\tau)$ population, where $\tau = 1/\sigma^2$ is the inverse of the variance, and suppose the prior information is vague and the Jeffreys-Lhoste prior $\xi(\mu, \tau) \propto 1/\tau$ is appropriate, then the posterior density of the parameters is

$$\xi(\mu, \tau \mid \text{data}) \propto \tau^{n/2-1} \exp-(\tau/2)\left[n\left(\mu - \bar{x}\right)^2 + \sum_{i=1}^{i=n} \left(x_i - \bar{x}\right)^2 \right] \tag{2.18}$$

Using the properties of the gamma density, τ is eliminated by integrating the joint density with respect to τ to give

$$\xi(\mu \,|\, \text{data}) \propto \left\{ \Gamma(n/2)n^{1/2}/(n-1)^{1/2}S\pi^{1/2}\Gamma(n-10/2) \right\} / \left[1 + n(\mu - \bar{x})^2/(n-1)S^2 \right]^{(n-1+1)/2} \tag{2.19}$$

which is recognized as a t-distribution with n-1 degrees of freedom, location $\bar{x}$ and precision n/S^2. Transforming to $(\mu - \bar{x})\sqrt{n}/S$, the resulting variable has a Student's t-distribution with $n-1$ degrees of freedom. Note the mean of μ is the sample mean, while the variance is $[(n-1)/n(n-3)]$, $n > 3$.

Eliminating μ from (12) results in the marginal distribution of τ as

$$\xi\left(\tau\,|\,S^2\right) \propto \tau^{[(n-1)/2]-1} \exp{-\tau}\,(n-1)S^2/2, \tau > 0, \tag{2.20}$$

which is a gamma density with parameters $(n-1)/2$ and $(n-1)S^2/2$. This implies the posterior mean is $1/S^2$ and the posterior variance is $2/(n-1)S^4$.

An example, consider the AR(1) (2.15) series where $\theta = .6$ and $\sigma^2 = 1$, then suppose R is used to generate a realization of $n = 50$ from thus series.

Our goal is to determine the posterior distribution of θ and $\tau = 1/\sigma^2$.

The R code used for the simulation is given below, namely:

RC 2.2

```
set.seed(1)
y<-w<-rnorm(50)
for ( t in 2:50){y[t]<-.6*y[t-1]+w[t]
time<-1:50
plot(time,y)
```

The vector y contains the 50 simulated values for the autoregressive time series.

```
Y=(-.62,-.1922,-.9509,1.0247,.9443,-.2538,.3351,.93938,1.13954,
.37826,1.73873,1.43308,.23861,-2.07153,-.1179,-.1157,
-.0856,.89246,1.3566,1.4079,1.763,1.8403,1.17878,-1.28207,
-.14942,-0.14578,-.24326,-1.6167,-1.4481,-.45096,1.0881,
.55007,.71771,.37682,-1.15096,-1.10557,-1.0576,.-.69389,
.6836,1.1733,.5395,.07034,.73916,1.000165,.-.08865,-.7606,
-.09183,.71343,.3157.1.07053).
```

The likelihood function is

$$L(\theta|y) = (\tau/2\pi)^{n/2} \exp{-(\tau/2)} \sum_{i=1}^{i=n} \left[y(t) - \theta y(t-1) \right]^2 \tag{2.21}$$

where y is the n by 1 vector of observations. Suppose one assumes the prior density of the parameters is

$$\zeta(\theta,\tau) = 1/\tau, \tau > 0, -\infty < \theta < \infty, \qquad (2.22)$$

Then it can be shown that the posterior density of θ is

$$\zeta(\theta|y) \propto \left\{1 + \lambda(\theta - v)^2 1\right\}^{-n/2} \qquad (2.23)$$

where

$$v = \sum_{t=2}^{t=n} y(t)y(t-1) / \sum_{t=2}^{t=n} y^2(t-1). \qquad (2.24)$$

Thus, the posterior distribution of θ is a univariate t with $n-1$ degrees of freedom, mean v, and precision $\lambda = (n-1)/c$, where

$$c = \sum_{t=1}^{t=n} y^2(t) - \left[\sum_{t=2}^{n} y(t)y(t-1)\right]^2 / \sum_{t=2}^{t=n} y^2(t-1). \qquad (2.25)$$

Using 50 observations of the vector y, it follows that

$$c = 28.581, \lambda = 1.71442, \text{ and } v = .6246$$

thus, the posterior distribution of θ is a t with 49 degrees of freedom, mean .6246, and precision 1.7144.

This section will introduce the way MCMC techniques are used to execute the posterior analysis for the AR(1) time series model which was analyzed analytically above. Remember the vector y of observations from the process with parameters $\theta = .6$ and $\tau = 1$, and consider the WinBUGS code below.

BC 2.1

```
model;

·v~dgamma(.01,.01)
#v is the precision τ with a noninformative gamma (.01,.01)
distribution
theta~beta(6,4)
# the prior distribution of theta is beta(6,4)
# the vector Y is the vector of 50 observations
# Y follows a multivariate normal distribution with mean mu
and variance covariance matrix Sigma. The matrix tau is the
inverse of the variance covariance matrix
Y[1,1:50]~dmnorm(mu[],tau[,])f
```

```
for( i in 1:50){mu[i]<-0}
tau[1:50,1:50]<-inverse(Sigma[,])

for (i in 1:50){Sigma[i,i]<-v/(1-theta*theta)}
for( i in 1:50){ for j in i+1:50
(Sigma[i,j]<-v*pow(theta,j)*1/(1-theta*theta)}}
for( i in 2:50){for j in 1:i-1)
{Sigma[I,j]<-v*pow(theta,i-1)*1/(1-theta*theta)}}
}
# the following list statement if for the 50 by 1 observation
vector
list(Y=structure (.Data=c(-.62,-.1922,-.9509,1.0247,.9443,
-.2538,.3351,.93938,1.13954, .37826,1.73873,1.43308,.23861,
-2.07153,-.1179,-.1157,-.0856,.89246,1.3566,1.4079,1.763,
1.8403,1.17878,-1.28207,-.14942,-0.14578,-.24326,-1.6167,
-1.4481,-.45096,1.0881,.55007,.71771,.37682,-1.15096,
-1.10557,-1.0576,-.69389, .6836,1.1733,.5395,.07034,.73916,
1.000165,-.08865,-.7606,-.09183,.71343,.3157.1.07053),.
Dim=c(1,50)))
# the following list statement specifies the initial values of
MCMC process
list(theta=.6, v=1)
```

Note that the WinBUGS analysis did not assume the same prior as was assumed in the analytical approach, nevertheless, the two analyses should agree because the MCMC approach assumed a noninformative gamma prior. Also note, that both analyses did not utilize the stationary restriction $|\theta| < 1$.

The Bayesian analysis is executed with 45,000 observations for the simulation with a 5,000 burn in and a refresh of 100. The results are reported in the following Table 2.1.

The Bayesian analysis for the AR(1) model shows that the posterior mean of the correlation coefficient θ is .6258, which compares quite favorable to the value .6 used to generate the data. Note the posterior mean of .6258 is computed via WinBUGS, whereas the analytical value computed earlier is .6246, and the two values agree to the nearest 100-th decimal.

Bayesian methods for autoregressive processes will be developed in more detail in Chapter 5.

TABLE 2.1

Posterior Analysis for AR(1) Series

Parameter	Mean	SD	Error	2 1/2	Median	97 1/2
θ	.6258	.1509	.002015	.3096	.6383	.8683
σ^2	.5724	.2138	.002894	.228	.552	1.043

2.4.3 The Poisson Distribution

The Poisson distribution often occurs as a population for a discrete random variable with mass function

$$f\left(x|\theta\right)=e^{-\theta}\theta^{x}/x!,\qquad(2.26)$$

where the gamma density

$$\xi\left(\theta\right)=\left[\beta^{\alpha}/\Gamma\left(\alpha\right)\right]\theta^{\alpha-1}e^{-\theta\beta},\qquad(2.27)$$

is a conjugate distribution that expresses informative prior information. For example, in a previous experiment with m observations, the prior density would be gamma with the appropriate values of alpha and beta. Based on a random sample of size n, the posterior density is

$$\xi(\theta\,|\text{data})\propto\theta^{\sum_{i=1}^{i=n}x_i+\alpha-1}e^{-\theta(n+\beta)},\qquad(2.28)$$

which is identified as a gamma density with parameters $\alpha'=\sum_{i=1}^{i=n}x_i+\alpha$ and $\beta'=n+\beta$. Remember the posterior mean is α'/β', median $(\alpha'-1)/\beta'$, and variance $\alpha'/(\beta')^2$.

One of the most important time series is the Poisson process. The Poisson process $N(t)$ with parameter $\lambda>0$ is defined as follows.

1. $N(t)$ is the number of events occurring over the time 0 to t with $N(0)=0$ and the process has independent increments.

2. For all $t>0$, $0<P[N(t)>0]<1$, that is to say for all intervals, no matter how small, there is a positive probability that an event will occur, but it is not certain an event will occur.

3. For all $t\geq0$, $\lim\{P[N(t+h)-N(t)\geq2]/P[N(t+h)-N(t)=1]\}$, where the limit is as h approaches 0. This implies that events cannot occur simultaneously.

The process has stationary independent increments, thus for all points $t>s\geq0$ and $h>0$, the two random variables $N(t+h)-N(s+h)$ and $N(t)-N(s)$ are identically distributed and are independent.

Based on these four axioms, one may show that for all $t>0$, there exists a $\lambda>0$ such that $N(t)$ has a Poisson distribution with mean λt. Thus the average number of events occurring over $[0,t)$ is λt and the average number of events occurring per unit time is λ. The Poisson process is a counting process (it counts the number of events occurring over time) and has many generalizations that will be introduced in Chapter 7. An interesting feature of the Poisson process is that the time between the occurrence of two adjacent events has an exponential distribution. In particular, if $N(t)$, $t \geq 0$ is a Poisson process with parameter λ, then the successive inter-arrival times are independent and have an exponential distribution with mean $1/\lambda$, thus the Poisson process can be simulated via the exponential distribution. For example consider a Poisson process with parameter $\lambda = 5$, and suppose a realization of 50 using the exponential distribution with mean $1/5 = .2$ is to be generated using the following WinBUGS code.

BC 2.2

```
model {
for (i in 1 : 1000) {
y[i] ~ dexp(.2)
}
}
```

The 50 successive inter-arrival times are given by the vector I.

```
I=(.403,11.00,23.11,1.92,.25,4.34,3.53,.10,1.59,.05,3.11,2.21,3.
03,5.96,7.22,.96,8.75,2.23,29.84,2.96,2.41,2.86,.5411.48,,2.10,1
.43,8.99,6.87,1.73,6.76,14.91,11.90,1.21,12.08,4.49,4.14,1.94,1.
30,1.86,4.86,.21,13.27,.42,1.60,3.38,3.39,2.97,9.97, 7.03,2.54)
```

The 50 corresponding waiting times are the components of the vector W below:

```
W=(.40,11.40,34.51,36.43,36.68,41.02,44.55,44.65,46.24,46.29,4
9.40,51.61,54.64,60.60,67.82,68.78,77.53,79.76,109.60,112.56,1
14.97,117.83,118.37,129.85,131.95,133.38,142.37,149.24,150.97,
157.73,172.64,184.54,185.75,197.83,202.32,206.46,208.40,209.70,
211.56,216.42,216.63,229.90,230.32,231.92,235.30,238.69,241.66,
251.63,258.66,261.20).
```

Thus, the first event occurred at time .403 time units and the second at 11.40 time units, and the last at 261.2 units.

Let T_n be the n-th inter-arrival time and W_n the corresponding waiting time, then

$$W_n = T_1 + T_2 + \cdots + T_n,\qquad(2.29)$$

where $n = 0,1,2,\ldots$, thus, we know that

$$T_n \sim \exp(\lambda)\qquad(2.30)$$

and

$$W_n \sim \text{gamma}(n,\lambda) \qquad (2.31)$$

That is the inter-arrival times have a common exponential distribution with parameter λ and n-th waiting time has a gamma distribution with parameters n and λ. In the next section on inference, based on the above inter-arrival and waiting times, Bayesian inferences for the intensity λ will be performed.

2.5 Inference

2.5.1 Introduction

In a statistical context, by inference one usually means estimation of parameters, tests of hypotheses, and prediction of future observations. With the Bayesian approach, all inferences are based on the posterior distribution of the parameters, which in turn is based on the sample, via the likelihood function and the prior distribution. We have seen the role of the prior density and likelihood function in determining the posterior distribution, and presently will focus on the determination of point and interval estimation of the model parameters, and later will emphasize how the posterior distribution determines a test of hypothesis. Lastly, the role of the predictive distribution in testing hypotheses and in goodness of fit will be explained.

When the model has only one parameter, one would estimate that parameter by listing its characteristics, such as the posterior mean, media, and standard deviation and plotting the posterior density. On the other hand, if there are several parameters, one would determine the marginal posterior distribution of the relevant parameters and as above, calculate its characteristics (e.g. mean, median, mode, standard deviation etc.) and plot the densities. Interval estimates of the parameters are also usually reported and are called credible intervals.

2.5.2 Estimation

Inferences for the normal (μ,τ) population are somewhat more demanding, because both parameters are unknown. Assuming the vague prior density $\xi(\mu,\tau) \propto 1/\tau$, the marginal posterior distribution of the population mean μ is a t-distribution with n-1 degrees of freedom, mean $\bar{x}$, and precision n/S^2, thus the mean and the median are the same and provide a natural estimator of μ, and because of the symmetry of the t-density, a $(1 - \alpha)$ credible interval for μ is $\bar{x} \pm t_{\alpha/2,n-1}S/\sqrt{n}$, where $t_{\alpha/2,n-1}$ is the upper $100\alpha/2$ percent point of the t-distribution with n-1 degrees of freedom. To generate values from the $t(n-1, \bar{x}, n/S^2)$ distribution, generate values from Student's t-distribution with n-1 degrees of freedom, multiply each by $S/\sqrt{n}$, and then add $\bar{x}$ to each. Suppose n =30,

```
x = (7.8902,4.8343,11.0677,8.7969,4.0391,4.0024,6.6494,8.4788,
0.7939,5.0689,6.9175,6.1092,8.2463,10.3179,1.8429,3.0789,2.847
0,5.1471,6.3730,5.2907,1.5024,3.8193,9.9831,6.2756,5.3620,5.32
97,9.3105,6.5555,0.8189,0.4713), then x = 5.57 and S = 2.92.
```

Using the same dataset, the following WinBugs code is used to analyze the problem.

BC 2.3

```
Model;
{ for( i in 1:30) { x[i]~dnorm(mu,tau) }
mu~dnorm (0.0,.0001)
tau ~dgamma( .0001,.0001)
sigma <- 1/tau }
list( x = c(7.8902,4.8343,11.0677,8.7969,4.0391,4.0024,6.6494,
8.4788,0.7939,5.0689,6.9175,6.1092,8.2463,10.3179,1.8429,3.078
9,2.8470,5.1471,6.3730,5.2907,1.5024,3.8193,9.9831,6.2756,5.36
20,5.3297,9.3105,6.5555,0.8189,0.4713))
list( mu = 0, tau = 1)
```

Note, that a somewhat different prior was employed here, compared with previous, in that μ and τ are independent and assigned proper but noninformative distributions. The corresponding analysis gives (Table 2.2):

Upper and lower refer to the lower and upper 2 ½ percent points of the posterior distribution. Note a 95% credible interval for mu is (4.47, 6.65) and the estimation error is .003566. See the appendix for the details on executing the WinBUGS statements above.

The program generated 30,000 samples from the joint posterior distribution of μ and σ using a Gibbs sampling algorithm, and used 29,000 for the posterior moments and graphs with a refresh of 100.

TABLE 2.2
Posterior Distribution of μ and $\sigma = 1/\sqrt{\tau}$

Parameter	Mean	Std dev	MC error	Median	Lower	Upper
μ	5.572	.5547	.003566	5.571	4.4790	6.656
σ	9.15	2.570	.01589	8.733	5.359	15.37

2.5.3 Testing Hypotheses

An important feature of inference is testing hypotheses. Often in stochastic processes, the scientific hypothesis can be expressed in statistical terms with a formal test implemented. Suppose $\Omega = \Omega_0 \cup \Omega_1$ is a partition of the parameter space, then the null hypothesis is designated as H_0: $\theta \in \Omega_0$ and the alternative by H_1: $\theta \in \Omega_1$, and a test of H_0 versus H_1 consists of rejecting H_0 in favor of H_1 if the observations $x = (x_1, x_2, ..., x_n)$ belong to a critical region C. In the usual approach, the critical region is based on the probabilities of type I errors, namely $\Pr(C|\theta)$, where $\theta \in \Omega_0$ and of type II errors, namely $1-\Pr(C|\theta)$, where $\theta \in \Omega_1$. This approach to testing hypothesis was developed formally by Neyman and Pearson and can be found in many of the standard references, such as Lehmann [20].

Lee [21] presents a good elementary introduction to testing and estimation in a Bayesian context.

In the Bayesian approach, the posterior probabilities

$$p_0 = \Pr(\theta \in \Omega_0| data) \tag{2.32}$$

and

$$p_1 = \Pr(\theta \in \Omega_1| data) \tag{2.33}$$

are required, and on the basis of the two, a decision is made whether or not to reject H in favor of A or to reject A in favor of H. Also required are the two corresponding prior probabilities

$$\pi_0 = \Pr(\theta \in \Omega_0) \tag{2.34}$$

and

$$\pi_1 = \Pr(\theta \in \Omega_1) \tag{2.35}$$

Now consider the prior odds π_0/π_1 and posterior odds p_0/p_1. In turn consider the Bayes factor B in favor of H_0 relative to H_1, namely

$$B = (p_0 / p_1)/(\pi_0 / \pi_1), \tag{2.36}$$

Then, the posterior probabilities p_0 and p_1 can be expressed in terms of the Bayes factor, thus:

$$p_0 = 1/\left[1+(\pi_1 / \pi_1)B^{-1}\right] \tag{2.37}$$

and the Bayes factor is interpreted as the odds in favor of H_0 relative to H_1 as implied by the information from the data.

When the hypotheses are simple, that is, $\Omega_0 = \{\theta_0\}$ and $\Omega_1 = \{\theta_1\}$, note that the odds ratio can be expressed as the likelihood ratio.

$$B = p(x|\,\theta_0)/p(x|\,\theta_1) \tag{2.38}$$

This interpretation is not valid when Ω_0 and Ω_1 are composite. Consider the restriction of the prior density $p(\theta)$ to Ω_0, namely

$$p_0(\theta) = p(\theta)/\pi_0, \quad \theta \in \Omega_0 \tag{2.39}$$

and its restriction to Ω_1, namely

$$p_1(\theta) = p(\theta)/\pi_1. \quad \theta \in \Omega_1 \tag{2.40}$$

Note the integral of $p_0(\theta)$ with respect to θ over Ω_0 is 1.

Now it can be shown that that the posterior probability of the null hypothesis is

$$p_0 = \pi_0 \int p(x|\,\theta) p_0(\theta) d\theta \tag{2.41}$$

where the integral is taken over Ω_0.

In a similar way, the posterior probability of H_1

$$p_1 = \pi_1 \int p(x|\,\theta) p_1(\theta) d\theta \tag{2.42}$$

where the integral is taken over Ω_1.

Now the Bayes factor can be expressed as

$$B = (p_0/p_1)/(\pi_0/\pi_1) = \int_{\theta \in \Omega_0} p(x|\,\theta) p_0(\theta) d\theta / \int_{\theta \in \Omega_1} p(x|\,\theta) p_1(\theta) d\theta \tag{2.43}$$

which is the ratio of weighted likelihood functions, weighted by the prior probability densities restricted to Ω_0 and Ω_1.

An important aspect of testing hypotheses is when the null hypothesis is a point null hypothesis and the alternative is composite, thus consider

$$H_0 : \theta = \theta_0 \tag{2.44}$$

versus

$$H_1 : \theta \neq \theta_0 \tag{2.45}$$

where θ_0 is known. How does one assign prior information to this case? A reasonable approach to assign a positive probability π_0 for the null hypothesis and for the alternative assign a prior density $\pi_1 p_1(\theta)$, where

$$\int_{\theta \neq \theta_0} p_1(\theta) d\theta = 1 \tag{2.46}$$

Thus, $\pi_0 + \pi_1 = 1$ and it is seen that the prior probability of the alternative is π_1, and for values $\theta \neq \theta_0$, p_1 is the density of a continuous random variable that expresses the prior knowledge one has for the alternative hypothesis.

Let

$$p(x) = \pi_0 p(x|\theta_0) + \pi_1 \int p_1(\theta) p(x|\theta) d\theta \tag{2.47}$$

where x is the vector of observations with conditional density $p(x|\theta)$ and where $p(x)$ is the marginal density of the observations.

By letting

$$p_1(x) = \int_{\theta \neq \theta_0} p_1(\theta) p(x|\theta) d\theta \tag{2.48}$$

The marginal density (2.58) can be expressed as

$$p(x) = \pi_0 p(x|\theta_0) + \pi_1 p_1(x) \tag{2.49}$$

and the posterior probabilities of the null and alternative hypotheses can be expressed as

$$p_0 = \pi_0 p(x|\theta_0) / [\pi_0 p(x|\theta_0) + \pi_1 p_1(x)] = \pi_0 p(x|\theta_0) / p(x). \tag{2.50}$$

In a similar manner

$$p_1 = \pi_1 p_1(x) / p(x) \tag{2.51}$$

for the posterior probability of the alternative hypothesis. If one desires to use the Bayes factor, then one may show

$$B = p(x|\theta_0) / p_1(x) \tag{2.52}$$

The above derivation of the posterior probabilities in the context of hypothesis testing closely follows Lee [21].

In summary, for testing hypotheses via the Bayesian approach, the following is required:

1. The prior probabilities of the null and alternative hypotheses, namely π_0 and π_1.

2. The prior density $p_1(\theta)$ for values of $\{\theta : \theta \neq \theta_0\}$.
3. The likelihood function, that is the joint conditional density of the observations $x = (x_1, x_2, ..., x_n)$ given θ, for all values of θ in the parameter space.

For the first example in testing hypotheses when the null is simple but the alternative is composite, consider the AR(1) process

$$Y(t) = \theta Y(t-1) + W(t), t = 1, 2, ...$$ (2.53)

where

$$W(t), t = 1, 2, ...$$ (2.54)

is a sequence of independent normal random variables with mean zero and precision τ, and $\tau > 0$.

Consider the following testing problem using a Bayesian approach, where the null hypothesis is

$$H : \theta = .6$$ (2.55)

versus the alternative

$$A : \theta \neq .6.$$

Recall that the null hypothesis value $\theta = .6$ is used to generate a sample of size n = 50 from the process, thus we will be testing to see if the null hypothesis is indeed supported by the data generated from the model.

Recall that the likelihood function for θ and τ is

$$L(\theta, | \tau, | data) = (\tau / 2\pi)^{n/2} \exp - (\tau / 2) \left\{ \sum_{t=1}^{t=n} y^2(t-1)[\theta - \mu]^2 + c \right\}$$

where and

$$c = \sum_{t=1}^{t=n} y^2(t) - \left[\sum_{t=1}^{t=n} y(t) y(t-1) \right]^2 / \sum_{t=1}^{t=n} y^2(t-1)$$ (2.56)

I use the marginal likelihood for θ

$$p(\theta | data) = \tau^{(n-1)/2} \left[(n-1)\pi \right]^{1/2} / (2\pi)^{n/2} c^{n/2} f(\theta | data)$$ (2.57)

where

$$f(\theta|data) = \left\{\tau^{1/2}\Gamma(n/2)/\left[(n-1)\pi\right]^{1/2}\Gamma((n-1)/2)\right\}\left\{1+(\tau/(n-1))\left[\theta-\mu\right]^2\right\}^{n/2}$$

and

$$\tau = (n-1)\sum_{t=1}^{t=n}y^2(t-1)/c. \qquad (2.58)$$

Note that $f(\theta|\ data)$ is the density of a t-distribution with n-1 degrees of freedom, location μ, and precision τ.

We now return to (2.47) and calculate the posterior probability p_0 of the null hypothesis.

Note that the posterior probability of the null hypothesis is

$$p_0 = \left[1 + \gamma_1 p_1(y)/\gamma_0 p(y|\ \theta_0)\right]^{-1} \qquad (2.59)$$

where γ_0 is the prior probability of the null hypothesis and $\gamma_1 = 1 - \gamma_0$. Also,

$$p(y|\ \theta) = \left\{\tau^{(n-1)/2}\left[(n-1)\pi\right]^{1/2}/(2\pi)^{n/2}c^{n/2}\right\}f(\theta|y) \qquad (2.60)$$

and $f(\theta|\ y)$ is the density of a univariate t-distribution with n-1 degrees of freedom, location μ, and precision τ.

Also

$$p_1(y) = \int p_1(\theta)p(y|\ \theta)d\theta = \tau^{n/2}\left[(n-1)\pi\right]^{1/2}/(2\pi)^{n/2}c^{n/2}, \qquad (2.61)$$

thus, when the observation is inserted into (2.60) the posterior probability of the null hypothesis can be calculated. The student will be asked to calculate this probability based on the 50 observations generated from the AR(1) series (2.15).

An earlier and more informal approach , see Lindley [8], to testing hypotheses is to reject the null hypothesis if the 95% credible region for θ does not contain the set of all θ such that $\theta \in \Omega_0$. In the special case that $H: \theta = \theta_0$ versus the alternative $A: \theta \neq \theta_0$, where θ is a scalar, H is rejected when the 95% confidence interval for θ does not include θ_0. However, there are some logical problems with this approach. If a continuous prior density is used for the entire parameter space, the prior probability of the null hypothesis is zero, which implies a posterior probability of zero for the null hypothesis, thus implying illogical reasoning for this approach to testing hypotheses.

In this book, hypothesis testing is an important component as does estimating the unknown parameters, however, when testing called for the formal approach developed above in this section will be conducted.

2.6 Predictive Inference

2.6.1 Introduction

Our primary interest in the predictive distribution is to check for model assumptions. Is the adopted model for an analysis the most appropriate?

What is the predictive distribution of a future set of observations Z? It is the conditional distribution of Z given X = x, where x represents the past observations, which when expressed as a density is

$$g(z|x) = \int_{\Omega} f(z|\theta)\xi(\theta|x)d\theta, z \in R^m \tag{2.62}$$

where the integral is with respect to θ, and $f(x|\theta)$ is the density of $x = (x_1, x_2..., x_n)$, given θ. This assumes that given θ, that Z and X are independent. Thus, the predictive density is posterior average of $f(z|\theta)$ with respect to the posterior distribution of θ.

The posterior predictive density will be derived for the binomial and normal populations.

2.6.2 The Binomial Population

Suppose the binomial case is again considered, where the posterior density of the binomial parameter θ is

$$\xi(\theta|x) = [\Gamma(\alpha+\beta)\Gamma(n+1)/\Gamma(\alpha)\Gamma(\beta)\Gamma(x+1)\Gamma(n-x+1)]\theta^{\alpha+x-1}$$
$$(1-\theta)^{\beta+n-x-1}, \tag{2.63}$$

a beta with parameters $\alpha + x$ and $n - x + \beta$, and x is the sum of the set of n observations. The population mass function of a future observation Z is $f(z/\theta) = \theta^z(1-\theta)^{1-z}$, and the predictive mass function of Z, called the beta-binomial, is

$$g(z|x) = \Gamma(\alpha+\beta)\Gamma(n+1)\Gamma\left(\alpha+\sum_{i=1}^{i=n}x_i+z\right)\Gamma(1+n+\beta-x-z) \tag{2.64}$$
$$\div \Gamma(\alpha)\Gamma(\beta)\Gamma(n-x+1)\Gamma(x+1)\Gamma(n+1+\alpha+\beta),$$

where $z = 0, 1$. Note this function does not depend on the unknown parameter, and that the n past observations are known, and that if $\alpha = \beta = 1$, one is assuming a uniform prior density for θ.

As an example for the predictive distribution of the binomial distribution, let

$$N = \begin{pmatrix} 1,7,4,6,2 \\ 5,3,4,6,5 \\ 3,6,2,3,1 \\ 5,7,2,5,4 \\ 6,1,3,3,4 \end{pmatrix} \tag{2.65}$$

be the transition counts for a five-state Markov chain and

$$\Phi = \begin{pmatrix} \phi_{11},\phi_{12},\phi_{13},\phi_{14},\phi_{15} \\ \phi_{21},\phi_{22},\phi_{23},\phi_{24},\phi_{25} \\ \phi_{31},\phi_{32},\phi_{33},\phi_{34},\phi_{35} \\ \phi_{41},\phi_{42},\phi_{43},\phi_{44},\phi_{45} \\ \phi_{51},\phi_{52},\phi_{53},\phi_{54},\phi_{55} \end{pmatrix} \tag{2.66}$$

as the one-step transition matrix.

Our focus is on forecasting the number of transitions Z_{11} from 1 to 1, that is the number of times the chain remains in state 1, assuming a total of m replications for the first row of the chain, that is $Z_{11} = 0, 1, 2, ..., m$. Using (2.66), one may show the predictive mass function of Z_{11} is equation (2.67)

$$g(z|n_{11} = 1) = \binom{m}{z} \Gamma(\alpha + \beta)\Gamma(n+1)\Gamma(\alpha+z+n_{11})\Gamma(\beta+n-z-n_{11})/ \tag{2.67}$$
$$\Gamma(\alpha)\Gamma(\beta)\Gamma(n_{11}+1)\Gamma(n-n_{11}+1)\Gamma(\alpha+\beta+n)$$

The relevant quantities of (2.67) are $n = 20$, $n_{11} = 1$. Also remember that α and β are the parameters of the prior distribution of ϕ_{11}, the probability of remaining in state 1 and that predictive inferences are conditional on $n = 20$, the total transition counts for the first row of the one-step transition matrix of the chain.

Another example of prediction is a binary time series is defined by

$$Y(t)|Y(t-1),Y(t-2),...,Z(t-1),Z(t-2),.... \sim Bern(\pi_t(\gamma))$$
$$g(\pi_t(\gamma)) = \gamma Z(t-1) \tag{2.68}$$
$$Z(t-1) = (Z_1(t-1),...,Z_p(t-p))$$

where $Z(t-1)$ is a regressor which can be independent of the previous binary observations or can be only autoregressive, namely

$$Z(t-1) = \big(Y(t-1), Y(t-2), \ldots, Y(t-p)\big)$$

It can also be a mixture of both. See Wilks and Wilby [22] and also Chapter 10 of Davis, Holan, Lund, and Ravishanker [23] for the article by Kirch and Kamgaing [24].

Returning to the autoregressive binary time series (2.63), let the function g be the canonical link $g(x) = \log(x/(1-x))$, then Bayesian inferences can be based on the partial likelihood function

$$L(\gamma) = \prod_{t-1}^{t=n} \pi_t(\gamma)^{y(t)} \big(1 - \pi_t(\gamma)\big)^{1-y(t)}, \qquad (2.69)$$

where γ is the 1 by p vector of regression parameters and the t-th binary observation is $y(t)$, $t = 1, 2, \ldots, n$.

2.6.3 Forecasting from a Normal Population

Moving on to the normal density with both parameters unknown, what is the predictive density of Z, with noninformative prior density

$$\xi(\mu, \tau) = 1/\tau, \quad \mu \in R \quad \text{and} \quad \sigma > 0 \qquad (2.70)$$

The posterior density is

$$\xi(\mu, \tau \mid data) = \Big[\big(\tau^{n/2-1}/(2\pi)^{n/2}\big)\Big]\exp{-(\tau/2)}\Big[n(\mu - \bar{x})^2 + (n-1)S_x^2\Big], \quad (2.71)$$

where $\bar{x}$ and S_x^2 are the sample mean and variance, based on a random sample of size n, $x = (x_1, x_2, \ldots, x_n)$. Suppose z is a future sample $z = (z_1, z_2, \ldots, z_m)$ of size m, then the predictive density of Z is

$$g(z \mid x) = \iint \Big[\tau^{(n+m)/2-1}/(2\pi)^{(n+m)/2}\Big]\exp$$
$$-(\tau/2)\Big[n(\mu - \bar{x})^2 + (n-1)S_x^2 + m(\bar{z} - \mu)^2 + (m-1)S_z^2\Big] \qquad (2.72)$$

where the integration is with respect to $\mu \in R$ and $\sigma > 0$.

m is the number of future observations, $\bar{z}$ is the sample mean of the m future observations, and S_z^2 is the corresponding sample variance.

It can be shown that the predictive density of z is   (2.73)

$$g(z|x) \propto \Gamma((n+m-1)/2)/\left[1+\zeta(\bar{z}-\bar{x})^2/(n+m-3)\right]^{(n+m-3+1)} \qquad (2.74)$$

where

$$\zeta = nm/(n+m)k(n+m-3) \qquad (2.75)$$

$$k = (n-1)S_x^2 + (m-1)S_z^2 + n^2(\bar{x})^2/(n+m) \qquad (2.76)$$

This density is recognized as a non-central t-distribution with n+m−3 degrees of freedom, location $\bar{x}$, and precision ζ.

The predictive distribution can be used as an inferential tool to test hypotheses about future observations, estimate the mean of future observations, and find confidence bands for future observations. In the context of stochastic processes, the predictive distribution for future normal observations will be employed to generate future values from a Wiener process.

Of interest in the context of time series is Brownian motion and the predictive distribution of the future observations z when $\mu = 0$, that is, when the posterior density is

$$g(\tau|x) \propto \left[\tau^{(n+m)/2-1}/(2\pi)^{(n+m)/2}\right] \exp\left(-(\tau/2)\left[\sum_{i-1}^{i=n}x_i^2 + \sum_{i=1}^{i=m}z_i^2\right]\right). \qquad (2.77)$$

This assumes the improper prior for τ,

$$\zeta(\tau) = 1/\tau, \tau > 0 \qquad (2.78)$$

For the Wiener process of Section 2.4, the process was sampled at times $t_1, t_2, ..., t_n$ with $t_1 < t_2 <, ..., < t_n$ and with independent increments

$$d_i = X_i - X_{i-1} \qquad (2.79)$$

and where

$$t_i - t_{i-1} = 1,$$

and $i = 1,2,..,n$.

Also

$$t_0 = 0.$$

Consider m future increments

$$z_i = x_i - x_{i-1} \qquad (2.80)$$

for $i = n+1, \ldots, n+m$. and time points satisfying

$$t_i - t_{i-1} = 1.$$

Now assume an improper prior density for τ, then the joint density of the d_i and z_i is

$$g(d, |z, | \tau) \propto \tau^{(n+m)/2-1} \exp(-\tau/2) \left[\sum_{i=1}^{i=n} d_i^2 + \sum_{i=n+1}^{i=n+m} z_i^2 \right], \quad \tau > 0. \qquad (2.81)$$

Thus, the predictive distribution of the m future independent increments is

$$g(z|d) \propto \Gamma\left((n+m)/2\right) / \left[1 + \left(\zeta / (n+m-1)\right) \sum_{i=n+1}^{i=n+m} z_i^2 \right]^{(n+m-1+1)/2} \qquad (2.82)$$

This is recognized as a non-central t-density with n+m−1 degrees of freedom, location the zero vector, and precision $\varsigma = (n+m-1)/\sum_{i=1}^{i=n} d_i^2$.

Recall the Brownian motion example with a variance of .01 and where 100 observations form the process designated by x. Using formula (2.79) with $m = 100$, $n = 100$, $\sum_{i=1}^{i=100} d_i^2 = 1.6458374, \zeta = 120.64514$, then based on **BUBS Code**

2.4, with the 100 predicted z values appear as the vector z.

BC 2.4

```
model {
for (i in 1 : 100) {
y[i] ~ dt(0, 120.645, 199)
}
}
z = c(-0.05473,-0.119,0.1056,-0.129,0.05168,-
0.06759,0.07575,0.04806,0.003992,  -0.1113,-0.154,-
0.009263,0.09279,-0.06837,-0.07757,-0.1289,0.03088,0.09818,
0.01693,-0.04028,-0.1602,0.09864,-
0.05848,0.002767,-0.1908,-0.1578,-0.004863,
0.04017,-0.05318,0.08215,-0.0231,0.1652,0.01179,0.151,-
0.2395,0.00945,-0.05023,-0.09512,-0.04164,0.09382,-
0.01882,-0.1193,0.03329,0.02761,-0.0716-
3,-0.05162,0.04595,0.108,0.01209,0.09053,-0.08401,0.08781,-
0.05834,-0.09858,0.1072,0.1007,0.04107,0.222,0.1023,-
0.003405,-0.002853,0.1584,
```

```
0.05611,0.05067,0.04823,0.02001,0.1747,-
0.1451,-0.0137,-0.1187,0.04217,-0.01667,-
0.04725,0.00841,0.09915,-0.05576,0.02669,0.04407,0.03509,
0.06624,0.05622,-0.05857,-0.1255,-0.03296,-0.128,-0.0193,-
0.05927,-0.1122, 0.06573,0.06395,0.044,0.04435,0.04717,-
0.1504,0.06941,-0.03644,-0.04695,-0.1194,-0.003718,-0.08247))
```

To see the accuracy of the above predicted values, the sample mean and variance should be computed. How close to zero is the sample mean and how close to .01 is the sample variance of the Brownian motion example?

2.7 An Example of Bayesian Inference in a Stochastic Epidemic

It is best to begin with the deterministic version of an epidemic model, because the basic concepts of the theory of epidemics are introduced.

2.7.1 Deterministic Model

Let $I(n)$ and $S(n)$ denote the number of infected and number of susceptible individuals at time n respectively, where the dynamics of the chain follow the system of difference equations:

$$S(n+1) = S(n) - \beta S(n)I(n)/N + I(n)(b+\gamma)$$
$$I(n+1) = \beta S(n)I(n)/N + I(n)(1-b-\gamma)$$

(2.83)

where, $n = 0, 1, 2, \ldots, S(0) > 0, I(0) > 0, S(n) + I(n) = N$.

These equations are interpreted as follows: The number of new susceptible individuals at time n+1 is the number of individuals that did not become infected $S(n)[1 - \beta I(n)/N]$, plus the number of infected individuals that recovered, namely $\gamma I(n)$, and plus the offspring (newborns) from the infected group $bI(n)$. Since the total population size is constant, the number of offspring from the susceptible class is the same as the number of susceptible people that die, namely, $bS(n)$. The restrictions on the unknown parameters are $0 < \beta \leq 1, 0 < b + \gamma \leq 1$.

In the second equation of (1.32), $S(n)$ is replaced by $N - I(n)$ giving

$$I(n+1) = I(n)[\beta(N-I(n))/N] + 1 - b - \gamma = I(n)[1 + \beta - b - \gamma - \beta I(n)/N] \quad (2.84)$$

There are two equilibrium solutions, that is where $I(n + 1) = I(n) = E$ which are $E = 0$ and $E = N[1 - (b + \gamma)/\beta]$.

The equilibrium point is a function of the reproduction number

$$R_0 = \beta/(b+\gamma), \tag{2.85}$$

which has an interesting meaning in epidemiology: It is when the whole population is susceptible and one infected and infectious person is introduced into the population, R_0 is the average number β of successful contacts during the period of infectivity, $1/(b+\gamma)$ will result in a new infected person.

2.7.2 The Stochastic Epidemic

Assume the facts about the simple model in the deterministic case, but where $I(n)$ is a random variable denoting the number of infected individuals at time n, where the population is of size $N = I(n) + S(n)$, and $S(n)$ is a random variable denoting the number of susceptible people at time n, $n = 0, 1, 2, \ldots$. Now assume that the time interval from n to $n + 1$ is small enough so that there is almost one change over that time period. For the Bayesian analysis focus will be on the number of infected people

$I(n)$ with state space $\{0, 1, 2, \ldots, N\}$, which has two classes $\{0\}$ and $\{1, 2, \ldots, N\}$, where state 0 is absorbing, denoting that the infection dies out. The transition matrix is defined by the following three equations:

$$\begin{aligned} P_{i,i+1} &= \Pr\left[I(n+1) = i+1 \mid I(n) = i\right] = \beta i (N-i)/N = \lambda_i \\ P_{i,i-1} &= \Pr\left[I(n-1) = i-1 \mid I(n) = i\right] = (b+\gamma)i, \end{aligned} \tag{2.86}$$

and

$$P_{i,i} = \Pr\left[I(n+1) = i \mid I(n) = i\right] = 1 - \lambda_i - (b+\gamma)i.$$

Thus, the one-step transition matrix of the number of infected people is

$$P = \begin{pmatrix} 1, 0, \ldots\ldots\ldots\ldots\ldots\ldots\ldots\ldots\ldots\ldots\ldots\ldots\ldots\ldots, 0 \\ b+\gamma, 1-b-\gamma-\lambda_1, \lambda_1, 0, \ldots\ldots\ldots\ldots, 0 \\ 0, 2(b+\gamma), 1-2(b+\gamma)-\lambda_2, 0, \ldots\ldots\ldots, 0 \\ \cdot \\ \cdot \\ \cdot \\ 0, \ldots\ldots\ldots\ldots\ldots 0, N(b+\gamma), 1-N(b+\gamma) \end{pmatrix}, \tag{2.87}$$

The goal as a Bayesian is to make inferences about the unknown parameters, the birth rate b, β the number of contacts, and γ the number of infected people that recover. I will begin with estimating the parameters b, γ, and β using as data transition counts for the first three entries of the second row of P, where the transition counts will be realizations generated via the multinomial distribution.

Consider the multinomial distribution with parameter
$p = (.005, .9851, .0099)$, then using the R function rmultinom, the following realization was generated with transition counts
$(n_{10}, n_{11}, n_{12}) = (3, 993, 4)$ corresponding to the transition probabilities

$$
\begin{aligned}
P_{10} &= b + \gamma, \\
P_{11} &= 1 - \lambda_1 - (b + \gamma), \\
P_{12} &= \lambda_1 = \beta (N-1)/N, \\
N &= 100, \\
b &= \gamma = .0025,
\end{aligned}
\tag{2.88}
$$

and

$$
\beta = .01.
$$

Therefore, the transition probabilities are estimated as
$P_{\tilde{1}0} = .003, P_{\tilde{1}1} = .973$, and $P_{\tilde{1}2} = .004$. Thus, using (5.9), the estimates for the parameters of the epidemic are .0040404 for β and .0015 for b and γ. What are the Bayesian estimates?

Assume that the prior distribution for the transition probabilities is the improper prior

$$
\zeta \left(P_{10}, P_{11}, P_{12} \right) = \sum_{j=0}^{j=2} P_{1j}^{-1},
\tag{2.89}
$$

where

$$
\sum_{j=0}^{j=1} P_{1j} = 1, \, 0 < P_{1j} < 1, \text{ and } j = 1, 2, 3.
$$

It can be shown that the posterior distribution of the transition probabilities is Dirichlet with parameter $(n_{10}, n_{11}, n_{12}) = (3, 993, 4)$, thus the marginal posterior distribution of P_{10} is beta(3,997), P_{11} is beta(993,7), and P_{12} beta(4,996).

The Bayesian analysis is executed with BUGS code 2.5 with 35,000 observations for the simulation and a burn in of 5,000. The step command g2 gives the posterior probability that $R_0 > 1$.

BC 2.5

```
model;
{
p10~dbeta(3,997)
p11~dbeta(993,7)
p12~dbeta(4,996)
bplusgamma<-p10
N<-100
beta<-p12*N/(N-1)
b<-bplusgamma/2
R0<-beta/bplusgamma
g1<-step(R0-.5)
g2<-step(R0-1)
}
```

As a result of the simulation, the Bayesian analysis for the simple epidemic model is reported in Table 2.3.

Note that the posterior probability that $R_0 > 1$ is .663, that is in symbols

$$g^2 = \Pr[R_0 > 1| data] = .663$$

The estimates of the other parameters P_{10}, P_{11}, and P_{12} are similar to the usual estimates given above. Recall that the transition probabilities $P_{10} = .005$, $P_{11} = .9851$, $P_{12} = .0099$ were used to generate the multinomial realization $(n_{10}, n_{11}, n_{12}) = (3, 993, 4)$ for the Bayesian analysis, and these values for the transition probabilities should be compared to the posterior means (.0029, .993, .0039) of Table 2.3. It appears that the posterior means are quite close to these values. See Chapter 5 for additional information about epidemics.

TABLE 2.3

Posterior Distribution of Epidemic Model

Parameter	Mean	SD	Error	2 1/2	Median	97 1/2
R_0	2.029	2.655	.0097	.2935	1.389	7.538
B	.00149	.000859	.0000032	.00031	.00133	.00361
$b + \gamma$	.002986	.001718	.0000064	.00062	.00267	.00722
P_{10}	.002986	.001718	.0000064	.00062	.00267	.00722
P_{11}	.993	.00262	.0000096	.987	.9933	.9972
P_{12}	.00399	.001992	.0000083	.0011	.00366	.00879
β	.004037	.002003	.0000112	.00113	.003705	.00886
g^2	.663	.4727	.002646	0	1	0

2.8 Comments

This chapter introduces the reader to the basic concepts of Bayesian inference. Of course, this consists of Bayes theorem, which involves the ideas of prior, posterior, and predictive distributions. Once these are given estimation, testing hypotheses, and forecasting easily follows. Many examples illustrate the basic ideas of this book, including Bayesian inference for stochastic epidemics.

2.9 Exercises

1. For the Beta density (2.8) with parameters α and β, show that the mean is $[\alpha/(\alpha+\beta)]$ and the variance is $[\alpha\beta/(\alpha+\beta)^2(\alpha+\beta+1)]$.

2. From equation (2.14), show the following. If the normal distribution is parameterized with μ and the precision $\tau = 1/\sigma^2$, the conjugate distribution is as follows: (a) the conditional distribution of μ given τ is normal with mean $\bar{x}$ and precision $n\tau$, and (b) the marginal distribution of τ is gamma with parameters $(n-1)/2$ and $\sum_{i=1}^{i=n}(x_i - \bar{x})^2/2 = (n-1)S^2/2$, where S^2 is the sample variance.

3. Verify Table 2.1, which reports the Bayesian analysis for the parameters of an AR(1) time series.

4. Verify the following statement: To generate values from the $t(n-1, \bar{x}, n/S^2)$ distribution, generate values from Student's t-distribution with n-1 degrees of freedom and multiply each by $S/\sqrt{n}$ and then add $\bar{x}$ to each.

5. Verify Equation (2.82), the predictive density of a future observations Z from a normal population with both parameters unknown.

6. Suppose x_1, x_2, .., x_n are independent and that $x_i \sim gamma(\alpha_i, \beta)$, and show that $y_i = x_i/(x_1 + x_2 + ... + x_n)$ jointly have a Dirichlet distribution with parameter $(\alpha_1, \alpha_2, ..., \alpha_n)$. Describe how this can be used to generate samples from the Dirichlet distribution.

7. Suppose $(X_1, X_2, ..., X_k)$ is multinomial with parameters n and $(\theta_1, \theta_2, ..., \theta_k)$, where $\sum_{i=1}^{i=k} X_i = n$, $0 < \theta_i < 1$ and $\sum_{i=1}^{i=k} \theta_i = 1$. Show that

$E(X_i) = n\theta_i$, $Var(X_i) = n\theta_i(1 - \theta_i)$, and $Cov(X_i, X_j) = -n\theta_i\theta_j$. What is the marginal distribution of θ_i?

8. Suppose $(\theta_1, \theta_2, ..., \theta_k)$ is Dirichlet with parameters $(\alpha_1, \alpha_2, ..., \alpha_k)$, where $\alpha_i > 0$,, and $\sum_{i=1}^{i=k} \theta_i = 1$. Find the mean and variance of θ_i and covariance between θ_i and θ_j, $i \neq j$.

9. Show the Dirichlet family is conjugate to the multinomial family.

10. Suppose $(\theta_1, \theta_2, ..., \theta_k)$ is Dirichlet with parameters $(\alpha_1, \alpha_2, ..., \alpha_k)$. Show the marginal distribution of θ_i is beta and give the parameters of the beta. What is the conditional distribution of θ_i given θ_j?

11. For the exponential density

$$f\left(x|\theta\right) = \theta \exp{-\theta x}, \quad x > 0$$

where x is positive and θ is a positive unknown parameter, suppose the prior density of θ is

$$g\left(\theta\right) \propto \theta^{\alpha-1} \exp{-\beta\theta}, \quad \theta > 0,$$

what is the posterior density of θ? In Markov jump processes, the exponential distribution is the distribution of the inter-arrival times between events.

12. Refer to Section 2.7.2. Based on BUGS code BC 2.1, generate 100 observations from an exponential distribution with mean 3.

13. Refer to Section 2.5.3. on testing hypotheses. Let θ be the autoregressive parameter of an AR(1) time series and consider a test of the null hypothesis $H_0 : \theta = .6$ versus the alternative $H_1 : \theta \neq .6$. Refer to Equations (2.53) through (2.58). Use the Bayesian approach of Lee [21] and use the data generated for the AR(1) series.

14. Verify the predictive probability mass function (2.63) for the binomial.

15. Verify the predictive distribution (2.82) of m future observations form a Brownian motion process.

16. Based on the multinomial mass function and R code

```
n<-1000
prob<-c(.2,.2,.2,.2,.2)
multinom(1,n,prob)
generate 1000 observations from the multinomial with
parameter
vector (.2,.2,.2,.2,.2). List the number of counts over
the five categories.
```

Do your results imply they were generated from a multinomial with the probabilities (.2,.2,.2,.2,.2)? How would you test the hypothesis that they were?

References

1. Bayes, T. (1764). An essay towards solving a problem in the doctrine of chances, *Phil. Trans. Roy. Soc. London*, 53, 370.
2. Laplace, P.S. (1778). Mémoire des les probabilities, Mémoires de l'Academie des sciences de Paris, 227.
3. Stigler, M. (1986). *The History of Statistics. The Measurement of Uncertainty Before 1900*, The Belknap Press of Harvard University Press, Cambridge, MA.
4. Hald, A. (1990). *A History of Mathematical Statistics From 1750-1930*, Wiley Interscience, London.
5. Lhoste, E. (1923). Le calcul des probabilities appliqué a l'artillerie, lois de probabilité à prior, *Revu d'artillirie*, Mai, 405.
6. Jeffreys, H. (1939). *An Introduction to Probability*, Clarendon Press, Oxford.
7. Savage, L.J. (1954). *The Foundation of Statistics*, John Wiley & Sons Inc., New York.
8. Lindley, D.V. (1965). *Introduction to Probability and Statistics from a Bayesian Viewpoint, Volumes I and II*, Cambridge University Press, Cambridge.
9. Broemeling, L.D. and Broemeling, A.L. (2003). Studies in the history of probability and statistics XLVIII: the Bayesian contributions of Ernest Lhoste, *Biometrika*, 90(3), 728.
10. Box, G.E.P. and Tiao, G.C. (1973). *Bayesian Inference in Statistical Analysis*, Addison Wesley, Reading, MA.
11. Zellner, A. (1971). *An Introduction to Bayesian Inference in Econometrics*, JohnWiley & Sons Inc., New York.
12. Broemeling, L.D. (1985). *The Bayesian Analysis of Linear Models*, Marcel-Dekker Inc, New York.
13. Leonard, T., and Hsu, J.S.J. (1999). *Bayesian Methods: An Analysis for Statisticians and Interdisciplinary Researchers*, Cambridge University Press, Cambridge UK.
14. Gelman, A., Carlin, J.B., Stern, H.S., and Rubin, D.B. (1997). *Bayesian Data Analysis*, Chapman & Hall/CRC, New York.
15. Congdon, P. (2001). *Bayesian Statistical Modeling*, John Wiley & Sons LTD, London.
16. Congdon, P. (2003). *Applied Bayesian Modeling*, John Wiley & Sons Inc., New York.
17. Congdon, P. (2005). *Bayesian Models for Categorical Data*, John Wiley & Sons Inc., New York.
18. Carlin, B.P. and Louis, T.A. (1996). *Bayes and Empirical Bayes for Data Analysis*, Chapman & Hall, New York.
19. Gilks, W.R., Richardson, S., Spiegelhalter, D.J. (1996). *Markov Chain Monte Carlo in Practice*, Chapman & Hall/CRC, Boca Raton, FL.

20. Lehmann, E.L. (1959). *Testing Statistical Hypotheses*, John Wiley & Sons Inc., New York.
21. Lee, P.M. (1997). *Bayesian Statistics, an Introduction*, second edition, Arnold, a member of the Hodder Headline Group, London.
22. Wilks, D. and Wilby, R. (1999). The weather generation game: a review of stochastic weather models. *Prog. Phys. Geography*, 23, 329–357.
23. Davis, R.A., Holan, S.H., Lund, R., and Ravishanker, N. (2016). *Handbook of Discrete -Valued Time Series*, CRC Press/Chapman & Hall, Boca Raton, FL.
24. Kirch, C. and Kamgaing, J.T. (2016). Detection of change points in discrete-valued time series. *Chapter 10 in Handbook of Discrete -Valued Time Series*, edited by Davis, R.A., Holan, S.H., Lund, R., and Ravishanker, N., CRC Press, Boca Raton FL.

3

Infectious Diseases

3.1 Introduction

This chapter presents a brief description of infectious diseases and should be understood before the student can appreciate the nature of the subject in this book.

Germs are all around us and when humans are involved it is called an infection. This book describes the statistical analysis of the evolution of infections, and this chapter is a brief introduction to the subject. According to Chapter 6 of Comptons' Encyclopedia [1, p. 167], the body has a special way of reacting to infections and has a system that fights off the first infectious bodies, and through memory gives the body a immunity against future attacks by the same type (same genetic properties) of invasion. Many substances can harm the body and are referred to as antigens, including bacteria, fungi, viruses. The body reacts by producing chemicals called antibodies.

Antibodies are proteins called immunoglobulins, where each is made up of a chain of chemical subunits, or amino acids, and a light chain of them. The light chains have special sites, where the amino acids can link with complements on an antigen molecule. When an antibody attaches to an antigen, it deactivates by covering a key portion of the harmful substance. In some cases, through a process called opsonization, antibodies "butter" the surface of the antigens in order to make them more susceptible to phagocytes, which then devour the antigens. Often an antibody attaches to a bacterial antigen but requires an intermediate or complement to actually devour the bacterium. As the antibody-antigen union circulates in the blood, the complex "fixes" the complement to it which then the complex produces enzymes to eat through the bacterial wall to make the organism burst.

There are several types of immunoglobulins, where the largest is designated as IgM and IgC, the most available and versatile. The next most plentiful is IgA which is especially adaptable to work areas where body secretions can injure other antibodies. Other immunoglobulins are associated with allergic reactions. IgM is produced at the first sign of an antigen. Later it is replaced by a more effective IgG.

When an infection first appears, the immune system appears not to respond, and antibodies in the blood cannot be detected. This is because the basic cells involved in the production of antibodies have been triggered by the presence of an antigen to multiply themselves. The amount of antibody begins to increase on approximately day two of infection, then exponentially grows. By day five the antibody level has increased by a thousand.

The first antibodies, the large IgM type, are not the best prepared to attack a wide range of antigens but, on the other hand, are very effective against bacteria. The more versatile IgG is a component of the blood on about the fourth day of infection, its production is stimulated by the increase of IgM. During this period, IgM levels off and the immune system begins to make IgG. This antibody attaches well to antigens and eventually envelopes then so that the antigens cannot prompt an immune response, and IgG production is terminated. This is an example of negative feedback control.

3.2 Antibody Production

Antibodies are made up of two types of cells: Plasma cells and a class of white blood cells, namely lymphocytes. Plasma cells originate from lymphocytes and are present throughout the lymphatic tissue. Lymphocytes stem from cells in the blood-forming sections of the bone marrow. When the bone marrow cells circulate in the thymus, a lymphatic structure in the chest, they are stimulated to become lymphocytes and to make antibodies. Most lymphocytes last only a few hours, but a small number can survive for several years. These lymphocytes develop a memory antigen that were encountered in the past, thus inducing the immune system to produce antibodies directed against those or similar antigens when they enter the body.

When people develop antibodies against a disease by the action of their immune system, they have active immunity. When a person is injected with another person's, passive immunity to that disease can be acquired by that individual. Passive immunity is temporary, and some people may get relief from a disease through injections of serum containing gamma globulin, a portion of the blood rich in antibodies.

Without protective antibodies, we would die from the first disease that is encountered. This would be true of newborn babies, except that they receive passive immunity from their mothers. During her lifetime, a mother accumulates a wide variety of antibodies against a variety of host diseases. Enough of them are passed to the developing baby in her womb to give it a temporary immunity to many diseases during the early months of its life, until it can develop its own antibodies.

3.3 How Drugs Fight Disease

With the advent of drug therapy in the 20th century, doctors began to use lifesaving drugs to fight diseases. The clinical use of sulfanilamide, the predecessor of sulfa drug in the thirties and the mass production of penicillin, the fist antibiotic in the forties gave medical doctors extremely powerful tools with which to attack infections. A disease-fighting drug never acts by itself. It works jointly with the body's immune system. In addition, it has become available for the prevention of viral diseases.

3.4 How Certain Drugs Attack Infections

Certain antibiotics such as penicillin, streptomycin, and tetracycline are very effective against bacterial infections. The designation "antibiotic" is based on the concept of antibiosis, or the use of substances made by one living thing to kill another. Antibiotics are made by bacteria and molds that are specially cultured by commercial drug laboratories. Antibiotics kill bacteria and other disease organisms in a variety of ways. For example, some destroy cell walls, while others interfere with the multiplication of bacteria or fatally alter the way the bacteria manufacture vital proteins. Still others mix up the genetic plan of the bacteria. Ordinarily, an antibiotic tricks bacteria into using the antibiotic's chemicals instead of closely related ones that organisms really need for making the key enzymes required for their growth and reproduction. With the antibiotic assimilated into their systems, instead of vital chemicals, an essential activity or structure of the pathogens is lacking and they die.

Sulfa drugs act in a similar fashion but less effective way. Weakened but not destroyed by the sulfa drugs, the pathogens fall prey to the body's scavenger cells. Drugs are also used against parasitic worms, infectious amoeba, and other pathogenic organisms. It should be noted that antibiotics are not usually effective against viruses, because of the drug's inability to enter the body cells, whereas viruses hide and multiply. However, the body does produce a protein called interferon that inhibits viral multiplication. A drug often recognizes the body's immune system as an antigen, thus initiating a severe reaction. In various cases, a person can suffer anaphylaxis, or extreme sensitivity to penicillin after repeated injections. Without quick medical intervention, severe cases of anaphylactic shock are often fatal.

3.5 Drug Resistance

Once in every several million cell divisions, a mutation produces immune bacteria, which is immune to an antibiotic drug. This occurs because the mutation changes the bacteria's genetic code, and consequently its ability to use certain chemicals for its activities. Some of the causes of mutations are radiation from space that enter the earth's environment, as well as some atmospheric chemicals. As a result of the mutation, all bacteria that stem from the immune germ will be resistant to the drug unless it mutates again to make the strain susceptible again. Thus, whenever a new antibiotic is developed, there is a small probability the bacteria will develop an immunity against it. Since mutations are fairly rare, there is a good chance of fighting a bacterial disease with another drug before future strains become resistant. Some members of the bacterial strain are resistant to certain drugs naturally. In time, they can eventually become selected via evolution and become the dominant drug-resistant forms of a pathogenic strain. More importantly, some bacteria can pass on their drug resistance to another stain by "infection". Since the passing of resistance factors does not depend upon the lengthy process of mutation, it poses a much greater problem of drug immunity. Thus, doctors must prescribe more than one antibiotic to fight certain diseases, in the hope that this will retard bacterial resistance.

3.6 Vaccine and Hormone Therapy

A person becomes artificially immune to some diseases by way of vaccination, which contain antigens that stimulate the yield of antibodies. Immunity to smallpox, polio, measles, rabies, and other viruses is induced by injecting a person with living by diminished disease organisms. A vaccine containing only dead organisms protects one against typhoid fever, whooping cough, measles, and polio. Vaccines containing toxins or poisons are used to prevent diphtheria and tetanus. When injected into a person, the production of antibodies is induced. The antibodies are called antitoxins. Some body disorders are caused by too much or has too little hormone yield. Hormones are body chemicals that affect many important biochemical reactions. When a person has a deficiency in hormones, the ailment is easy to treat with hormone shots.

3.7 Infectious Diseases

Infectious diseases can be transmitted in several ways. For example, they can be spread in droplets through the air when infected people sneeze or cough. Whoever inhales the droplets can then be infected. Some diseases can be passed through contaminated food or drinking utensils. On the other hand, some can be spread by sexual activity, while others transmitted during medical or surgical interventions. An source of infection is the use of contaminated needles by drug dealers or users. Once the infection is well established in the body, the infective agent begins to thrive and multiply throughout the body. Its proliferation can be fast or slow depending on the type of organism. For example, the symptoms of the common cold appear within days of the infection, but on the other hand the symptoms of kuru, an uncommon malady of the nervous system, appear on the average three years after the person was infected. Every infectious disease has an incubation period, the length of time the pathogen is established until the appearance of symptoms of the disease. Several factors also determine whether a person will become a victim after becoming infected. The quantity of invading germs, the dose of the infection all influence the outbreak of the disease. The virulence of the infection also plays a part, in addition to the condition of the body's immune system ability to fight the infection.

3.8 Contagious Diseases

Many infectious diseases are contagious; that is, the disease can be passed between people. To contract certain infectious diseases someone only needs to be in contact with someone who has the disease, or one can catch the disease by eating or drinking from contaminated utensils. Someone can be a carrier in several ways. One can be an asymptomatic carrier or have a disease without ever developing its symptoms. It is possible for one to be an incubatory carrier and pass on the pathogens at any time during the hidden incubation period. One can be a convalescent carrier and transmit some of the infectious organisms remaining in the body even after recovery. It stands to reason that anyone suffering the frank symptoms of a contagion can pass it on to others while the disease is running its course. The following tables

TABLE 3.1

Some Important Infectious Diseases

Name	Cause	Typical Sources	Incubation Period	Common Symptoms	Usual Treatment	Preventive Measures
AIDS	HIV-1	Sexual contact with a carrier, contaminated blood and hypodermic needles	6 Months to several years	Sever viral, fungal, protozoal, and bacterial infections	Antimicrobial agents, radiotherapy for Kaposi syndrome.	Avoid sexual contact with carriers, and avoid contaminated blood and hypodermic equipment
Amebiasis	*Entamoeba hystolytica*	Contaminated water, raw vegetables and flies	Variable; commonly 2–4 weeks	Stomach pain, fever, chills, bloody diarrhea	Tinidazole, metronidazole, Dehydroemetine	Improved sanitation and food handling, health education
Bacillary dysentery (shigelliosis)	*Shigella* bacteria	Contaminated food or water	1–7 days	Diarrhea, fever, stomach pain, and vomiting	Fluids and antibiotics	Food protection and improved sanitatioin
Chicken Pox (Varicella)	*Varicella zoster* (herpes virus)	Airborne droplets	2–3 weeks	Slight fever, small red bumps on skin	Lotion to relieve itching	Isolation of high-risk individuals
Cholera	*Vibrio cholerae*	Contaminated food and water	A few hours to 5 days	Profuse watery diarrhea, vomiting, and dehydration	Tetracycline, oral and intravenous fluids	Improved sanitation and food handling, water purification
Common cold	At least 100 rhinoviruses can cause a cold	Airborne droplets	1–3 days	Sneezing, sore throat, runny nose, headache, and coughing	Rest, pain relievers, cough syrup	None effective
Diphtheria	*Corynebacterium diptheriae* (a bacterium)	Contact with carrier	2–5 days	Sore throat, fever, swollen neck glands	Diphtheria antitoxin and antibiotics	Immunization

(Continued)

TABLE 3.1 (Continued)

Name	Cause	Typical Sources	Incubation Period	Common Symptoms	Usual Treatment	Preventive Measures
Rubella (German Measles)	*Rubella* virus	Airborne droplets	14–21 days	Headache, stiff joints, and rash	Lotion to relieve itching	Immunization
Gonorrhea	*Neisseria gonorrhoeae*	Sexual contact with carrier	2–7 days	Pus discharge from sex organs	Penicillin and other antibiotics	Prostitution control, condom use, and sex education
Hepatitis (types A,B,C and unidentified strains	Hepatitis virus and other pathogens	Contaminated for and water, blood syringes, and sexual contact	2–39 weeks	Fever, drowsiness, loss of appetite, and jaundice	Special diet and rest	Sterilized injection equipment, screening for infected blood, and vaccine for type B
Herpes simplex (fever blister cold sore)	Herpes simplex virus types 1 and 2	Contact with saliva of carrier	2–12 days	Small blisters about the mouth, lips, or genitals	Keep lesions clean and dry	Personal hygiene and health education
Influenza	Influenza viruses A,B, and C	Airborne droplets	2–3 days	Chills, fever, muscle pain, and sore throat	Fluids, bed rest, and pain relievers	Vaccines for some virus strains
Legionnaire's disease	*Legionella* bacteria	Airborne transmission	2–10 days	Appetite loss, muscle pain, headache, high fever and cough	Erythromycin	Disinfecting cooling-tower water air conditioners
Leprosy	*Mycobacterium leprae*	Long exposure to carrier	7 months to 6 years	Bumpy skin, nodules, sores, muscle weakness, and numbness	Dapsone acedapsone, rifampicin	Acedapsone, BCG vaccine
Malaria	Single-cell *Plasmodium* parasites	*Anopheles* mosquito bite	12 days -10 months	Chills, fever headache, and sweating	Quinine-based drugs	Drugs for treatment are also used for prevention

(Continued)

TABLE 3.1 (Continued)

Name	Cause	Typical Sources	Incubation Period	Common Symptoms	Usual Treatment	Preventive Measures
Measles (rubeola)	*Morbillivirus*	Airborne droplets, and contact with carrier	7–14 days	Fever, cough, spots on gums, skin rash	Lotion to relieve itching and bed rest	Immunization
Mononucleosis	Epstein-Barr virus	Contact with carrier's saliva	4–6 weeks	Fever, sore throat, fatigue, swollen lymph nodes	Fluids, bed rest, and pain relievers	None known
Mumps	Paramyxovirus	Airborne droplets and contact with carrier	2–3 weeks	Painfully swollen salivary glands	Soft diet, bed rest, and pain relievers	Immunization
Poliomyelitis	Poliovirus, types 1, 2, and 3	Contact with carrier	3–35 days	Headache, stiff neck, and back fever and paralysis	Mechanical respirators for some patients	Immunization
Rabbit fever	*Francisella tularensis* (a bacterium)	Contact with infected animals	2–10 days	Ulcer at entry site, swollen and burst lymph glands	Antibiotics	Rubber gloves while handling animals, and immunization
Rabies (human hydrophobia)	Rabies virus	Bite by infected animal	10 days-more than one year	Headache, fever, painful throat spasms	Antirabies serum followed by rabies vaccine series	Vaccination of all dogs and cats
Rheumatic fever	*Streptococcus pyrogens* (a bacterium)	Contact with 'strep throat' or scarlet fever carrier	7–21 days after first strep infection	Painful joints, inflamed heart bumps near joints, and rash	Aspirin, steroid drugs, and rest	Antibiotic treatment to kill strep germs
Salmonella infection (Salmonellosis)	Numerous strains of salmonella bacteria	Contaminated food, egg, and dairy products	6–72 hours	Stomach pain, diarrhea, nausea, fever, and vomiting	fluids	Thorough cooking of animal-derived food stuffs, refrigerate food, and avoid raw eggs

(Continued)

TABLE 3.1 (Continued)

Name	Cause	Typical Sources	Incubation Period	Common Symptoms	Usual Treatment	Preventive Measures
Scarlet fever (scarlatina)	*Streptoccus pathogens* (a bacteria)	Contact with carriers of strep throat	1-5 days	Sore throat, red bumps on tongue, skin rash	Antibiotics and pain relievers	Antibiotic treatment to kill strep bacteria
Smallpox (variola)	*Variola virus*	Contact with carrier	7-17 days	Fever, headache, and skin lesions	Antibiotics to hinder other infections	Immunization no longer necessary
Syphilis	*Treponema pallidum*	Sexual contact with carrier	10 days-10 weeks	Painless chancre rash, lethargy, and gummy tumors	Penicillin and other antibiotics	Health and sex education, condoms, and control of prostitution
Tetanus	*Clostridium tetani* (a bacterium)	Wounds containing contaminated soil or other matter	4-21 days	Stiff and painful jaw and neck muscles	Cleaning wound, antibiotics, tetanus immune globulin	Immunization
Toxic shock syndrome	A strain of *Staphylococcus aureus* (a bacterium)	Associated with use of vaginal tampons	1-2 days	High fever, vomiting, rash, diarrhea, and shock	Hospitalization, fluid replacement, and antibiotics	Avoid vaginal tampons, or use intermittently during each menstrual cycle
Tuberculosis	*Mycobacterium tuberculosis*	Airborne droplets	4-12 weeks	Cough, bloody sputum, chest pain, and weight loss	Isoniazid antibiotics and/or surgery	Improvement of social conditions, tuberculin tests, and chest X-rays
Typhoid fever	*Salmonella typhi* (a bacterium)	Contaminated food or water	1-3 weeks	Fever, headache, appetite loss, and red skin spots	Chloramphenicol antibiotics	Improved sanitation, and immunization
Whooping Cough (Pertussis)	*Bordetella pertussis*	Airborne droplets	7-21 days	Spasmodic cough ending in a "whoop" breath, and vomiting	Hospitalization of infants, small, frequent meals, fluids	Erythromycin, immunization (vaccine has some associated risk)

Source: Table based on an article taken from Compton's Encyclopedia Volume Six, pages 171-172.

contain information about many of the present and now common global infections. As in the case of all diseases, certain symptoms may or may not be present. In addition, the tables are for general information and not for self-diagnosis of any disease (Table 3.1).

We now present an introduction to emerging infectious diseases followed by detailed information about smallpox, malaria, and tuberculosis. Smallpox is now eradicated, but tuberculosis and malaria are still with us, the former taking approximately some one billion lives in the past, and the later malaria taking approximately 30,000 lives yearly.

3.9 Emerging Infections

According to Drexler [2], infections are part of life, and all creatures feast on one another, and in turn are feasted upon. When humans are the meal, it is called infectious diseases, this book in part pertains to new and emerging infections: those that have increased in rate of virulence and geographic range, or threaten to do so. This book attempts to explain why the infections are materializing and why they will remain with us. Also, this book tells the stories of scientists are racing for a cure to conquer these invisible enemies. Different threats will be examined, including animal and insect-borne diseases, food-borne pathogens, antibiotic resistance, pandemic influenza, and infectious causes of chronic disease.

The list is not unique. At any time, new and old infectious diseases are present. For example, in the mid-1970s to the early 1980s. For example, first came swine flu in February of 1976. The government prepared for a repeat of the epidemic, similar to the 1918 influenza pandemic, but it did not happen. However, in the summer of 1976, a new infection appeared, Legionnaires' disease, which took place in Philadelphia and caused 34 deaths. Since it was new, for a time it presented a challenge to the public health experts but was finally identified as a bacterial infection. Soon to follow, was the occurrence of Lyme disease, toxic shock syndrome, *E. coli* O157:H7, sexually transmitted diseases, and the most series threat Ebola virus. The Centers for Disease Control, in June 1981, described a mysterious cluster of fatal among five gay men in Los Angeles: This was later identified as acquired immunodeficiency syndrome (AIDS), where approximately 250,000 had been infected in the U.S.

The same puzzles of biology and convergence of habits as well as mistakes in monitoring that resulted in AIDS are constantly drawing new diseases. At the 20th anniversary of the CDC report, other infections were being introduced into the environment. A staph infection had turned very virulent which was not expected and was resistant to the most powerful drugs commonly used to treat staph. Four healthy children and a college student suddenly died, and many more infected. *E. coli* killed a juvenile girl after consuming watermelon at a restaurant in Milwaukee, one of the 5,000 deaths yearly from foodborne pathogens. Mosquitos and birds carried West Nile virus in New York and the southern states. People enjoying the outdoors as well as city dwellers were contracting tickborne Lyme disease. In the fall of 2001, bioterrorism first appeared with the appearance of anthrax spores.

The scientist Hans Zinsser [3, p. 3], is remembered for this 1934 citation: "However secure a well-regulated civilized life may become, bacteria Protozoa, infected fleas, mosquitoes, and bedbugs will always lurk in the shadows ready to pounce when neglect, poverty, famine, or war lets down the defenses. And even in normal times they prey on the weak, the very young, and the very old, living among us, in mysterious obscurity waiting their opportunities," Through media coverage and often sensationalism reportage and false statements, Americans have become aware of the threat of infections. The CDC has been confronting such tales as bananas carrying flesh-eating bacteria, drug addicts placing HIV-contaminated needles in pay phone coin-return boxes, virus-soaked sponge arriving in the mail, and other outrageous reports. Later in 2001, there were reports of war-germ warfare. One felt helpless and at the mercy of a wayward world out of control with puzzling health threats that took hold of the public's imagination.

In order to offer a local view of a universal and true danger, this chapter emphasized primarily the U.S. It should be noted that the distinction between national and global threats is somewhat arbitrary. Pathogens do not require a visa, and secret agents shadow environmental change everywhere, and the pace of change is accelerating. Health officials in America observe the field outside of our national border, partly because many of these diseases can be transported in people or goods or animals to this country. A good example of this is the present infection of coronavirus which has its origins in the vicinity of Wuhan, China. Investigators must also build up a surveillance infrastructure to keep up to date of the many pathogens that are abroad, because genetically associated may already be here, lying in wait ready to infect the people. Recall in 1993, the appearance of the dangerous pulmonary syndrome that originated in the Southwest. Initially, scientists were baffled by this infectious disease until diagnostic tests were developed by the U.S. Department of Defense. It turned out that this pestilence was related to a virus encountered in Korea which was later identified as the genus Hantavirus.

What is encountered presently is what is always occurring: one plague after the other, and usually several at once. Think of the coronavirus and its relative influenza which is currently attacking the population. Indeed, U.S. intelligence agencies describe infectious disease as a "nontraditional" threat, both to individuals and to countries.

Before the recent headlines about avian flu, a hepatitis C epidemic, parasite-contaminated water slides, a new type of Creutzfeldt-Jakob disease, and anthrax, there was typhus, smallpox, polio, cholera, rabies, and the Black

Death of the middle ages. They are still with us, none has been eradicated, and in some cases are deadly and intractable today. Horrible news of flesh-eating bacteria are still with us. For example, in the fifth century BC, Hippocrates described a condition in which the flesh, muscles, and sinews fell from the bones, leaving a skeleton. There were many deaths, and the path of the disease was the same, regardless of what part of the body was involved.

Small human populations suffer the oldest diseases of mankind: chronic ailments such as leprosy, or herpes, or that have room in animals and the soil, such as yellow fever, the virus of which is found in monkeys. On the other hand, when the population is dense and filthy enough to keep to enhance the spreading of germs and sufficiently large to supply the susceptibles do such infections as measles, smallpox, typhoid fever, and influenza – so called crowd diseases or "zymotics" remain in circulation.

The shattering plagues of history bespoke *Homo sapiens* immunological naivete. It is believed that malaria contributed to the fall of Rome, and that the plague of Antoninus (AD166-180), most likely smallpox, induced between one-fourth to one-third of the population of Italy. Also, the plague of Justinian (AD 542-543) is thought to be one of the first cases of rat spread bubonic plague where it is believed that the whole human race was close to total annihilation. The historian Procopius reported that the disease killed approximately 10,000 people daily in Byzantium, and spread from Constantinople to Denmark.

Over the following centuries, the infections emerged in wave. It is reported that between 1346 and 1350 AD, one-third of the European population fell to bubonic plague spread from Asia to Europe by the Mongol armies, which were followed by another army of rodents carrying infected fleas that bit humans. In the sixteen and seventeenth centuries, slave ships from West Africa brought yellow fever and its mosquito vector *Aedes aegypti* to the New World. Smallpox hitched a ride to the Americas by the Spanish conquistadors, killing approximately one-third of the non-immune natives, which was in turn followed by similarly lethal attack by measles. Diseases introduced by European people, decimated an estimated 95% of the pre-Columbian population. To a lesser extent, exotic infections attacked in reverse killing Europeans. European settlers succumbed to malaria, yellow fever, and other endemic infections in tropical Africa, India, Southeast Asia, and New Guinea. Syphilis, a bacterial scourge that relies on a mobile population and indiscriminate sexual contact, appeared in 1494, perhaps with Columbus's returning soldiers.

The industrial revolution of the 19th century amplified such ancient diseases as tuberculosis, a bacterial infection that thrives in crowded housing. Illnesses from contaminated food and water , such as typhoid fever and cholera increased in virulence. But, life expectancy increased during the 19th century, perhaps the historian argued that the improvement was based on strong resistance, and from sanitation measures such as sewage disposal, which of course, reduced a person's exposure to disease-causing pathogens. Also, it is apparent that personal hygiene and health practices, such as boiling water and isolating sick relatives, may have made some difference.

A new discipline called bacteriology began in the late 1870s and this scientific effort found the microbes that caused cholera, tuberculosis, gonorrhea, typhoid, and scarlet fever. Needless to say, this was a revolution that used the science of biology to study the cause of these diseases. By 1900, scientists unanimously agreed that microorganisms, spread by casual contact, food and water contamination, insects, and by asymptomatic human carriers, in the case of typhoid and tuberculosis, were the cause of communicable diseases. The discoveries expanded government health initiatives such as water purification, food inspection, rodent control, and more awareness of individual hygiene actions, such as covering a cough and washing hands before eating. Of course, most relevant during these times of the coronavirus is "social distance", recommended by the CDC as a person being at least six feet away from other people.

The years 1890–1930 are now referred to as the golden era of American public health movement. An optimistic declaration was made in a 1924 issue of Scientific American editorial that commented " the natural outcome of the struggle between mankind and microbe has always favored man."

The microbiologist René Dubos described life itself as emergence in an ongoing evolution and adaptation. In this manner of understanding, emerging infections are merely episodes in a Darwinian saga stretching over thousands of years from or in the distant past. Conditions endlessly shift, that is, temperatures rise and fall, habitats flourish and perish, food supplies grow lush and decrease, and all living things transform themselves and die.

In the unending drama of emerging infections, nature's undercover operatives are the same: viruses, bacteria, fungi, protozoa, known collectively as microorganisms. The plot of this story has not changed, similar to an author of mysteries which usually have several plots running simultaneously throughout the story. In a similar manner, biologists have discovered very few pathogenic plots which are breathtaking when the story is elucidated.

Microorganisms play the survival game very well indeed, because they adapt far more rapidly than humans as the scene shifts in front of them. Among humans each generation is approximately 20 years, but for bacteria a generation ranges from 20–30 min, and in the case of viruses, a generation is much smaller. Richard Krause, former director of the National Institute of Allergy and Infectious Disease (NIAID) calls this rapidity a millennium in a fortnight. The current director of this agency is Dr. Fauci, who appears with President Trump on the daily briefings of the Coronavirus Task Force. An important aspect of evolution is natural selection, the process by which genetically adapted individuals leave more offspring and in the process transmit more favorable characteristics, and thus operate far more efficiently in the setting of microorganisms. Since these aggregate in large numbers, bacteria and viruses do support a considerable variety in their communities, including mutations that may be expressed when the environment changes. A thimble can contain a billion bacteria, can disappear on Tuesday, and appear in the same quantity on Wednesday.

According to the epidemiologist David Morens, when one looks at the association between bugs and humans, it is important to concentrate on bugs. For example, when an enterovirus like polio transits the gastrointestinal tract in three days, its genome mutates. This level of mutation has taken *Homo sapiens* about 8 million years to accomplish. So who is going to adapt to whom? Pitted against such nimble competition, the human capacity to evolve may be dismissed as almost inconsequential. This observation was made by Joshua Lederberg, Robert Shope, and Stanley Oaks [4]. Lederberg was Professor emeritus at Rockefeller University and won the Noble Prize in 1959.

With microorganisms less is more. Consider the word, virus, where the word comes from the term for "poisonous substance" and consists of nucleic acid DNA or RNA, encapsulated by a shell of protein and some fatty material referred to as lipids. The biologist Peter Medawar observed that a virus "is a piece of bad news wrapped in a protein." Viruses are tiny ranging from 20 to 400 nm in diameter and millions would fit in the period at the end of this sentence. They can be observed only with an electron microscope. Some are rod shaped while others are 20-sided. Others have strange forms with multisided heads and cylindrical tails. Outside of a living cell, a virus is a dormant particle and lacking in raw materials that are necessary for synthesis. It enters a host cell that it captures and takes over the cell's metabolic machinery to produce copies of itself that sometimes bursts out of the captured cell. This behavior implies that he or it cannot be cultured in artificial media. However, it can be propagated in live cells, fertilized eggs, tissue cultures, or bacteria. It is thought that viruses were originally fragments of genetic material derived from cellular organisms, perhaps bare nucleic acid, or pieces of DNA from bacteria or higher animals.

Viruses make us sick by killing the host cell or by skewing the cell's function, and our bodies respond with fever, the secretion of a chemical called interferon, or by marshalling the immune system's because the immune system is too late to make an efficient response. For example, the virus that causes AIDS is very adept at attacking the immune system itself. Also, because the virus takes over the machinery of living cells to replicate, it is very difficult to develop drugs that struggle against the infection without harming the cells.

Bacteria are about 1,000 times larger than viruses and are more independent. Single-cell organisms that are visible under a microscope are known as "prokaryotic", and they are quite primitive that they lack a membrane-bound nucleus with linear chromosomes inside. Instead, bacteria usually have a tangled necklace of DNA joined at the extremities, and often smaller rings of DNA referred to as plasmids, which contain genes that allow the bacteria to manufacture proteins beyond its usual repertoire. Unlike more advanced organisms, bacteria carry one set of chromosomes instead of two, an arrangement that implies that every gene is needed, and every selective advantage must be maintained. By taking in new genetic material instead of slowly adapting over millions of years, they evolve sporadically in quantum bursts. Bacteria appear on three forms: spherical (coccus), rodlike (bacillus), and curved (vibrio, spirillum, or spirochete). They are ancient and found as fossils in layers more than three million years ago. Over that time, bacteria have developed a wide range of behaviors over a large variety of environments.

Over such a long period of time, because they have adapted by attaching to cells, making paralyzing toxins in order to evade our body's defense system and also to shrug off drugs and antibodies. They incorporate foreign genes from almost anywhere: from other bacteria, viruses, plants, yeasts, and in a 24-hour flea market. For example, the pneumococcus bacterium, which causes pneumonia and other inflictions, soaks up DNA that has spilled out of dead or dying "relatives", that is, inheritance via cannibalism that has left, among other things, antibiotic resistance.

When a virus acquires a toxin gene from deadly *Shigella dysenteriae* and inserts it into harmless *E. coli 0157:H7* a dangerous bacterial hybrid that clings to mucosal surfaces in the intestine and in turn produces additional toxins that have the effect of triggering hemolytic uremic syndrome, which is the most common of kidney failure in children. Such a phenomena is an example of genetic engineering, according to Stanford University molecular biologist Lucy Shapiro. They also use a stealthy strategy called phase variation, hiding their immunity-provoking surface proteins and sugars to trick the body's defenses. According to Joshua Lederberg they have a memory, that is, they are carrying about bits of their evolutionary experience in unexpressed forms, waiting to be expressed.

Bacteria inflict damage in a different way than viruses by multiplying so rapidly they crowd out the host tissues and destroy their routine function. Often, they kill cells outright, but sometimes they produce toxins that can paralyze, destroy metabolic pathways, or generate a massive immune response that in itself is toxic. Drug-resistant bacteria sometimes manufacture an enzyme that can destroy antibiotics and eliminates them altogether. Special virulence factors enable bacteria to penetrate cells, gather nutrients for growth and survival, and evade the host's defenses by evading the immune response. In addition, bacteria do not attack until their numbers are sufficiently high to establish an infection. This is a communication system called "quorum sensing", that enables the microbes to coordinate their activities. The bacteria that join together in the slimy biofilms such as dental plaque assume individual specialized tasks. Despite these feints and stratagems, bacteria are easier to treat than viruses. Because they are independent and because their morphology differs from that of mammalian cells, they are more susceptible to drugs delivered via the blood stream.

A more puzzling class of infectious agents: are animal and human brain diseases, such as bovine spongiform encephalopathy and its human counterpart, the new variant Creutzfeldt-Jakob disease that apparently violate the laws of biology. A different kind of protein called prions are folded in a very unique way, that is to say when they come in contact with other proteins, they turn them into prions, thus setting of or off a chain reaction that results in the brain being riddled with holes. A cow can contact this disease by eating one gram of prion infected tissue, the size of a pepper corn from another cow. Unlike viruses or bacteria, prions cannot reproduce and evoke no immune response. They also resist heat, ultraviolet light, radiation, and sterilization.

The common idea about emerging infections is that they are noxious because they are new, that is, they are ill adapted to the human host. Since their damaging power is supposedly a tip off to their recent arrival and to a bad biological fit. Animal viruses, such as Ebola or Sin Nombre that cause hantavirus pulmonary syndrome, often trigger bizarre symptoms ranging from hemorrhagic breakdown to acute respiratory failure, because the immune response has not evolved with that of the virus. In the long run, microorganisms and people usually reach a subtle understanding. Humans acquire resistance to the infectious agent while the parasite becomes milder, which permits us to survive its assault while allowing it to transmit its gene to someone else. Microorganisms need their hosts to survive, indeed a dead host is a dead in. The reason the lethal spore-forming bacillus *Clostridium botulus*, the cause of botulism, has not leveled our species is because when it kills us with toxins, its future is doomed.

In unlocking microbes' secrets, investigators have gained respect for these hidden foes. It is agreed that an encumbered species are composed of too many working parts, which are fragile when enduring stress. Bacteria have been evolving for at least 3 billion years and are very well adapted and stripped down. Stanford University microbiologists Stanley Falkow says : "I am aware of the minute creatures, they know more about the biology of the human cell than most cell biologists. They know how to tweak it and how to exploit it."

Viruses may be more clever. "Some viruses are enormous and have a large number of genes that do a lot of things. But other viruses are streamlined, and those are the ones that I really admire," say molecular biologist and composer Jeffrey Taubenberger, who has studied the 1918 flu virus. He continues "These viruses are so tightly packed that several different genes can be coded from the same sequence by starting at different places-the sequences actually overlap to conserve space. Genetically, they work like a Bach fugue. In a purely biological sense, they're incredibly beautiful."

In what follows are brief explanations of tuberculosis, malaria ..., coronavirus, foodborne pathogens and animal threats to humans.

3.10 Tuberculosis

The following definition of tuberculosis is taken from https://en.wikipedia.org/wiki/Tuberculosis

Tuberculosis (TB) is an infectious disease usually caused by Mycobacterium tuberculosis (MTB) bacteria. Tuberculosis generally affects the lungs but can also affect other parts of the body. Most infections do not have symptoms, in which case it is known as latent tuberculosis.

3.11 Malaria

The following description of malaria is based on https://en.wikipedia.org/wiki/Malaria:

Malaria is a mosquito-borne infectious disease that affects humans and other animals. Malaria causes symptoms that typically include fever, tiredness, vomiting, and headaches. In severe cases, it can cause yellow skin, seizures, coma, or death.

3.12 Coronavirus

Presently, the coronavirus is sweeping the country. Below is a brief description.

Coronaviruses are a group of related viruses that cause diseases in mammals and birds. In humans, coronaviruses cause respiratory tract infections that can range from mild to lethal. Mild illnesses include some cases of common cold, while more lethal varieties can cause SARS, MERS, and COVID-19. Symptoms in other species vary: in chickens, they cause an upper respiratory tract disease, while in cows and pigs they cause diarrhea. There are yet to be vaccines or antiviral drugs to prevent or treat.

3.13 Foodborne Pathogens

The April 22 issue of the Spokesman Review has an interesting article about a foodborne pathogen Los Angeles. It appears on page 1 of the Business/

Sports section of the paper. Its headline is "Chipolte agrees to record $25 million fine." The article continues as "Chipolte Mexican Grill Inc. agreed Tuesday to pay a record $25 million fine to resolve criminal charges that it served tainted food that sickened more than 1,100 people in the U.S. from 2015–2018."

3.14 Animal Virus Threats to Humans

Francovich [5] who writes for the Spokesman Review in Spokane, Washington, had an interesting article appearing in the Sunday May 3rd edition. He reports the following. "Imagine walking through a market teeming with humans and nonhuman animals: monkeys, pigs, bats pangolins, beavers, rats, deer, and other creatures unknown and unappetizing to most Americans. Smashed into this small area, half-a-million square feet-slightly more than 10 acres, is a dizzying kaleidoscope of species. There are animals that under more natural circumstances would rarely, if any, interact. You are perusing, like all other humans filtering in and out. Everything is for sale and you are looking for food, fulfilling an evolutionary imperative that provides rhythm to our days. "The article continues by describing the virus interacting between humans and animals. For example, the malaria virus between mosquitos and humans. Consider the wet markets found in China and other countries in Asia. It is in these kind of places that investigators believe SARS-CoV-2 virus, which causes COVID-19 make the jump from bats to pangolins (Asian and African mammals) before transforming to humans. Another example is chronic wasting disease, CWD, which is a neurological malady that kills deer and elk. The infected animal stumble, drool, shed weight, and also lose their fear of people, then die. The disease is now in 26 U.S. states and three Canadian provinces. Although there is no evidence that it has passed to humans, there is always the possibility. For additional information, the reader is referred to the Francovich article in the Spokesman Review.

References

1. Compton's Encyclopedia. (1997). *Some Notable Infectious Diseases. Compton's Learning Company*, A Wholly Owned Subsidiary of Softkey International, Inc, Chicago, IL, Vol. 6, 171-172.
2. Drexler, M. (2002). *Secret Agents, the Menace of Emerging Infectious Diseases.* Penguin Books Publishers, New York, NY.

3. Zinsser, H. (1934). *Rats, Lice, and History*, Little Brown and Company, Boston, MA.

4. Lederberg, J. Shope, R., and Oaks, S.C. (1992). *Emerging Infections: Microbial Threats to Health in the United States*, National Academy Press. Washington, DC.

5. Francovich, E. (2020). Animal virus threat grows. Front page of the May 3rd edition of the Spokeman Review.

4

Bayesian Inference for Discrete Markov Chains: Their Relevance to Infectious Diseases

4.1 Introduction

This chapter presents the necessary information in order to understand the analysis of infectious diseases presented in chapters 5 and 7.

This chapter begins with the formal approach to using Bayesian methods of making inferences for infectious diseases, modeled as time series in particular those processes with a countable number of states and an index over discrete time units. In Chapter 5 the stochastic epidemics will be modeled as a discrete time processes with a finite number of states for the number of susceptible individuals, the number of infected individuals, and the number of individuals removed. Bayesian methods of inference consist of estimation, testing hypotheses, and making predictions (of future observations), and these methods were introduced in Chapter 2 for several well-known processes.

In general Bayesian inferences will be provided for each case of a Markov chain introduced in the following sections of the chapter. The chapter begins with a brief review of the definition of a Markov chain, followed by the presentation of many examples, including the example given by Andreyevich Markov [1], a birth and death process with a countable number of states, and the idea of weighted directed graph with associated examples and transition matrices.

This is followed by an explanation of how to compute the n-step transition probabilities illustrated by examples including the gamblers ruin problem and an example involving a chain that explains the status of the weather. In order to determine the long-term behavior of a chain, the integer powers of the one-step transition matrix P are needed and it is at this point the R code for computing such powers of P is presented. The long-term behavior using R to compute the powers of P is illustrated with several examples, including stochastic epidemics. For each example, Bayesian inferences are provided by simulating the states of the chain thus estimating the associated transition matrix P, testing hypotheses about the entries of the transition matrix, and generating future observations from the chain based on the estimated transition matrix P.

Next to be considered is the limiting behavior of a Markov chains, thus the idea of a limiting distribution and a stationary distribution is explained. It is shown that the long-term probability of a particular state is the same as the proportion of the time the chain is in that state. Both analytical and computation methods using R illustrate ways of determining the limiting probabilities for some interesting cases of Markov chains, including the general two-state chain. Closely associated with the liming distribution of a chain is the stationary distribution of the chain. The stationary distribution of a chain is defined and demonstrated that the limiting distribution of a chain is a stationary distribution π and one that satisfies

$$\pi = \pi P \tag{4.1}$$

where P is the transition matric of the chain.

The chapter continues with the definition of a regular transition matrix and finding the stationary distribution of such chains. Computational methods for determining the stationary distribution of regular chains are introduced and involve using R. The details of computing the stationary distributing with R are made clear by referring to the following examples: a random walk on a graph, a random walk on a weighed directed graph, and a random walk on a hypercube.

In order to fully understand the long-term behavior of a chain, one must know how often the states of a chain are visited, and this in turn relates to the idea of a communicating class, the ideas of recurrent and transient states, and finally the idea of an irreducible chain. In order to understand the idea of a recurrent and transient state, the associated graph showing the transition probabilities of the chain provides an invaluable tool. The definition of recurrence and transient depends on the long-run behavior of the chain: A state is recurrent if the probability is one if it is eventually revisited, but the state is transient, if the probability is less than one if it is eventually revisited. Also presented is the R code which computes the expected return to the states of a Markov chain. The period of a state of a chain is also a class property as is recurrence. That is, consider a class of states that all communicate, then if one state of the class is recurrent all are recurrent, and if one in the class has period 2 they all have period 2. For some of these examples, simulations provide realizations that will illustrate the period of a state, the recurrence and transience of a state, then, Bayesian inferences for the unknown transition matrices determined. In general, the communicating classes of a chain will be determined, then for each class the states of that class will be examined as to their nature, that is, are they recurrent, transient, and what are their periods?

This can be a challenge if all one has the number of transition pairwise among the states of the chain, and is consequently a challenge in providing Bayesian inferences for the chain. A chain is called periodic if it is irreducible (all the states communicate), and all states have period greater than one, if not, the chain is said to be aperiodic, that is, if the states have period 1.

The last important idea considered in this chapter is ergodic Markov chains, namely those chains that are irreducible and aperiodic. For such chains, it is known that they have a unique stationary distribution which is its limiting distribution. The stationary command in R easily computes the stationary distribution of an ergodic chain. From the perspective of the Bayesian, realizations will be generated from the transition matrix, then the transition probabilities of the chain estimated from the posterior distribution.

Absorbing chains is the last topic to be discussed in Chapter 4. A state is called absorbing if the probability of remaining in the state over one time period is one. Of course, a good example is the gambler's ruin chain with transition matrix

$$P = \begin{pmatrix} 0,.6,0,0,.4,0 \\ .4,0,.6,0,0,0 \\ 0,.4,0,.6,0,0 \\ 0,0,.4,0,0,.6 \\ 0,0,0,0,1,0 \\ 0,0,0,0,0,1 \end{pmatrix}. \tag{4.2}$$

Assuming the gambler starts with \$2 with a chance of winning \$1 on each round of .6 and either gains \$5 or loses, then the absorbing states are 0 and 5. When P is arranged into the canonical form, one is able to compute the probability of eventual ruin using R. From a Bayesian approach, I will generate realizations from the chain with transition matrix P, then test the hypotheses that the probability of winning one dollar is .6.

4.2 Examples of Markov Chains with Biased Coins

Recall the definition of a Markov chain: Consider a sequence of random variables $X(n)$, $n = 0, 1, 2, \ldots$ then this sequence is said to be a Markov chain if for a positive integers and states $i, j, i_{n-1}, \ldots, i_0$

$$P\left[X(n+1) = j \,|\, X(n) = i \,|\, X(n-1) = i_{n-1} \,|\, \ldots \,|\, X(0) = i_0\right]$$
$$= P\left[X(n+1) = j \,|\, X(n) = i\right]. \tag{4.3}$$

The states are assumed to be non-negative integers, and the first example is taken form Diaconis [2], who studied the results of a large number of coin tosses resulting in the one-step transition matrix

$$P = \begin{pmatrix} .51, .49 \\ .49, .51 \end{pmatrix}. \qquad (4.4)$$

This shows evidence of a slight bias, where if the previous toss results in heads, the current toss results in heads with probability .51, and if the previous toss resulted in a head, the current toss occurs with a tail with probability .49. Also, if the previous toss resulted in a tail, the current toss results in a head with probability .49. Suppose we generate a realization from this chain with transition matric P using the following R code given by Dobrow [3]. Note this is a Markov chain where $X(n) = 1$ denotes a head and $X(n) = 2$ signifies a tail.

R Code 4.1

```
> markov <- function(init,mat,n,labels) {
+ if (missing(labels)) labels <- 1:length(init)
+ simlist <- numeric(n+1)
+ states <- 1:length(init)h
+ simlist[1] <- sample(states,1,prob=init)
+ for (i in 2:(n+1))
+ {simlist[i] <- sample(states,1,prob=mat[simlist[i-1],])}
+ labels[simlist]
+ }
> P<-matrix(c(.51,.49,.49,.51),nrow=2,ncol=2,byrow=TRUE)
> init<=c(1,0)
```

Markov is a function with inputs init, P, and n. init is initial distribution, where c(1,0) denotes the initial toss is head while c(0,1) denotes the initial toss is a tail.

The following realization was based on the following inputs for the Markov function given by R Code 4.1: init=c(1,0), P given by 4.3, and n=100.

```
1 2 1 2 1 2 2 2 2 1 1 1 2 1 2 2 2 2 2 2 2 1 2 1 1 1 1 2 2 2 2 2
2 1 1 1 2 1 2 1 2 2 1 2 2 1 1 1 2 2 1 2 1 2 1 2 2 1 1 2 1 1 2 2 1
2 2 1 2 1 1 2 2 1 1 1 2 2 1 1 2 1 2 1 2 1 1 2 2 2 2 2 2 1 1 2 2 2
2 2 1 1 1 1 1 2.
```

Thus, the usual estimated values of the transition probabilities for P_{11} and P_{12} are .4545 and .5454, respectively, and are .4363 and .5636 for P_{21} and P_{22}, respectively. Consider the Bayesian approach to estimating P_{11}, then one must place a prior distribution on this parameter, which in turn depends on the count n_{11} that has a binomial distribution with parameters P_{11} and $n_{1.} = n_{11} + n_{12}$. I am assuming noninformative prior information about P_{11} with the improper prior density

$$\pi\left(P_{11}\right) \propto P_{11}^{-1}\left(1-P_{11}\right)^{-1}, 0 < P_{11} < 1. \tag{4.5}$$

Thus, the posterior density of

$$\pi\left(P_{11}| n_{1.}\right) \propto P_{11}^{n_{11}-1}\left(1-P_{11}\right)^{n_{12}-1}, 0 < P_{11} < 1, \tag{4.6}$$

which is a beta distribution with parameters n_{11} and n_{12}. If one employs the posterior mean to estimate P_{11}, then the estimator is $E(P_{11} | n_{1.}) = n_{11}/(n_{11} + n_{12}) = 20/(20 + 24) = .4545$, which is the usual maximum likelihood estimator of P_{11}. It should be noted that if one uses the uniform prior for P_{11}, the posterior mean of this parameter is

$$E(P_{11} | n_{1.}) = (n_{11} + 1)/(n_{11} + n_{12} + 2) = .4565,$$

which is not much different than the estimate based on the prior distribution (4.6). Of course, it is of interest to know the 95% credible interval for P_{11}, which is left as an exercise for the reader.

4.3 Fundamental Computations

This section will explore how to compute the n-step transition probabilities of a Markov process, the joint distribution of such a process at arbitrary time points, and the marginal distribution of the process at a given time point. Also presented are the R routines that will be used to compute the n-step transition probabilities and the associated Bayesian inference procedures. For example, estimation of the n-step transition probabilities of a Markov process is a primary goal, but other inference procedures such as testing hypotheses and prediction procedures will also be described. This will entail the simulation of realizations for interesting examples from biology.

Let us now consider the n-step transition matrix with ij-th element

$$P_{ij}^{n} = P\left[X(n) = j | X(0) = i\right], \tag{4.7}$$

where $P_{ij}^{0} = P\left[X(0) = j | X(0) = i\right] = 1, i = j$ and 0 otherwise. We now show that the n-step transition matrix is the n-th power of the one-step transition matrix P. Note in (4.7) that P_{ij}^{n} is not the n-th power of P_{ij}, and that the n-th power of P is denoted by $(P_{ij})^{n}$.

Consider

$$P\big[X(n)=j|\,X(0)=i\big]=\sum_k P\big[X(n)=j|\,,X(n-1)=k|\,,X(0)=i\big]$$
$$\times P\big[X(n-1)=k|\,X(0)=i\big]$$
$$=\sum_k P\big[X(n)=j|\,X(n-1)=k\big]$$
$$\times P\big[X(n-1)=k|\,X(0)=i\big]$$
$$=\sum_k P_{kj}P\big[X(n-1)=k|\,X(0)=i\big],$$

(4.8)

which is valid because of the Markov property and the fact the process is time homogenous, thus, for n=3

$$P\big[X(3)=j|\,X(0)=i\big]=\sum_k P_{kj}P\big[X(2)=k|\,X(0)=i\big]=\sum_k P_{kj}P_{ik}^2=\big(P^3\big)_{ij},\quad (4.9)$$

which is the ij-th element of the third power of the first-step transition matrix P, as was to be shown.

Consider the following example of a random walk on a cycle graph consisting of five vertices labeled 0,1,2,3,4, then the one-step transition matrix is

$$P=\begin{pmatrix}0,.5,0,0,.5\\.5,0,.5,0,0\\0,.5,0,.5,0\\0,0,.5,0,.5\\.5,0,0,.5,0\end{pmatrix}$$

(4.10)

That is the starting at vertex zero (the initial state), the probability of remaining in that state is 0, but is ½ of moving to the vertex to the right is ½. Note that the probability of remaining in the initial state is always zero. What is the transition matrix after six moves? It can be shown to be

$$P^6=\begin{pmatrix}0.312500 & 0.109375 & 0.234375 & 0.234375 & 0.109375\\0.109375 & 0.312500 & 0.109375 & 0.234375 & 0.234375\\0.234375 & 0.109375 & 0.312500 & 0.109375 & 0.234375\\0.234375 & 0.234375 & 0.109375 & 0.312500 & 0.109375\\0.109375 & 0.234375 & 0.234375 & 0.109375 & 0.312500\end{pmatrix}$$

(4.11)

Note the pattern of the six-step transitions as follows: the probability of a return to the initial position is .312500 and the probability of moving one vertex to the right is .109375 as is the probability of moving one vertex to the left etc. Also, the probability of moving two units to the right or left is .234375.

The following code is used to generate the n-step transition probabilities, where the function matrixpower has two arguments: the matrix-labeled mat of one-step transition probabilities given by (4.10) and the desired power k, which refers to the k-step transition probabilities, where k=6. This example is from Dobrow [3]. See the R Code 4.2 below.

R Code 4.2

```
matrixpower <- function(mat,k) {
        if (k == 0) return (diag(dim(mat)[1]))
        if (k == 1) return(mat)
        if (k > 1) return( mat %*% matrixpower(mat, k-1))
```

Of interest to the Bayesian is to estimate the probabilities of the one-step transition matrix (4.9), then use those estimates to estimate the six-step transition probabilities (4.10) and compare them to the entries of the matrix (4.10). Consider the first row of (4.10) which is the conditional distribution of the five states (vertex number) given the initial state 0, then I will assume the distribution of the number of transitions is multinomial with probabilities 0,.5,0,0,.5,0 and will generate four realizations assuming a total of 50 transitions with the following R statement for generating observations from the multinomial distribution.

```
> rmultinom(4,50,prob)
        [1]     [2]     [3]     [4]
[0]     0       0       0       0
[1]     22      32      23      18
[2]     0       0       0       0
[3]     0       0       0       0
[4]     28      18      27      32
```

Thus, the first realization generates 22 transitions from state 0 to state 1, and 28 one-step transitions from state 0 to state 4, while there are zero transitions from 0 to the other three states 0, 2, and 3. The obvious estimates for the transition probabilities are $22/50 = .44$ and $28/50 = .56$ for P_{01} and P_{04}, respectively. Based on the first realization, what are the Bayesian estimates for these two transition probabilities? To perform the Bayesian analysis, I assumed that there were 50 transitions, that the conditional distribution of observed transitions had a Bernoulli distribution with probability $P_{01} = .5$. Fifty observations were generated using WinBUGS, then using those 50 simulated observations, P_{01} was estimated based on BC 4.1. Note that the 50 simulated observations are included in the list statement and that the prior distribution of P_{01} is uniform. The Bayesian analysis is executed with 35,000 observations generated from the posterior distribution and initially with 5,000 observations.

BC 4.1

```
model {
        p01~dbeta(1,1)
           for (i in 1: 50) {
               y[i] ~ dbern(p01)
           }
        }
list(
y = c(
1.0,0.0,0.0,1.0,1.0,
0.0,0.0,1.0,1.0,1.0,
1.0,1.0,1.0,0.0,0.0,
1.0,0.0,1.0,0.0,1.0,
1.0,1.0,1.0,0.0,1.0,
1.0,0.0,0.0,1.0,0.0,
0.0,0.0,1.0,0.0,0.0,
0.0,1.0,1.0,1.0,0.0,
1.0,0.0,1.0,1.0,1.0,
1.0,1.0,0.0,0.0,1.0))
```

The following table presents the posterior distribution of P_{01}.

Based on the posterior mean and median, the estimate of P_{01} is .5769 with a posterior standard deviation of .06797 and the Monte Carlo Markov Chain (MCMC) error is quite small implying that the estimate of .5769 is within .000385 units of the actual posterior mean. The 95% credible interval of P_{01} varies from .4433 to .7066. The posterior mean of .5769 is different for the value .50 of P_{01} used to generate the 50 transitions given in the list statement of BC 4.1. Recall that the goal of this section is to provide estimates of the six-step transition matrix (4.11). I will use R code 4.2 to generate the sixth power of

$$\hat{P} = \begin{pmatrix} 0,.5769,0,0,.4321 \\ .5769,0,.4321,0,0 \\ 0,.5769,0,.4321,0 \\ 0,0,.5769,0,.4321 \\ .5769,0,0,.4321,0 \end{pmatrix}. \tag{4.12}$$

Note that I used $\hat{P}_{01} = \hat{P}_{10} = \hat{P}_{21} = \hat{P}_{32} = \hat{P}_{40} = .5769$ for estimates of the one-step transition probabilities in the matrix (4.10). As a consequence of using R code 4.2, the estimated six-step transition probabilities are given by

$$\hat{P}^6 = \begin{pmatrix} 0.40965410 & 0.1149245 & 0.2626511 & 0.1819211 & 0.08607882 \\ 0.09515764 & 0.4294210 & 0.1058457 & 0.1819211 & 0.24288429 \\ 0.35066753 & 0.1149245 & 0.3216377 & 0.1058457 & 0.16215428 \\ 0.24288429 & 0.3242767 & 0.1149245 & 0.2409077 & 0.13223654 \\ 0.14131536 & 0.3242767 & 0.2164934 & 0.1058457 & 0.26729857 \end{pmatrix} \quad (4.13)$$

One should compare the estimated six-step transition probabilities given by (4.11) with the corresponding entries of matrix (4.13), the matrix of "actual" six-step transition probabilities.

A computation of interest in this section is that of the marginal distribution of $X(n)$. It is easy to show that the marginal distribution is

$$P[X(n) = j] = (\alpha P^n)_j \; n \geq 0 \quad (4.14)$$

namely, the j-th component of the vector αP^n, where α is the row vector denoting the initial distribution of the process, that is the j-th component of α is $P[X(0) = j]$ and P^n is the n-th power of the one-step transition matrix P. In order to explain this idea, suppose that $P[X(6) = 1]$ is to be estimated assuming that $\alpha = (1,0,0,0,0)$, that is the initial state is 0. Note that the estimated value of P^6 is given by (4.13), thus $P[X(6) = 1]$ is estimated by the first component of the 1 by 5 vector

$$\hat{P}[X(6) = 0]$$
$$= (1,0,0,0,0) \begin{pmatrix} 0.40965410 \; 0.1149245 \; 0.2626511 \; 0.1819211 \; 0.08607882 \\ 0.09515764 \; 0.4294210 \; 0.1058457 \; 0.1819211 \; 0.24288429 \\ 0.35066753 \; 0.1149245 \; 0.3216377 \; 0.1058457 \; 0.16215428 \\ 0.24288429 \; 0.3242767 \; 0.1149245 \; 0.2409077 \; 0.13223654 \\ 0.14131536 \; 0.3242767 \; 0.2164934 \; 0.1058457 \; 0.26729857 \end{pmatrix}, \quad (4.15)$$

which is the first component of $(.4096,.1149,.2626,.1819,.0860)$, namely .4096. Thus, at time six the estimated probability that the process returns to the first state (the starting vertex of the cycle graph) is .4096. The student will be asked to estimate $P[X(6) = 0]$ given other initial distributions α. Refer to the exercises at the end of the chapter.

Lastly to be considered is the Bayesian estimation of the joint distribution of the process at an arbitrary number of time points, but for now I consider the following example based on the cycle graph with estimated one-step transition matrix (4.15). For example, it can be shown that

$$P\left[X(5) = i, X(6) = j, X(9) = k, X(17) = l \right] = P_{kl}^8 P_{jk}^3 P_{ij} \left(\alpha P^5 \right)_i \quad (4.16)$$

for states i, j, k, and l =0,1,2,3,4. How does one estimate this joint probability from a Bayesian viewpoint? Note that this probability depends on the one-step transition matrix P and its powers of order 8, 3, and 5. This probability will be estimated by

$$\hat{P}\left[X(5)=i,X(6)=j,X(9)=k,X(17)=l\right]=\hat{P}_{kl}^{8}\hat{P}_{jk}^{3}\hat{P}_{ij}\left(\alpha\hat{P}^{5}\right)_{i}, \qquad (4.17)$$

where $\hat{P}$ is given by (4.23) and i, j, k, and l=0,1,2,3,4. Recall that the entries of $\hat{P}$ are Bayesian estimates. Consider a special case of (4.15), namely

$$\hat{P}\left[X(5)=0,X(6)=1,X(9)=2,X(17)=3\right], \qquad (4.18)$$

that is, the probability that the process begins at the vertex 0 and is at 0 at time 5, moves to the right at the next step, and at time 9 is at vertex 2, and at time 17 is at vertex 3. Suppose it is assumed that the initial state is at vertex 0, thus let $\alpha=(1,0,0,0,0)$. Using the matrixpower function of R, it can be shown that Bayesian estimates of the powers of $\hat{P}$ are

$$\hat{P}^{3}=\begin{pmatrix} 0.0000000, & 0.4796177, & 0.1077132, & 0.1077132, & 0.33219956 \\ 0.4796177, & 0.0000000, & 0.3592352, & 0.1077132, & 0.08067757 \\ 0.1077132, & 0.4796177, & 0.0000000, & 0.2961040, & 0.14380876 \\ 0.1920002, & 0.1438088, & 0.3953308, & 0.0000000, & 0.29610404 \\ 0.4435222, & 0.1438088, & 0.1438088, & 0.2961040, & 0.00000000 \end{pmatrix}, \quad (4.19)$$

$$\hat{P}^{5}=\begin{pmatrix} 0.06269902, & 0.42559064, & 0.13651139, & 0.13651139, & 0.28450488 \\ 0.42559064, & 0.06269902, & 0.31876879, & 0.13651139, & 0.10224748 \\ 0.13651139, & 0.42559064, & 0.06269902, & 0.23875887, & 0.18225740 \\ 0.24333324, & 0.18225740, & 0.31876879, & 0.06269902, & 0.23875887 \\ 0.37984463, & 0.18225740, & 0.18225740, & 0.23875887, & 0.06269902 \end{pmatrix}, \quad (4.20)$$

and

$$\hat{P}^{8}=\begin{pmatrix} 0.3712193, & 0.1560907, & 0.2545221, & 0.1772599, & 0.1152173 \\ 0.1359664, & 0.3913436, & 0.1370367, & 0.1772599, & 0.2327027 \\ 0.3375513, & 0.1560907, & 0.2881902, & 0.1330784, & 0.1593988 \\ 0.2396826, & 0.3129464, & 0.1508060, & 0.2109279, & 0.1599465 \\ 0.1806956, & 0.3129464, & 0.2097930, & 0.1330784, & 0.2377960 \end{pmatrix}. \quad (4.21)$$

This is sufficient information to estimate the desired probability as:

$$\hat{P}_{23}^{8}\hat{P}_{12}^{3}\hat{P}_{01}\left(\alpha\hat{P}^{5}\right)_{0}=(.2387)(.3592)(.5769)(.0626)=.00309. \qquad (4.22)$$

Thus, the joint probability of the three events (going from the initial vertex 0 to the final vertex 3, at times 5, 6 7, and 19) is .00309.

Of course, different initial distributions α could have been used resulting in different probabilities of the event. Referring to the exercises at the end of the chapter, the student is invited to explore the use of various initial distributions and their effect on the primary event of interest described above. Also, left as an exercise to develop a Bayesian test of the hypothesis that $P_{01} = .5$ versus the alternative.

4.4 Limiting Distributions

It is very important to know the long-term behavior of an epidemic. In the long run, what are the possible states of a Markov chain, and how do they depend on the initial state? Such problems come under the subject of limiting probabilities. The R Code 4.2 (matrixpower) will be employed to determine the long-term behavior of a Markov chain. An example, based on a study of Martell [4], reveals the long-term behavior of the Canadian Forest Fire Weather Index. A five-state transition matrix is based on data taken over 26 years at 15 weather stations. The time unit is a day and the following matrix, taken from one location in the early summer, gives the probability of daily changes in the fire index (the states of the chain). The fire index has five values: nil, low, moderate, high, and extreme.

$$P = \begin{pmatrix} .575, & .118, & .172, & .109, & .026 \\ .453, & .243, & .148, & .123, & .033 \\ .104, & .343, & .367, & .167, & .019 \\ .015, & .066, & .381, & .505, & .096 \\ .000, & .060, & .149, & .567, & .224 \end{pmatrix}. \tag{4.23}$$

Thus, the probability of going from nil risk to low risk, in a one day period, is.118, and the probability of remaining at a nil risk (over one day) is .575, etc. On the other hand, the probability of a daily change from a nil risk to an extreme risk is only .026. It is interesting to note that the probability of a daily change from an extreme risk to a nil risk is essentially 0 to three decimal places. Of interest to the forest service is the long-term behavior of the daily risk index, that is, what is the long-term chance of risk on a typical day in late summer?

This will be answered by using R Code 4.2 to compute powers of the one-step transition matrix P (4.23). Thus, consider powers 3,10,17, and 18;

$$P^3 = \begin{pmatrix} 0.3317973 & 0.1762260 & 0.2353411 & 0.2111096 & 0.04552595 \\ 0.3263579 & 0.1753868 & 0.2352439 & 0.2160688 & 0.04694271 \\ 0.2830784 & 0.1922351 & 0.2466504 & 0.2293466 & 0.04868947 \\ 0.1579034 & 0.1832159 & 0.2798370 & 0.3123858 & 0.06665790 \\ 0.1177433 & 0.1654309 & 0.2858074 & 0.3532858 & 0.07773251 \end{pmatrix}, \quad (4.24)$$

$$P^{10} = \begin{pmatrix} 0.2643504 & 0.1812413 & 0.2518115 & 0.2491008 & 0.05349592 \\ 0.2642635 & 0.1812455 & 0.2518332 & 0.2491513 & 0.05350655 \\ 0.2640283 & 0.1812567 & 0.2518919 & 0.2492878 & 0.05353532 \\ 0.2625915 & 0.1813257 & 0.2522504 & 0.2501214 & 0.05371100 \\ 0.2618765 & 0.1813600 & 0.2524288 & 0.2505362 & 0.05379840 \end{pmatrix}, \quad (4.25)$$

$$P^{17} = \begin{pmatrix} 0.2636889 & 0.1812730 & 0.2519766 & 0.2494847 & 0.05357682 \\ 0.2636880 & 0.1812731 & 0.2519768 & 0.2494852 & 0.05357692 \\ 0.2636856 & 0.1812732 & 0.2519774 & 0.2494866 & 0.05357722 \\ 0.2636711 & 0.1812739 & 0.2519810 & 0.2494950 & 0.05357899 \\ 0.2636639 & 0.1812742 & 0.2519828 & 0.2494992 & 0.05357987 \end{pmatrix}, \quad (4.26)$$

and

$$P^{18} = \begin{pmatrix} 0.2636856 & 0.1812732 & 0.2519774 & 0.2494866 & 0.05357721 \\ 0.2636852 & 0.1812732 & 0.2519775 & 0.2494869 & 0.05357727 \\ 0.2636839 & 0.1812733 & 0.2519778 & 0.2494876 & 0.05357742 \\ 0.2636764 & 0.1812736 & 0.2519797 & 0.2494919 & 0.05357834 \\ 0.2636727 & 0.1812738 & 0.2519806 & 0.2494941 & 0.05357880 \end{pmatrix}. \quad (4.27)$$

This demonstrates that the day 17 and day 18 probability of a change agrees to at least four decimal places, and implies that the long-run probability of risk in late summer is nil: .2636, low: .18127, moderate: .25197, high: .24984, and extreme: .05257.

Of course, the three long-run probabilities of Table 4.1 are somewhat misleading because the one-step transition matrix P (4.24) gives only an estimate

TABLE 4.1

Long-Term Behavior of Risk of Forest Fire

Nil	Low	Moderate	High	Extreme
.2636	.1812	.2519	.2494	.0535

of the transition probabilities. What should be remembered is that these probabilities are based on the number of observed transitions from one state to the other, which is not available. Thus, I will generate transition counts corresponding to the transition probabilities of (4.23) with the R command:

> rmultinom(5,100,prob)

where prob = (.575.118,.172,.109,.026) is the first row of the one-step transition matrix P.

Thus, for the first realization, there were 60 transitions over one day from a nil to a nil risk, 9 daily changes from a nil to a low risk, 16 daily changes from a nil to a moderate, 12 from a nil to a high risk, and 3 from a low to an extreme risk. One can see the transition counts do indeed follow the transition probabilities given by the first row of (4.22).

The multinomial mass function for the transition counts is

$$f\left(n_{11},n_{12},n_{13},n_{14},n_{15}\mid p_{11},p_{12},p_{13},p_{14},p_{15}\right)=\left[n!/\prod_{j=1}^{j=5}n_{1j}\right]\prod_{j=1}^{j=5}p_{1j}^{n_{1j}}. \qquad (4.28)$$

where $n = \sum_{j=1}^{j=5} n_{1j}$ is the total number of transition counts with initial fire index nil, the transition probabilities are unknown, and $\sum_{j=1}^{j=5} p_{1j} = 1$. Assuming the improper prior density

$$\xi\left(p_{11},p_{12},p_{13},p_{14},p_{15}\right)\propto\left[1/\prod_{j=1}^{j=5}p_{1j}\right], \qquad (4.29)$$

for $0 < p_{1j} < 1, j = 1, 2, 3, 4, 5$ and $\sum_{j=1}^{j=5} p_{1j} = 1$, it is seen that the posterior distribution of the five transition probabilities is Dirichlet $(n_{11}, n_{12}, n_{13}, n_{14}, n_{15})$=Dirichlet$(60,9,16,12,3)$.

Thus, the various posterior means are:

$$\begin{aligned} E\left(P_{11}\mid data\right) &= 60/100 = .6, \\ E\left(P_{12}\mid data\right) &= 9/100 = .09, \\ E\left(P_{13}\mid data\right) &= 16/100 = .16, \\ E\left(P_{14}\mid data\right) &= 12/100 = .12, \end{aligned} \qquad (4.30)$$

and

$$E(P_{15}\mid data) = 3/100 = .03.$$

72

Bayesian Analysis of Infectious Diseases

TABLE 4.2

Five Realizations of Forest Fire Index Risk

Transitions	R1	R2	R3	R4	R5
n_{11}	60	64	65	61	57
n_{12}	9	12	7	6	17
n_{13}	16	12	11	20	17
n_{14}	12	10	15	9	8
n_{15}	3	2	2	4	1

The posterior means should be compared to the corresponding transition probabilities .575, .118, .172, .109, and .026 respectively used to generate the multinomial realizations of Table 4.2. It is seen that the agreement is quite good. How do we construct credible intervals for these parameters?

For P_{11} it can be shown that (5027, .6934) is a 95% credible interval, where .5049 is the 2 ½ percentile and .694 is the 97 ½ percentile. In a similar manner (.04241, .15327) is a 95% credible interval for P_{12}. The exercises at the end of the chapter will involve finding credible intervals for the other transition probabilities for the evolution of the forest fire index.

The following R command was used to compute the p-th 100 percentile of the beta distribution with parameters alpha = shape 1 and beta = shape 2:

qbeta(p, shape1, shape2, ncp = 0, lower.tail = TRUE, log.p = FALSE)

In particular for the posterior distribution of P_{11}, the following command was employed to find the 97 ½ percentile, which gives an answer of .6934.

qbeta(.975,60,40, = 0, lower.tail = TRUE, log.p = FALSE).

Also, one needs the posterior variance of the transition probabilities, thus, recall that if a random variable has a beta distribution with parameters α and β, then its variance is $\alpha\beta/[(\alpha + \beta)^2(\alpha + \beta + 1)]$, therefore,

$$VAR(P_{11}| data) = (60)(40)/\left[(60+40)^2(60+40+1)\right] = .002376237. \quad (4.31)$$

We now develop a Bayesian method of predicting future transitions for the forest fire index model with transition matrix P given by (4.24). The Bayesian predictive density is defined as follows:

Let $m_{1j}, j = 1, 2, 3, 4, 5$ be the future transitions counts corresponding to the first row of the transition matrix P of (4.33) and assume the transition counts follow a multinomial distribution with density

$$f(m_{11},m_{12},m_{13},m_{14},m_{15},p) = [m!/ m_{11},m_{12},m_{13},m_{14},m_{15}]\prod_{j=}^{j=5} p_{1j}^{m_{1j}}. \quad (4.32)$$

That is, a multinomial mass function with parameters $p = (p_{11}, p_{12}, p_{13}, p_{14}, p_{15})$ and $m = \sum_{j-1}^{j=5} m_{1j}$. Therefore, the posterior density of the transition probabilities P_{1j}, $j = 1, 2, 3, 4, 5$ is Dirichlet $(n_{11}, n_{12}, n_{13}, n_{14}, n_{15})$ with density

$$\xi(p|n) = \left[\Gamma(n) / \prod_{j=1}^{j=5} \Gamma(n_{1j}) \right] \prod_{j=1}^{j=5} p_{1j}^{n_{1j}-1} \tag{4.33}$$

where $n = \sum_{j=1}^{j=5} n_{1j}$ and $1 = \sum_{j=1}^{j=5} p_{1j}$.

The Bayesian predictive mass function of the m_{1j}, $j = 1, 2, 3, 4, 5$ is

$$g(m|n) = E[f(m|p)], \tag{4.34}$$

where $m = \sum_{j-1}^{j=5} m_{1j}$ is the total number of transitions, m_{1j} is the number of transitions form state 1 to state j, and j = 1,2,3,4,5.

Here the E of (4.34) denotes the expectation of the conditional mass function (4.33) of the future transitions (given the transition probabilities) with respect to the posterior distribution of the transition probabilities with density (4.33). It can be shown that the predictive mass function (4.33) reduces to

$$g(m_{11}, m_{12}, m_{13}, m_{14}, m_{15}, n_{11}, n_{12}, n_{13}, n_{14}, n_{15})$$
$$= \left[m! \Gamma(n) \prod_{j=1}^{j=5} \Gamma(n_{1j} + m_{1j}) \right] / \left[\prod_{j=1}^{j=5} m_{1j}! \prod_{j=1}^{j=5} \Gamma(n_{1j}) \Gamma(m+n) \right], \tag{4.35}$$

where $m = \sum_{j-1}^{j=5} m_{1j}$ is the total number of transitions, m_{1j} is the number of transitions form state 1 to state j, and j = 1,2,3,4,5.

Note that (4.35) is the conditional mass function of the future transition counts given the past transition counts. The following WinBUGS code generates 1,000 observations from the predictive mass function (4.35) where the posterior distribution of the transition probabilities is the Dirichlet with parameters (60,9,16,12,3). This assumes the prior density of the transition probabilities is the improper prior given by (4.39). The 100 transition counts are given by the list statement with matrix y. Note that the first vector of predicted transition counts is (59,16,9,14,2), that is the number of transitions from state 1(nil) to state 1(nil) is 59, the number of predicted transitions from state 1(nil) to state 5 (extreme) is 2, etc. Also note the variation across the 100 prediction vectors of the counts of the fire index.

BC 4.2

```
{
alpha[1]<-60
alpha[2]<-9
alpha[3]<-16
alpha[4]<-12
alpha[5]<-3

for( i in 1:100){

y[i,1:5]~dmulti(p[i,1:5],100)
p[i,1:5]~ddirch(alpha[1:5])

}}

List(y = structure(.Data = c(      "
58.0,16.0,9.0,14.0,3.0,
69.0,8.0,7.0,15.0,1.0,
60.0,3.0,22.0,13.0,2.0,
77.0,4.0,9.0,8.0,2.0,
53.0,8.0,18.0,17.0,4.0,
48.0,8.0,26.0,16.0,2.0,
63.0,5.0,11.0,16.0,5.0,
64.0,8.0,21.0,7.0,0.0,
62.0,8.0,7.0,22.0,1.0,
70.0,6.0,9.0,13.0,2.0,
56.0,10.0,16.0,13.0,5.0,
52.0,13.0,17.0,15.0,3.0,
63.0,12.0,16.0,9.0,0.0,
58.0,3.0,20.0,15.0,4.0,
64.0,6.0,14.0,16.0,0.0,
64.0,9.0,19.0,7.0,1.0,
59.0,5.0,20.0,14.0,2.0,
64.0,7.0,14.0,13.0,2.0,
70.0,12.0,11.0,6.0,1.0,
59.0,7.0,3.0,27.0,4.0,
61.0,9.0,14.0,16.0,0.0,
72.0,7.0,15.0,6.0,0.0,
53.0,11.0,13.0,20.0,3.0,
63.0,8.0,14.0,11.0,4.0,
57.0,9.0,18.0,13.0,3.0,
68.0,13.0,11.0,6.0,2.0,
70.0,7.0,14.0,7.0,2.0,
47.0,18.0,12.0,14.0,9.0,
60.0,12.0,16.0,12.0,0.0,
58.0,8.0,12.0,14.0,8.0,
```

```
57.0,6.0,26.0,10.0,1.0,
71.0,10.0,6.0,11.0,2.0,
44.0,21.0,24.0,5.0,6.0,
63.0,10.0,16.0,4.0,7.0,
60.0,8.0,17.0,9.0,6.0,
65.0,6.0,12.0,15.0,2.0,
63.0,6.0,20.0,9.0,2.0,
52.0,12.0,28.0,7.0,1.0,
65.0,5.0,20.0,9.0,1.0,
47.0,11.0,25.0,15.0,2.0,
50.0,13.0,21.0,14.0,2.0,
61.0,2.0,16.0,15.0,6.0,
61.0,9.0,12.0,12.0,6.0,
71.0,2.0,15.0,9.0,3.0,
66.0,2.0,9.0,16.0,7.0,
69.0,10.0,13.0,6.0,2.0,
55.0,2.0,16.0,24.0,3.0,
61.0,14.0,14.0,11.0,0.0,
65.0,7.0,14.0,13.0,1.0,
53.0,2.0,27.0,9.0,9.0,
74.0,8.0,5.0,12.0,1.0,
63.0,10.0,13.0,14.0,0.0,
49.0,8.0,15.0,23.0,5.0,
80.0,5.0,4.0,6.0,5.0,
55.0,5.0,28.0,7.0,5.0,
58.0,10.0,16.0,14.0,2.0,
53.0,10.0,19.0,16.0,2.0,
69.0,7.0,13.0,7.0,4.0,
62.0,9.0,14.0,15.0,0.0,
67.0,5.0,16.0,11.0,1.0,
55.0,20.0,14.0,10.0,1.0,
58.0,6.0,19.0,16.0,1.0,
60.0,5.0,15.0,15.0,5.0,
61.0,10.0,16.0,10.0,3.0,
68.0,11.0,6.0,14.0,1.0,
57.0,10.0,21.0,9.0,3.0,
71.0,6.0,11.0,10.0,2.0,
55.0,15.0,14.0,8.0,8.0,
43.0,12.0,21.0,21.0,3.0,
70.0,3.0,13.0,14.0,0.0,
60.0,10.0,12.0,11.0,7.0,
45.0,14.0,10.0,21.0,10.0,
49.0,10.0,28.0,13.0,0.0,
51.0,8.0,22.0,15.0,4.0,
38.0,8.0,28.0,22.0,4.0,
68.0,5.0,14.0,12.0,1.0,
51.0,8.0,30.0,8.0,3.0,
62.0,8.0,21.0,9.0,0.0,
46.0,9.0,30.0,14.0,1.0,
```

```
63.0,9.0,19.0,8.0,1.0,
67.0,11.0,10.0,9.0,3.0,
67.0,8.0,12.0,11.0,2.0,
45.0,23.0,17.0,12.0,3.0,
54.0,18.0,12.0,9.0,7.0,
56.0,18.0,14.0,9.0,3.0,
63.0,7.0,14.0,10.0,6.0,
52.0,14.0,16.0,14.0,4.0,
55.0,8.0,10.0,19.0,8.0,
65.0,12.0,14.0,8.0,1.0,
67.0,3.0,12.0,15.0,3.0,
62.0,8.0,16.0,12.0,2.0,
60.0,12.0,20.0,7.0,1.0,
70.0,8.0,8.0,13.0,1.0,
54.0,8.0,19.0,14.0,5.0,
70.0,4.0,12.0,10.0,4.0,
50.0,9.0,15.0,23.0,3.0,
58.0,19.0,10.0,12.0,1.0,
54.0,8.0,8.0,27.0,3.0,
49.0,13.0,18.0,14.0,6.0,
56.0,6.0,17.0,18.0,3.0),
.Dim = c(100,5)))
```

The student will be asked to verify the list of predicted transition counts given by the matrix y of the above list statement in BC 4.2.

Consider the following test of hypotheses concerning the first row of the transition matrix of the fire index sample.

$$H_0 : P_{11} = .575, P_{12} = .118, P_{13} = .172, P_{14} = .109, P_{15} = .026. \qquad (4.36)$$

versus

$$H_1 : H_0 \text{ is not true} \qquad (4.37)$$

How does one assign prior information to this case? A reasonable approach is to assign a positive probability π_0 for the null hypothesis and for the alternative assign a prior density $\pi_1 \zeta_1(P)$, where

$$\int_{P:H_1} \zeta_1(P)dP = 1. \qquad (4.38)$$

Thus, $\pi_0 + \pi_1 = 1$ and it is seen that the prior probability of the alternative is π_1 and for values of the alternative, ζ_1 is the density of the continuous random vector P that expresses the prior knowledge one has for the alternative hypothesis. Note that $P = (P_{11}, P_{12}, P_{13}, P_{14}, P_{15})$ is the first row of the transition matrix and $P_0 = (.575, .118, .172, .109, .026)$ is the hypothesized value under the null hypothesis.

Let

$$\zeta\left(n_{obs}\right) = \pi_0 \zeta\left(n_{obs} \mid P_0\right) + \pi_1 \int \zeta_1(P) p\left(n_{obs} \mid P\right) dP. \tag{4.39}$$

where $n_{obs} = (n_{11}, n_{12}, n_{13}, n_{14}, n_{15})$ is the vector of observations with conditional mass function $\zeta(n_{obs} \mid P)$ and where $\zeta(n_{obs})$ is the marginal mass function of the observations.

By letting

$$\zeta_1\left(n_{obs}\right) = \int_{P \neq P_0} \zeta_1(P) \zeta\left(n_{obs} \mid P\right) dP \tag{4.40}$$

The marginal density (4.40) can be expressed as

$$\zeta\left(n_{obs}\right) = \pi_0 \zeta\left(n_{obs} \mid P_0\right) + \pi_1 \zeta_1\left(n_{obs}\right) \tag{4.41}$$

and the posterior probabilities of the null and alternative hypotheses can be expressed as

$$p_0 = \pi_0 \zeta\left(n_{obs} \mid P_0\right) / \zeta\left(n_{obs}\right). \tag{4.42}$$

In a similar manner, the posterior probability of the alternative hypothesis is

$$p_1 = \pi_1 \zeta_1\left(n_{obs}\right) / \zeta\left(n_{obs}\right). \tag{4.43}$$

In order to compute the probability of the null and alternative hypotheses, the following distributions are relevant.

First, the probability mass function of the observations given the unknown parameters is multinomial

$$\zeta\left(n_{obs} \mid P\right) = \left[n! / \prod_{j=1}^{j=5} n_{1j}! \right] \prod_{j=1}^{j=5} P_{1j}^{n_{1j}}, \tag{4.44}$$

where $\sum_{j=1}^{j=5} P_{1j} = 1$ and $\sum_{j=1}^{j=5} n_{1j} = n$. Also, the prior density of unknown parameters under the alternative is Dirichlet, namely

$$\zeta_1(P) = \left[\Gamma\left(\sum_{j=1}^{j=5} \alpha_{1j}\right) / \prod_{j=1}^{j=5} \Gamma\left(\alpha_{1j}\right) \right] \prod_{j=1}^{j=5} P_{1j}^{\alpha_{1j}-1} \tag{4.45}$$

where $\sum_{j=1}^{j=5} P_{1j} = 1$. To compute the posterior probability of the null hypothesis, the relevant information required is $n_{obs} = (60, 9, 16, 12, 3)$ and for the parameters of the prior I used

$\alpha = (23, 4.72, 6.88, 4.36, 1.04)$. Now one can show that

$$\zeta\left(n_{obs}\mid P_0\right) = \left[100! / 60!9!16!12!3!\right](.575)^{60}(.118)^{9}(.172)^{16}(.109)^{12}(.026)^{3} \quad (4.46)$$
$$= .00025145477.$$

and

$$\zeta_1(n_{obs}) = .001114$$

Therefore, the probability of the null hypothesis is

$$p_0 = .184599, \quad (4.47)$$

thus, the evidence suggests the null hypothesis is not true. The hypothesized values were those used to generate various realizations (depicted in Table 4.2) from the fire index example with transition matrix (4.33). The student will be asked to repeat this hypothesis testing example using the second realization of Table 4.3, consequently one would expect a different (different than .18459) posterior probability of the null hypothesis.

Of course, the limiting probabilities of a stochastic process are related to the stationary distribution of the process, and this will be explored in the next section.

TABLE 4.3

Five Realizations for Social Mobility Study

Transition Count	1	2	3	4	5
n_{21}	14	11	10	12	8
n_{22}	139	128	148	141	157
n_{23}	47	61	42	47	4
n_{11}	98	82	86	86	81
n_{12}	84	105	106	99	107
n_{13}	18	13	8	15	13
n_{31}	4	3	6	3	3
n_{32}	99	102	101	99	109
n_{33}	97	95	93	98	88

4.5 Stationary Distributions

The objective of this section is to provide Bayesian inferences for the stationary distribution of a stochastic process. It is interesting to consider what will happen if the limiting distribution of a Markov chain $\{X(n), n = 0, 1, \ldots\}$ is assigned as the initial distribution of the chain.

Consider the two-state chain with transition matrix

$$P = \begin{pmatrix} 1-p, p \\ q, 1-q \end{pmatrix}, \tag{4.48}$$

where $0 < p < 1$ and $0 < q < 1$, then, it can be shown the limiting distribution is given by the vector

$$\theta = \big(q/(p+q), p/(p+q)\big). \tag{4.49}$$

Also, it can be shown that the distribution of $X(1)$ is given by $\theta P = \theta$. A vector π that satisfied the set of equations $\pi P = \pi$ sets the stage for the concept of a stationary distribution of a Markov chain. The definition of a stationary distribution is as follows:

For a Markov chain with transition matrix P, the stationary distribution of the chain is given by the vector π that satisfies

$$\pi = \pi P$$

which is the system of equations

$$\pi_j = \sum_i \pi_i P_{ij}, \forall j. \tag{4.50}$$

Bayesian inferences for the stationary probability vector π will be the principal topic of this section. Consider the following example of a Markov chain with transition matrix

$$P = \begin{pmatrix} .45, .48, .07 \\ .05, .70, .25 \\ .01, .50, .49 \end{pmatrix}, \tag{4.51}$$

where the three states represent the social class of a person, namely: 1 denotes lower class, 2 signifies middle class, 3 represents the upper class. The transition probabilities denote class mobility of a family member. Thus .48 is the probability, a person with lower class parents will be a member of the middle class, while the probability is .07, the person will have a higher occupation class. See Ross [5,p154] for additional details. The stationary distribution π satisfies the following system of equations:

$$\pi_1 = .45\pi_1 + .05\pi_2 + .01\pi_3$$
$$\pi_2 = .48\pi_1 + .70\pi_2 + .50\pi_3$$
$$\pi_3 = .07\pi_1 + .25\pi_2 + .49\pi_3 \qquad (4.52)$$
$$\pi_1 + \pi_2 + \pi_3 = 1.$$

It can be shown that the solution is $\pi_1 = .07$, $\pi_2 = .62$, and $\pi_3 = .31$, thus, in the long term 7% will be in the lower class, 62% in the middle, and 31% in higher class occupations. The R code below computes the stationary distribution of a Markov chain with a given transition matrix mat.

RC 4.3

```
stationary <- function(mat) {
x = eigen(t(mat))$vectors[,1]
as.double(x/sum(x))
}
mat<-matrix(c(.45,.48,.07,.05,.70,.25,.01,.50,.49),
nrow=3,ncol=3,byrow=TRUE)
```

π_1=0.06238859, π_2= 0.62344029, and π_3= 0.31417112 is the solution given by R.

Remember in practice what one knows are the transition counts of the chain, from which the transition probabilities are computed, thus in reality the transition probabilities (4.61) are only estimates.

In order to make Bayesian inferences, I will generate several realizations from the chain which will provide one with transition counts, then using those counts as the sample information, Bayesian inferences are possible. Table 4.3 portrays five realizations from a multinomial distribution with three classes and probabilities (.05, .70, .25) for a total of n=200 outcomes. The following R code was used to generate the five realizations from the second row of the transition matrix (4.51) of the social mobility example. Note this routine generates samples from the appropriate multinomial distribution.

```
> rmultinom(5,100,prob)
```

where prob = (.05,.70,.250) is the second row of the one-step transition matrix P(4.51).

Consider the second row of the transition matrix, then using the first realization, there are 14 transitions form a middle to a lower class occupation,

139 people with middle class occupations and whose parents have middle class occupations, and 47 people with higher class occupations and whose parents are middle class.

Thus, for the first realization, there are 14 transitions from a middle to a lower class occupation, 139 people with middle class occupations and whose parents had middle class occupations, and 47 people with higher class occupations and whose parents are middle class. Notice the similarity from realization to realization as well as the variation. For the first realization, one would estimate P_{21} by $14/200=.07$, P_{22} by $139/200= .695$, and P_{23} with $47/200=.235$. I arbitrarily set n=200, which should be a large enough sample size to efficiently estimate the transition probabilities. How should the Bayesian estimate the stationary distribution of the social mobility example? Obviously, one needs the estimates of all the nine transition probabilities. Two sources of information are needed for the Bayesian analysis: the information prior to the study (the prior density for the transition probabilities) and the information from the sample, the transition counts of Table 4.3, expressed as a multinomial mass function for the transition counts given the vector of transition probabilities. Using an improper prior for the transition probabilities for the first row of P, the prior density is

$$\xi\left(P_{11},P_{12},P_{13}\right) \propto \prod_{j=1}^{j=3} P_{1j}^{-1}, \qquad (4.53)$$

where for the first row of transition probabilities $\sum_{j=1}^{j=3} P_{1j} = 1$.

Assume the transition counts for the first row follow a multinomial distribution with mass function

$$g\left(n_{11},n_{12},n_{13},P_{11},P_{12},P_{13}\right) = \left[200!/98!84!18!\right] P_{11}^{98} P_{12}^{84} P_{13}^{18}, \qquad (4.54)$$

where $\sum_{j=1}^{j=3} P_{1j} = 1$. Thus, by Bayes theorem, the posterior distribution of the transition probabilities of the first row is Dirichlet(98,84,18). In a similar manner, the posterior distribution of the transition probabilities of the second row is Dirichlet(14,139,47), and for the third is Dirichlet(4,99,97). This is sufficient information to provide estimates of the transition probabilities. See DeGroot [6] for the formulas for the moments of the Dirichlet distribution.

Consider first estimating the transition probabilities and stationary distribution via Bayes theorem. Based on the first realization for the social mobility example, I will generate samples from the posterior distribution of the nine transition probabilities as well as the posterior distribution of the stationary distribution. In general, the solution (π_1, π_2, π_3) is the stationary distribution of the mobility example.

The constraint is imposed by solving an associated system of equations:

$$P_{11} + P_{21}x_2 + P_{31}x_3 = 1$$
$$P_{12} + P_{22}x_2 + P_{32}x_3 = x_2$$

(4.55)

with solution $x = (1, x_2, x_3)$, where

$$x_2 = \left[P_{32}(1 - P_{11}) + P_{12}P_{31} \right] / \left[P_{32}P_{21} - P_{31}(P_{22} - 1) \right]$$

(4.56)

$$x_3 = \left[1 = P_{11} - P_{21}x_2 \right] / P_{31}.$$

Let $T = 1 + x_2 + x_3$ be the sum of the components of x, then the stationary distribution is

$$\pi = (1/T)(1, x_2, x_3).$$

(4.57)

The following BUGS code generates the posterior distribution of the transition probabilities and the stationary distribution and the code statements are similar to those expressed by equations (4.56) and (4.57). A total of 35,000 observations are generated from the posterior distribution with a burn in of 500.

BC 4.3

```
model;
{
# transition probabilities social mobility
p11~dbeta(98,102)
p12~dbeta(84,116)
p13~dbeta(18,182)
p21~dbeta(14,186)
p22~dbeta(139,61)
p23~dbeta(47,153)
p31~dbeta(4,196)
p32~dbeta(99,101)
p33~dbeta(97,103)

x2<-(p32*(1-p11)+p12*p31)/(p32*p21-p31*(p22-1))
x3<-(1-p11-p21*x2)/p31
tot<-1+x2+x3
# stationary distribution
pi1<-(1/tot)
pi2<-x2*(1/tot)
pi3<-x3*(1/tot)

}
```

TABLE 4.4

Posterior Distributions for the Social Mobility Example

Parameter	Mean	SD	Error	2 1/2	Median	97 ½
P_{11}	.4903	.0353	.0002103	.4219	.4901	.5589
P_{12}	.4199	.0347	.0002319	.353	.4194	.4886
P_{13}	.0897	.0201	.000127	.0544	.0883	.1329
P_{21}	.0699	.0179	.0001153	.0386	.0684	.1089
P_{22}	.6953	.0326	.0001996	.6296	.6958	.7577
P_{23}	.2349	.0299	.000188	.1788	.2342	.2956
P_{31}	.0200	.0098	.0000624	.0055	.0184	.0134
P_{32}	.4947	.0353	.000249	.4254	.495	.5636
P_{33}	.4885	.0355	.000211	.4162	.4854	.5555
π_1	.0955	.0224	.000144	.0565	.0939	.1446
π_2	.6103	.0282	.000180	.5557	.6102	.6661
π_3	.2942	.0368	.000237	.2212	.295	.3645

The Bayesian analysis is reported in Table 4.4.

Table 4.4 reveals a lot of information for estimating the stationary distribution of a Markov chain. Thus, in the long run, one would expect that 9 ½ percent of the participants would be in a lower class occupation with a 95% credible interval of (.0565, .1446), from 5 ½ percent to 14.4 percent. The Bayesian estimates of the stationary distribution should be compared to the stationary distribution (.0623, .6234, .3144), which was based on the reported transition probabilities of (4.61). On the other hand, the Bayesian stationary distribution is based on one realization generated from the transition matrix (4.61). The Bayesian medians of the stationary distribution are quite close: .0565 compared to .0955, .6103 compared to .6234, and .2942 compared to .3144.

4.6 Where is that Particular State?

4.6.1 Introduction

How is a Bayesian analysis developed for a Markov chain with several communicating classes? The long-term behavior of a Markov chain involves many topics of interest, including knowing how often a particular state is visited, and this all depends on the concepts of the accessibility of a state from the other states of the chain. Recall the key concept of accessibility, which is defined as follows: state j is accessible from state j if there exists a $n \geq 0 \ni P_{ij}^n > 0$. Refer to section 3.4.2 for additional information about accessible states. Accessibility leads to the idea of communication between states namely, two states communicate if j is accessible from i and i is accessible from j and this relation is designated by $i \leftrightarrow j$. Remember the communication relation $i \leftrightarrow j$ is reflexive, symmetric, and transitive, and partitions the state space into various communication classes. The member of a class communicates with itself and all other states in that class, but not with states outside of that class. The following example demonstrates how the communication relation partitions a chain with six states into three classes. Let the six-by-six transition matrix with states 1,2,3,4,5, and 6 be

$$P = \begin{pmatrix} 1/6,1/3,0,0,1/2,0 \\ 0,1,0,0,0,0, \\ 0,0,0,0,3/4,1/4 \\ 1,0,0,0,0,0, \\ 4/5,0,0,1/5,0,0 \\ 0,0,1/2,0,1/2 \end{pmatrix}. \tag{4.58}$$

Thus, the probability that 1 communicates with itself is 1/6, while the probability of going from state 3 to state 5 is 3/4, etc.

The following R code develops a transition graph that shows the partitioning of the six states into three communication classes.

RC 4.4

```
library(igraph)
P<-matrix(c(1/6,1/3,0,0,1/2,0,
+ +            0,1,0,0,0,0,
+ +            0,0,0,0,3/4,1/4,
+ +            1,0,0,0,0,0,
+ +            4/5,0,0,1/5,0,0,
+ +            0,0,1/2,0,1/2,0),nrow=6,ncol=6,byrow=TRUE)
> g<-graph.adjacency(P,weighted=TRUE)
> plot(g)
```

For example, for this chain, the probability of a transition from state 1 to state 2 is 1/3 but once the state is in state 2, it stays there, thus, 2 is an absorbing state. When all the states of a chain form one communicating class, the chain is called irreducible. A communicating class is closed if it is impossible to transition to a state outside of the communicating class.

4.6.2 Irreducible Chains

An example of an irreducible chain with states 1,2, and 3 is one with transition matrix

$$P = \begin{pmatrix} 1/2,1/2,0 \\ 1/2,1/4,1/4 \\ 0,1/3,2/3 \end{pmatrix}, \tag{4.59}$$

where one can easily show that each state communicates with each of the other two. The corresponding transition graph is represented by Figure 4.4 and demonstrates the chain is irreducible. The graph was executed using a suitable modification of R code 4.4

A total of 1000 observations were generated from the chain with transition matrix P (4.59). Using only those simulations starting with the three state, I found the following number of transitions from the conditional distribution of the third row of P. There were 0 transitions from 3 to 1, 76 transitions from 3 to 2, and 175 from 3 to state 3; thus, the fraction of 3 to 2 transitions is $76/251 = .302$, and for 3 to 3, the fraction is $175/251 = .697$. Note based on the third row of P, $P_{32} = 1/3$ (compared to .302) and $P_{33} = 2/3$ (compared to .697), and it appears the Markov chain simulation is believable. Another way to generate observations from the conditional distribution is to assume a multinomial distribution with parameters 0,1/3,2/3 and use the R code

```
prob<-c(0,1/3,2/3)
> rmultinom(3,100,prob)
```

which produces three multinomial realizations with parameter vector(P_{31}, P_{32}, P_{33}).

Bayesian inferences are made the usual way: (a) assume the distribution of the transition counts of Table 4.5 is a multinomial with unknown parameter vector (P_{31}, P_{32}, P_{33}), (b) assign a uniform prior distribution to these three unknown parameters, and (c) determine the parameters of the posterior Dirichlet distribution of (P_{31}, P_{32}, P_{33}). Using the first realization of Table 4.6

TABLE 4.5

Three Multinomial Realizations

	R1	R2	R3
P_{31}	0	0	0
P_{32}	30	27	28
P_{33}	70	70	72

TABLE 4.6

Posterior Distribution of Transition Probabilities of Irreducible Chain

Prob	Mean	SD	Error	2 1/2	Median	97 1/2
P_{31}	.00972	.009502	.00004776	.000251	.006879	.006879
P_{32}	.3012	.04501	.0002719	.2176	.2998	.3932
P_{33}	.6895	.04561	.000249	.5955	.691	.7745

and assigning the uniform prior to the unknown parameters results in a Dirichlet posterior with parameter vector $(1,31,71)$. Thus, the marginal posterior mean vector of (P_{31}, P_{32}, P_{33}) is $(1/103, 31/103, 71/103) = (.0097, .3009, .6893)$. Are these reasonable estimates? The following WinBUGS code pertains to estimating the transition probabilities for the third row of the transition probability matrix and is executed with 35,000 observations for the simulation and 5,000 for the burn in,

```
model;

{
# transition probabilities irreducible chain
p31~dbeta(1,102)
p32~dbeta(31,72)
p33~dbeta(71,32)
}
```

The posterior distributions of P_{32} and P_{33} appear to be symmetric about the posterior mean, and the MCMC errors imply the simulation was successful for estimating the posterior means. Note that estimation of P_{31} could have been ignored because it is known to be zero. Was the information in the first realization sufficient to accurately estimate the transition probabilities P_{32} and P_{33}? It will be left as an exercise to execute the Bayesian estimation of these two transition probabilities based on the other two realizations of Table 4.5.

As a last example consider the random walk with sate space $\{1,2,...,N\}$ and transition matrix

$$P = \begin{pmatrix} 1,0,0,0.........0 \\ q,0,p,0,.......0 \\ 0,q,0,p,0,....0 \\ \vdots \\ 0,0,0,......0,p,0 \\ 0,0,0,......q,0,p \\ 0,0,0,......0,0,1 \end{pmatrix}, \qquad (4.60)$$

where $0 \le p \le 1, 0 \le q \le 1, p + q = 1$.

Notice that the walker starts at state x, where x = 2, 3,4,5,6,7, or 8, and the walker stops walking when x = 1 or when x = 9.

The probability of moving to the right one step is p = .5 and the probability moving to the left is also .5. The states of 1 and 9 represent absorbing states, that is the walker stops moving when x = 1 or x = 9.It is seen from the graph and the transition matrix that there are three communicating classes: {1}, {2,3,4,5,6,7,8} and {9}.

4.6.3 Bayesian Analysis of Transient and Recurrent States

It is well-known that a Markov chain has two types of states: transient and recurrent. To demonstrate this, consider the chain with transition matrix

$$P = \begin{pmatrix} .34,.66,0.0 \\ 1.0,0.0,0.0 \\ .25,.50,.25 \end{pmatrix}, \tag{4.61}$$

where from 1, the chain either returns to state 1 in one step, or first moves to 2 and then returns to 1 at the second step. From 1 the chain revisits 1 with certainty.

On the other hand, for the chain that begins with 2, the chains first moves to 1 and it may continue to revisit 1 for many steps, but finally will return to 2, because the probability it will remain at 1 forever is the chance that it repeatedly transitions from 1 to 1, which is the probability of the limit as $n \to \infty$

$$\lim(P_{11})^n = \lim (.34)^n = 0$$

Therefore, it follows that from 2, the chain revisits 2 with probability 1.

Now consider the case where the process starts in state 3, then the chain may revisit 3 in successive steps, but with positive probability will eventually be in state 1 or 2; thus, from state 3 there is a positive chance that the chain that starts in 3 will never revisit 3, and this probability is ¾ = 1 − (1/4).

It is easily seen that 1 is a recurrent state, that is, it will occur an infinite number of times with certainty. For example, consider a simulation of 200 transitions, starting with state 1.

How well does the simulation follow the first row of the transition matrix, where one would expect 1/3 of 200 transitions to be from state 1 to state 1, 2/3 from state 1 to state 2, and zero from state 1 to state 3? How many times does the chain revisit state 1? It is revisited 120 times out of 200. Of course, we know that 1 is a recurrent state. Also, of course, the states 1 and 2 form a communicating class. A similar situation exists with state 2, which is also recurrent, on the other hand the state 3 is transient; thus, of interest is a simulation of 200 transitions starting with state 3.

It is seen that state 3 is revisited only once, since once the transition to the state 2 occurs, it is impossible the chain will return to state 3. Recall a state is transient if there is a positive probability the chain that starts with state 3, never returns to 3.

For the Bayesian, it would be of interest to test the hypothesis

H: $P_{31} = 1/4, P_{32} = 1/2, P_{33} = 1/4$ versus the alternative that H is not true.

The data will be based on simulating realizations from the multinomial with parameter vector $(1/4,1/2,1/4)$, thus one is interested in determining if the generated values actually came from the appropriate transition probabilities for the third row of P (4.72). This corresponds to the conditional distribution of the chain with initial value $X(0) = 3$. This is left as an exercise for the student. Refer to section 2.5.3 of Chapter 2 for relevant information on testing hypotheses from a Bayesian viewpoint.

One last topic to consider is a Bayesian estimator of the average return time (to a particular state) of an irreducible Markov chain. The analysis is based on the relationship between the stationary probability π_j (of the stationary distribution π of the chain) to the average number of steps between visits to the state j. To be more precise let

$$T_j = \min\{n : n > 0, X(n) = j\} \tag{4.62}$$

and let

$$\mu_j = E\left(T_j \mid X(0) = j\right) \tag{4.63}$$

be the expected return time to state j, then it can be shown that μ_j is finite and that

$$\pi_j = 1/\mu_j \tag{4.64}$$

and

$$\pi_j = \lim(1/n) \sum_{m=0}^{m=n-1} P_{ij}^m \tag{4.65}$$

Recall that the stationary distribution of the chain is determined by solving a linear system of equations involving the transition probabilities P_{ij} of the chain; thus, the Bayesian analysis is easily executed once one knows the posterior distribution of these transition probabilities. See Dobrow [2,*p*103] for the details on the verification of (4.65).

Recall the example of determining the stationary distribution of an irreducible chain involving and transition matrix

$$P = \begin{pmatrix} .45, .48, .07 \\ .05, .70, .25 \\ .01, .50, .49 \end{pmatrix}$$ with three states 1,2, and 3, where state 1 denotes lower

class, 2 middle, and 3 upper. This is an example of social mobility, where .48 is the probability of moving for the lower to the middle class in one generation. The Bayesian estimation of the stationary distribution was based on equation (4.50) which expressed the stationary probabilities in terms of the one-step transition matrix (4.61). Data for this example was generated via the multinomial distribution (see Table 5.4) and Bugs Code 4.6, which is used to execute the Bayesian analysis reported in Table (5.5). In order to estimate the first return times of the three states of the example of social mobility, the following code was amended to Bugs Code 4.3:

```
mui1<-1/pi1
mui2<-1/pi2
mui3<-1/pi3 .
```

with Table 4.7 reporting the Bayesian estimation of the first return times. An improper prior was used for the prior distribution of the transition probabilities. See equation (4.50).

Therefore, the posterior mean for the average return time to the lower class is 11.1 generations, 1.642 for the middle class, and 3.454 generations for the upper class. This appears plausible and is reflected in the transition matrix (4.61). It should be remembered that for each row of the transition matrix, the data was generated assuming a multinomial distribution and then assuming an improper prior, the posterior distribution was Dirichlet for each row, and hence for each cell a beta posterior density.

The average first return times are estimated with the following R program:

TABLE 4.7

First Return Times for Social Mobility Example

Parameter	Mean	SD	Error	2 1/2	Median	97 1/2
μ_1	11.1	2.766	.01619	6.91	10.68	17.69
μ_2	1.642	.0762	.0004363	1.501	1.639	1.799
μ_3	3.454	.4639	.00269	2.744	3.387	4.518

RC 4.5

```
> markov <- function(init,mat,n,labels) {
+ if (missing(labels)) labels <- 1:length(init)
+ simlist <- numeric(n+1)
+ states <- 1:length(init)
+ simlist[1] <- sample(states,1,prob=init)
+ for (i in 2:(n+1))
+ {simlist[i] <- sample(states,1,prob=mat[simlist[i-1],])}
+ labels[simlist]
+}
> P<-matrix(c(0,1,0,
+           .5,0,.5,
+           .333,.333,.333),nrow=3,ncol=3,byrow=TRUE)
> init<-c(1,0,0)
> markov(init,P,25)
 [1] 1 2 3 3 1 2 3 3 3 1 2 3 2 3 3 3 2 3 1 2 1 2 1 2 1 2
> trials<-10000
> simlist<-numeric(trials)
> for ( i in 1:trials){path<-markov(init,P,25)
+ returntime<-which(path=="1")-1
+ simlist<-returntime}
> mean(simlist)
[1] 11.85714
```

and the average return time to state 1 is computed as 11.85714, which is the usual average based on a run of 10,000 simulations. Note how much more informative the Bayesian analysis is as reported in Table 4.8. For example, in addition to the posterior mean (one's estimate of the return time), the posterior standard deviation, posterior median, and the 95% credible interval are given. See Dobrow [2,p106] for additional information about using R to estimate the average return times of the states of a Markov chain.

This section is concluded noting that recurrence and transience are class properties, that is, for a communicating class, all the states are recurrent or all are transient. For additional information about recurrence see section 3.5.4 of Chapter 3. Also, it is important to remember that for an irreducible finite chain that all the states are recurrent.

TABLE 4.8

Posterior Analysis for the Period of State 1

Parameter	Mean	SD	Error	2 1/2	Median	97 1/2
P_{11}^2	.5351	.00496	.0000294	.5254	.5351	.5449

4.7 Period of a Markov Chain

Also, it is important to remember that for an irreducible finite chain that all the states are recurrent. The goal of this section is to provide Bayesian inferences about the period of the states of an irreducible Markov chain. In particular, this will involve testing hypotheses using the Bayesian approach where the main interest is to test the hypothesis that a particular state has a stated period. Recall that the period of state i is defined as

$$d(i) = \gcd\{n > 0 : P_{ii}^n > 0\} \tag{4.66}$$

where P_{ii}^n is the n-step transition probability that the chain will return to state i in n time units. Thus, it is possible for the chain to return to state i in multiples of d(i). Consider the chain with states 1,2,3, and 4 and transition matrix

$$P = \begin{pmatrix} 0,.5,0,.5 \\ .5,0,.5,0 \\ 0,.5,0,.5 \\ .5,0,.5,0 \end{pmatrix}, \tag{4.67}$$

then, each state has period 2. Consider state 1, then the chain can return to 1 by first going to state 2, then returning to 1, or it can first go to 2 , then 3, then 4, and then return to 1, for a total of four transitions. The greatest common divisor of 2 and 4 is 2. Of course, there are other paths of returning to state 1, but they are multiples of 2. The following R statements generate the graph, then using the R matrix power code, it can be shown that all powers of P (4.67) are P, that is,

$$P^n = P, n = 1, 2, 3, \dots$$

Therefore, in particular

$$P_{11}^n = P_{11} = .5 > 0, \qquad n = 2, 4, 6. \tag{4.68}$$

This further confirms that the period of state 1 is 2, and of course the period of the other three states is also 2.

RC 4.6

```
P<-matrix(c(0,.5, 0,.5,
            .5, 0,.5, 0,
            0,.5, 0,.5,
            .5, 0,.5, 0),nrow=4,ncol=4,byrow=TRUE)
g<-graph.adjacency(P,weighted=TRUE)
plot(g)
```

Suppose that we want to estimate the probability of the return to state 1 has period 2.

For this example, $P_{11} = P_{11}^n = .5$, thus it is obvious that the period of state 1 is 2.

However, in practice one does not know the actual values of the transition probabilities; thus, transition counts will be generated using the transition matrix (4.50) and based on those counts, the posterior distribution of the $P_{11}^n, n = 2, 4, 6, \ldots$ will be determined.

Based on the transition matrix P, I generated 100 observations from the appropriate multinomial distribution for each of the four conditional distributions resulting in the following transition counts:

$$Q = \begin{pmatrix} 0, 48, 0, 52 \\ 48, 0, 52, 0 \\ 0, 52, 0, 48 \\ 47, 0, 53, 0 \end{pmatrix}, \tag{4.69}$$

and from this one can verify that the corresponding estimated transition matrix is

$$\hat{P} = \begin{pmatrix} 0, .48, 0, .52 \\ .48, 0, .52, 0 \\ 0, .52, 0, .48 \\ .47, 0, .53, 0 \end{pmatrix}. \tag{4.70}$$

Now consider the following powers of the estimated transition matrix:

$$\hat{P}^2 = \begin{pmatrix} .4748, 0, .5252, 0 \\ 0, .5008, 0, .4992 \\ .4752, 0, .5248, 0 \\ 0, .5012, 0, .4985 \end{pmatrix}, \tag{4.71}$$

$$\hat{P}^4 = \begin{pmatrix} .47501,0,.5249899,0 \\ 0,.50009978,0,.4990003 \\ .4750090,.5249901,0 \\ 0,.50000995,0,.499005 \end{pmatrix}, \qquad (4.72)$$

and it can be shown that higher even powers of $\hat{P}$ are essentially the same as $\hat{P}^2$, thus, since all the even powers of $\hat{P}$ are the same, it is sufficient to estimate only P_{11}^2.

Estimation will be done via the Bayesian approach which is to estimate the probability that the chain returns to state 1 in two transitions.

Consider the first row of P_{11}^2, then generate 100 observations to complete these four cell counts. Assuming the transition counts follow a multinomial distribution with mass function

$$f\left(n_{11},n_{12},n_{13},n_{14}|\ P_{11}^2,P_{12}^2,P_{13}^2,P_{14}^2\right)$$
$$= [100!/\ n_{11}!,n_{12}!,n_{13}!,n_{14}!]\prod_{j=1}^{j=4}P_{1j}^2 \qquad (4.73)$$

where $\sum_{j=1}^{j=4}P_{1j}^2 = 100$ and $\sum_{j=1}^{j=4}n_{1j} = 100$, the 100 cell counts were generated using the R function rmultinom(1,100,prob) with prob = c(.53,0,.47,0), and the resulting realization is $n_{11} = 54$, $n_{12} = 0$, $n_{13} = 46$, $n_{14} = 0$. This implies that the marginal distribution of n_{11} is binomial $\left(100,P_{11}^2\right)$ with mass function

$$f\left(n_{11}|\ P_{11}^2\right) = \binom{100}{n_{11}}\left(P_{11}^2\right)^{n_{11}}\left(1-P_{11}^2\right)^{100-n_{11}}, \qquad (4.74)$$

Where $0 < P_{11}^2 < 1$.

How should P_{11}^2 be estimated? If one assumes a uniform prior for the unknown parameter, the posterior distribution of P_{11}^2 is beta with parameter vector $(n_{11} + 1, 100 - n_{11} + 1)$, thus substituting $n_{11} = 54$, the posterior mean is $55/102 = .5392$. Remember that P_{11}^2 is the probability of a two-step transition to return to state 1, not the probability of the square of P_{11}.

Using WinBUGS to execute the Bayesian analysis, I generated 35,000 observations for the MCMC simulation with a burn in of 5,000 observations and a refresh of 100 with the following results:

Thus, the posterior mean is .5351 and the 95% credible interval is (.5254, .5449), which implies that state 1 has period 2. That is to say, the credible interval indicates that $P_{11}^2 > 0$. Because higher even powers of the matrix P^2 do not change, one would expect the Bayesian analysis for $P_{11}^n, n = 4,6,..$ to be the same as that portrayed in Table 4.8; thus, one is confident that state 1 has period 2. Also shown in the table are the posterior mean and median which imply a symmetric posterior density for P_{11}^2.

The WinBUGS code below generates the Bayesian analysis.

BC 4.4

```
model;
{
for (i in 1:100){
p[i]~dbin(p11,100)}
p11~dbeta(1,1)
}

list(
p = c(
56.0,53.0,48.0,55.0,50.0,
50.0,60.0,47.0,61.0,57.0,
56.0,49.0,48.0,55.0,54.0,
56.0,58.0,59.0,61.0,51.0,
50.0,48.0,43.0,52.0,51.0,
57.0,55.0,57.0,47.0,56.0,
56.0,54.0,60.0,50.0,53.0,
59.0,53.0,50.0,53.0,55.0,
50.0,58.0,47.0,61.0,56.0,
54.0,60.0,43.0,50.0,52.0,
57.0,57.0,60.0,53.0,63.0,
49.0,46.0,52.0,56.0,59.0,
58.0,54.0,46.0,51.0,49.0,
61.0,48.0,50.0,57.0,55.0,
57.0,59.0,51.0,43.0,58.0,
58.0,55.0,53.0,56.0,58.0,
46.0,56.0,54.0,52.0,53.0,
46.0,44.0,50.0,56.0,59.0,
49.0,50.0,57.0,57.0,53.0,
60.0,44.0,56.0,53.0,53.0))
```

The list statement contains the data of 100 values generated from a binomial distribution with parameters (.54, 100), and the code shows a beta uniform prior placed on the unknown parameter P_{11}^2.

4.8 Ergodic Chains and Time Reversibility

Time reversibility is an interesting property of some Markov chains. The type of Markov chain we are interested in is the so-called ergodic chains, which are irreducible, aperiodic (all states have period 1), and have a finite average return time. All finite chains are ergodic if they are aperiodic and irreducible. Such chains are of interest because they possess a unique positive stationary distribution π. Such processes can exhibit the time reversibility property

$$\pi_i P_{ij} = \pi_j P_{ji}, i, j = 1, 2, \ldots k, \tag{4.75}$$

where $(\pi_1, \pi_2, \ldots, \pi_k)$ is the stationary distribution and P_{ij} is the one-step transition probability. Such processes have no directional bias, such as a random walk where the chain moves one unit to the right with probability q and one unit to the left with probability 1-q with q = 1/2. If q > 1/2, the chain exhibits a bias that propels the process to the right and the process has a directional bias. Time reversibility, as defined by (4.85), implies a process such that its behavior in the future is the same as the process moving backwards, one cannot tell the difference.

Such processes invite many inferential challenges. For example, given the data from a finite, irreducible, and aperiodic Markov chain, is the process time reversible? In practice the data would consist of transition counts of the chain, from which one can estimate the one-step transition probabilities and stationary distribution. For the Bayesian, our main interest will be in determining if the chain is time reversible, where inferences will be either the posterior estimation of the parameters

$$\zeta_{ij} = \pi_i P_{ij} - \pi_j P_{ji}, i, j = 1, 2, \ldots, k$$

or a test of the hypotheses

$$H_o: \zeta_{ij} = 0 \text{ versus } H_1 : \zeta_{ij} \neq 0.$$

Two examples are described, where the first involves a chain which is known to be not time reversible while the other will be chain which is time reversible. Consider the example of social mobility described in section 4.4 with transition matrix

$$P = \begin{pmatrix} .45, .48, .07 \\ .05, .70, .25 \\ .01, .50, .49 \end{pmatrix}$$

In this example, the posterior distribution of the stationary transition was determined with BUGS code 4.4, with the results appearing in Table 4.4. The data consists of realizations generated from the multinomial distribution with 200 observations for each row of (4.50). An improper prior distribution (4.53) induces a Dirichlet posterior distribution for each row and a beta posterior for each transition probability. BUGS code 4.6 contains the equations (4.66) and (4.68) for determining the stationary distribution of the chain. In order to specify the posterior distribution of the relevant parameters, ζ_{ij}, a slight modification of the BUGS code is necessary. The modified code appears as BC 4.8. I used 35,000 observations for the simulation, with a burn in of 5,000. The relevant parameters are denoted by d11,d12, and d13, and the posterior analysis reported in Table 4.9.

TABLE 4.9

Posterior Analysis for a Time Reversible Chain

Parameter	Mean	SD	Error	2 1/2	Median	97 1/2
ζ_{12}	−00369	.01212	.000067	−02767	−.00360	.01987
ζ_{13}	−04937	.00967	.0000578	−06842	−.04941	−03036
ζ_{23}	−00362	.01228	.0000649	−02744	−.00362	.00694
P_{12}	.4602	.03516	.0002931	.3921	.4599	.5285
P_{13}	.5403	.03513	.0000235	.4707	.5402	.6088
P_{21}	.5747	.03479	.000185	.5066	.5748	.6429
P_{22}	.2046	.02857	.000164	.1515	.204	.2631
P_{23}	.2198	.02933	.000157	.1647	.219	.2798
P_{31}	.4752	.03545	.0002102	.4053	.4751	.5448
P_{32}	.175	.02685	.0001583	.1255	.1738	.2309
P_{33}	.3496	.03368	.0001988	.2856	.3488	.4174
π_1	.3432	.01183	.000063	.3195	.3434	.3658
π_2	.2812	.01903	.0001176	.2443	.2809	.3185
π_3	.3757	.02516	.0001478	.3265	.3758	.4249

BC 4.5

```
model;
{
p11~dbeta(98,102)
p12~dbeta(84,116)
p13~dbeta(18,182)
p21~dbeta(14,186)
p22~dbeta(139,61)
p23~dbeta(47,153)
p31~dbeta(4,196)
p32~dbeta(99,101)
p33~dbeta(97,103)

x2<-(p32*(1-p11)+p12*p31)/(p32*p21-p31*(p22-1))
x3<-(1-p11-p21*x2)/p31
tot<-1+x2+x3
pi1<-(1/tot)
pi2<-x2*(1/tot)
pi3<-x3*(1/tot)

d12<-pi1*p12-pi2*p21
d13<-pi1*pi3-pi3*p31
d23<-pi2*p23-pi3*p32
}
```

For the most part, the posterior distributions appear symmetric about the posterior mean. It is interesting to note that the 95% credible interval for ζ_{13} excludes zero. Is this chain time reversible?

The second example involves a transition matrix of a chain which is time reversible. See example 3.22 of Dobrow [2,p115], where the transition matrix is

$$P = \begin{pmatrix} 0,2/5,3/5 \\ 1/2,1/4,1/4 \\ 1/2,1/6,1/3 \end{pmatrix} \tag{4.76}$$

It can be verified that the chain is time reversible. In order to perform the Bayesian analysis, multinomial observations will be generated for each row of (4.74), then based on these realizations, the estimated transition probabilities and estimated stationary distribution will be determined using BUGS code 4.8. Using the improper prior the posterior distribution of the transition probabilities, stationary distribution, and the time reversible parameters ζ_{ij} will be available and reported in a way similar to Table 4.10.

Two hundred multinomial observations are generated for each row of (4.75) to give the transition count matrix Q, where

$$Q = \begin{pmatrix} 0,92,108 \\ 115,41,44 \\ 95,35,70 \end{pmatrix}. \tag{4.77}$$

The Bayesian analysis is executed with BUGS code 4.9 with 5,000 observations for the simulation, a burn in of 5,000, and a refresh of 100. The posterior analysis is reported in Table 4.11.

TABLE 4.10

Bayesian Analysis for Time Reversibility of Social Mobility

Parameter	Mean	SD	Error	2 1/2	Median	97 1/2
ζ_{12}	−.00253	.005433	.0000322	−.01347	−.00249	.00817
ζ_{13}	.02171	.00522	.0000324	.01181	.02161	.03218
ζ_{23}	−.00173	.0282	.000167	−.05476	−.00261	.05587

TABLE 4.11

Posterior Analysis for a Time–reversed Chain. Size 50 Multinomial Realizations

Parameter	Mean	SD	Error	2 1/2	Median	97 1/2
ζ_{12}	−.01573	.0244	.000116	−.01538	.03106	.03106
ζ_{13}	−.0456	.0192	.0000892	−.08319	−.04577	−.00811
ζ_{23}	−.0145	.02565	.000119	−.06306	−.01498	.03805
π_1	.3382	.02407	.000106	.2886	.3391	.383
π_2	.2818	.03643	.000182	.2125	.2812	.3548
π_3	.3801	.04833	.000232	.2854	.3798	.4742

BC 4.7

```
model;
{
p11~dbeta(1,99)
p12~dbeta(92,108)
p13~dbeta(108,92)
p21~dbeta(115,85)
p22~dbeta(41,159)
p23~dbeta(44,156)
p31~dbeta(95,105)
p32~dbeta(35,165)
p33~dbeta(70,130)

x2<-(p32*(1-p11)+p12*p31)/(p32*p21-p31*(p22-1))
x3<-(1-p11-p21*x2)/p31
tot<-1+x2+x3
pi1<-(1/tot)
pi2<-x2*(1/tot)
pi3<-x3*(1/tot)
d12<-pi1*p12-pi2*p21
d13<-pi1*pi3-pi3*p31
d23<-pi2*p23-pi3*p32
```

The stationary distribution estimated by the posterior mean is

$$\hat{\pi} = (.3432, .2812, .3757) \tag{4.78}$$

and the main parameters of interest, the ζ_{ij}, $i < j$, are estimated with the posterior median as −.00360, −.04941, and −.00362 respectively. Also, the posterior distribution of these parameters is evidently symmetric about the posterior mean and their 95% credible intervals imply the chain is time reversible. In order to show the uncertainty when using a smaller sample size for the multinomial realization, the example is repeated with a much smaller sample size of 50 (smaller than 200) for each row of (4.86). The

TABLE 4.12

Posterior Probability
of Time Reversibility

ν	ω_0
1	.9991
3	.99801
5	?
10	?
100	.9979
.0024	.9931

multinomial realizations for the three rows of the transition matrix (4.86) is portrayed in matrix

$$R = \begin{pmatrix} 0, 21, 29 \\ 28, 10, 12 \\ 23, 11, 16 \end{pmatrix}. \tag{4.79}$$

The Bayesian analysis is reported in Table 4.11 and should be compared to the results of Table 4.9. The latter analysis is based on realizations of size 50, whereas the results of the former posterior analysis is based on realizations of size 200.

Comparing Tables 4.9 and 4.11, one sees the posterior means are approximately the same, but that the posterior standard deviations are much smaller for Table 4.9, and as a consequence the 95% credible intervals are wider for Table 4.11. Overall, the conclusion about time reversibility based on Table 4.11 would be the same as those based on Table 4.9. The student will be asked as an exercise to repeat the analysis with multinomial simulations of size 20 and compare those results to Table 4.12. Will the Bayesian analysis imply time reversibility?

Our next phase of inference for time reversibility is to test the null hypothesis $H_o: \zeta_{ij} = 0$ versus $H_1 : \zeta_{ij} \neq 0$, where $\zeta_{ij} = \pi_i P_{ij} - \pi_j P_{ji}$, $i, j = 1, 2, ..., k$.

First consider $\zeta_{12} = \pi_1 P_{12} - \pi_2 P_{21}$ and a test of

$$H_0 : \zeta_{12} = 0 \text{ versus } H_1 : \zeta_{12} \neq 0,$$

where the test is based on the data generated with 200 multinomial observations for each row of the transition matrix (4.87), and the Bayesian analysis is recorded in Table 4.9. Note that the posterior mean and standard deviation are

$$E(\zeta_{12} | \text{data}) = -.00253 \text{ and } \sigma(\zeta_{12} | \text{data}) = .005433, \text{ respectively.}$$

Therefore, I will assume that $\zeta_{12} \sim normal(\mu, \sigma^2)$, where $\mu = -.00253$ and $\sigma^2 = .000029517$. Using BUGS code 4.8, one can show the density of ζ_{12} appears to be in the shape of a normal density; thus, for the purpose of testing H_0 versus H_1, it is assumed that ζ_{12} is indeed normally distributed.

For reviewing the Bayesian approach to testing hypotheses, the reader is referred to section 2.5.3 of Chapter 2. For the Bayesian approach it is assumed that $\zeta \sim normal(\mu, \sigma^2)$, where $\mu \sim normal(0, \nu^2)$ and ν^2 is known; thus, the test will be described as

$$H_0 : \mu = 0 \text{ versus } H_0 : \mu \neq 0.$$

The Bayesian test is implemented by computing the posterior probability of the null and alternative hypotheses. The test is based on the predictive density of $\zeta = \pi_1 P_{12} - \pi_2 P_{21}$, where $\zeta \sim normal(\mu, \sigma^2)$ and $\mu \sim normal(0, \nu^2)$; therefore, the predictive density is

$$f(\zeta) = \rho_0 f(\zeta | \mu = 0) + \rho_1 \int f(\mu) f(\zeta | \mu) d\mu \qquad (4.80)$$

where ρ_0 is the prior probability of the null hypothesis and ρ_1 is the prior probability of the alternative hypothesis, and $\rho_0 + \rho_1 = 1$. In addition the prior density of μ under the alternative is

$$f(\mu) = [1/\sqrt{2\pi\nu}]\exp{-(1/2\nu^2)}\mu^2 \qquad (4.81)$$

and

$$f(\zeta | \mu) = \left[1/\sqrt{2\pi}\sigma\right]\exp(1/2\sigma^2)(\zeta - \mu)^2, \qquad (4.82)$$

is the conditional density of γ given μ. Thus, it can be shown that the predictive density is

$$f(\zeta) = \rho_0\left[1/\sqrt{2\pi}\sigma\right]\exp(-1/2\sigma^2)\zeta^2$$
$$+ \rho_1\left[\nu\sigma/\sqrt{2\pi(\sigma^2 + \nu^2)}\right]\exp\left(-1/\left[2(\sigma^2 + \nu^2)\right]\right)\zeta^2. \qquad (4.83)$$

and that the posterior probability of the null hypothesis is

$$\omega_0 = \rho_0\left[1/\sqrt{2\pi}\sigma\right]\exp(1/2\sigma^2)\zeta^2 \div f(\zeta)$$

Using the information from Table 4.11, $\zeta = -.01573$ and letting $\rho_0 = \rho_1 = .5$, the posterior probability ω_0 of the null hypothesis is computed for various values of ν, the standard deviation of the prior distribution for μ and reported in Table 4.13. I am assuming that σ and ν are known. For example, when $\nu = 3$, the probability of null hypothesis (time reversibility) is .99801. This is not surprising since the observed value of the parameter

TABLE 4.13

Posterior Distribution of Epidemic Model

Parameter	Mean	SD	Error	2 1/2	Median	97 1/2
R_0	2.029	2.655	.0097	.2935	1.389	7.538
B	.00149	.000859	.0000032	.00031	.00133	.00361
$b + \gamma$	.002986	.001718	.0000064	.00062	.00267	.00722
P_{10}	.002986	.001718	.0000064	.00062	.00267	.00722
P_{11}	.993	.00262	.0000096	.987	.9933	.9972
P_{12}	.00399	.001992	.0000083	.0011	.00366	.00879
β	.004037	.002003	.0000112	.00113	.003705	.00886
n g2	.663	.4727	.002646	0	1	0

that measures time reversibility is $-.01573$ with a standard deviation of .0244. It is seen the evidence is very strong for the conclusion that the chain is time reversible regardless of what is used for the prior distribution of μ (4.93) under the alternative. The reader is invited to verify the values of ω_0 for Table 4.12 and to complete the entries designated.

The effect of ν on ω_0 is negligible.

4.9 Stochastic Epidemic

The following example is found in Bailey [7] and introduce the reader to the idea of a stochastic epidemic and will be revisited in Chapter 5.

Assume the facts about the simple model in the deterministic case, but where $I(n)$ is a random variable denoting the number of infected individuals at time n, where the population is of size $N = I(n) + S(n)$, and $S(n)$ is a random variable denoting the number of susceptible people at time n, n = 0,1,2,.... Now assume that the time interval from n to n + 1 is small enough so that there is at most one change over that time period. For the Bayesian analysis. focus will be on the number of infected people

$I(n)$ with state space $\{0,1,2,...,N\}$, which has two classes $\{0\}$ and $\{1,2,...,N\}$, where state 0 is absorbing, denoting that the infection dies out. The transition matrix is defined by the following three equations:

$$P_{i,i+1} = \Pr[I(n+1) = i+1 \mid I(n) = i] = \beta i(N-i)/N = \lambda_i$$
$$P_{i,i-1} = \Pr\left[I(n-1) = i-1 \mid I(n) = i\right] = (b+\gamma)i, \tag{4.84}$$

and

   Thus the one-step transition matrix of the number of infected people is

$$
P = \begin{pmatrix}
1,0,\dots\dots\dots\dots\dots\dots\dots\dots\dots\dots\dots\dots\dots,0 \\
b+\gamma,1-b-\gamma-\lambda_1,\lambda_1,0,\dots\dots\dots\dots,0 \\
0,2(b+\gamma),1-2(b+\gamma)-\lambda_2,0,\dots\dots\dots,0 \\
\vdots \\
0,\dots\dots\dots\dots0,N(b+\gamma),1-N(b+\gamma)
\end{pmatrix}.
$$

(4.85)

   The goal as a Bayesian is to make inferences about the unknown parameters: the birth rate b, β the number of contacts, and γ the number of infected people that recover. I will begin with estimating the parameters b, γ, and β using as data transition counts for the first three entries of the second row of P, where the transition counts will be realizations generated via the multinomial distribution.

   Consider the multinomial distribution with parameter p = (.005,.9851,.0099), then using the R function rmultinom, the following realization was generated with transition counts $(n_{10}, n_{11}, n_{12}) = (3,993,4)$ corresponding to the transition probabilities

$$
\begin{aligned}
P_{10} &= b+\gamma, \\
P_{11} &= 1-\lambda_1 -(b+\gamma), \\
P_{12} &= \lambda_1 = \beta(N-1)/N, \\
N &= 100, \\
b &= \gamma = .0025,
\end{aligned}
$$

(4.86)

and

$$
\beta = .01.
$$

   Therefore, the transition probabilities are estimated as

$$
\tilde{P_{10}} = .003, \tilde{P_{11}} = .973, \text{ and } \tilde{P_{12}} = .004.
$$

   Thus the estimates for the parameters of the epidemic are .0040404 for β and .0015 for b and γ. What are the Bayesian estimates?

   Assume that the prior distribution for the transition probabilities is the improper prior

$$
\zeta(P_{10},P_{11},P_{12}) = \sum_{j=0}^{j=2} P_{1j}^{-1}
$$

(4.87)

where

$$\sum_{j=0}^{j=1} P_{1j} = 1, 0 < P_{1j} < 1, \text{ and } j = 1, 2, 3.$$

It can be shown that the posterior distribution of the transition probabilities is

Dirichlet with parameter $(n_{10}, n_{11}, n_{12}) = (3,993,4)$, thus the marginal posterior distribution of P_{10} is beta(3,997), of P_{11} is beta(993,7), and of P_{12} beta(4,996).

The Bayesian analysis is executed with BUGS code 4.7 with 35,000 observations for the simulation and a burn in of 5,000. The step command g2 gives the posterior probability that $R_0 > 1$.

BC 4.7

```
model;
{
p10~dbeta(3,997)
p11~dbeta(993,7)
p12~dbeta(4,996)
bplusgamma<-p10
N<-100
beta<-p12*N/(N-1)
b<-bplusgamma/2
R0<-beta/bplusgamma
g1<-step(R0-.5)
g2<-step(R0-1)
}
```

As a result of the simulation, the Bayesian analysis for the simple epidemic model is reported in Table 4.13.

4.10 Tracking the Coronavirus

During the writing this book, the coronavirus pandemic has made news daily since its arrival in the United States sometime in January of 2020. The origin of the epidemic was China sometime during the month of December 2019. Of course, it took some time before the virus was identified as a novel contagion, related genetically to the common cold. According to the *IN Brief* section of *Significance* page 4 , Volume 17, issue 3, "Wall-to-wall media coverage of the pandemic plus fast and furious debate among statisticians and data scientists in various online discussion groups, addressing different aspects of the outbreak and the response left very little attention for other topics. A tweet (bit.ly/2xm5noa) from Hanselman (@shanselman) expressed the situation by drawing an analogy to computing": Life right now feels like I opened taskmaster and there is some rogue process called COVID that is using 20% of my CPU. One article getting a lot of attention was a blog post by Thomas Pueyo with the title

"Coronavirus: Why you must act now." In the article, Pueyo urged political leaders to implement social distancing, stressing the fast growth of cases in Italy and Iran. On March 16, a report from University College London reported the likely effect of multiple public health measures on retarding the blow of the disease. Assuming no effort is made to suppress the outbreak, team of investigators from University College London predicted half a million deaths in Great Britain and 2 million in the United States. On the other hand, a plan to slow the spread with home isolation of cases, home quarantine, social distancing would reduce to 250,000 the number of fatalities in the UK, and to a little over one million in the US. It appears that the only useful plan implies wide social distancing, home isolation of cases, and the closure of schools and universities.

For those who must stay at home, they would receive news from daily government briefings of new confirmed cases and deaths. It should be noted that the numbers being reported were not always what they appear to be, as was pointed out by statisticians and other scientists involved in investigating the pandemic. Professors Sylvia Richardson and David Spiegelhalter co-chairs of the Royal Statistical Society's new covid-19 task force(bit.ly/2yRuCyQ) wrote in an Observer story that the number of new cases need not be an accurate account of the actual number of cases who have been infected. This is because on how well the testing of cases is actually carried out. On the other hand, Professor Shiela Bird, who is also a member of the task force as well as a member of the editorial board of *Significance* told the BBC program **More or Less** to explain the reporting delays made daily announcements of new corona virus deaths very misleading. On April 19, *Significance* begin to publish its own online collection of articles that discuss topics including the modeling of pandemics, problems with testing, and possible solutions. A selection of these articles is featured in the present issue (volume 17 issue 3) of *Significance*.

4.11 Comments and Conclusions

A brief review of Chapter 4 is now presented and begins with an example from Diaconis [2] about biased coin tossing. The transition probability matrix is given by (4.4). The next example is based on information about rainy days, that is, if today it rains, what are the chances it will rain tomorrow, and if it didn't rain today what is the probability it will rain tomorrow etc. The transition matrix (4.7) is used to generate future realizations using the R function markov. Bayesian inferences consist of testing the hypothesis $P_{11} = .7$, which is the actual value used to generate samples from the chain. Assuming an improper prior for P_{11}, the posterior distribution of P_{11} is beta, and it is shown that the posterior probability of the null hypothesis is $P_0 = .98$. The Bayesian predictive mass function was derived and used to forecast future observations for the transition counts of the chain. BUGS code 4.3 was used generate the future observations.

Next to be considered is how to compute the n-step transition probabilities from the one-step transition matrix. This computation was illustrated with the random walk and implemented with the R function matrixpower, which computes the n-th power of the one-step transition matrix P. Multinomial simulations are used to generate transition counts for the one-step transition matrix, which in turn provides estimates of the one-step transition matrix of the random walk. The function matrix power then computes the six-step transition matrix with entries that estimate the six-step transition matrix. Assuming an improper prior for the one-step transition matrix, and assuming multinomial distributions for the cell counts of each row of P, it is known that the distribution of each row of P is Dirichlet. The challenge for the Bayesian is to determine that the posterior distribution of the entries of the sixth power of P. Section 4.3 is concluded with a specification of the Bayesian estimate of a joint probability of several random variables of the chain involving times 5, 6, 9, and 17 of the process.

Section 4.4 emphasizes the limiting distribution of a chain and illustrated with the forest fire index example. The R function matrixpower computes the limiting distribution of the chain by computing higher and higher powers of the one-step transition matrix P. If the limiting distribution exists the entries of higher powers of P will stabilize. Bayesian inferences consist of testing hypotheses about the fire index transition matrix, and predicting future observations with the Bayesian predictive density.

If a chain has a stationary distribution, it is of interest to be able to estimate it from sample data. If one knows the one-step transition matrix P, and if a stationary solution exists, it is known to be the solution of a system of linear equations. The primary goal of this section was to provide estimates of the stationary distribution and this was illustrated with the social mobility example. For information from the data, multinomial realizations were generated for each row of the chain, then assuming an improper prior, the marginal posterior distribution of each transition probability is determined to be a beta. The system of equations (4.61) determines the stationary distribution as a function of the nine cell entries of P. BUGS code implements the Bayesian estimation of the stationary distribution and the results are reported in Table 4.5. Also a R program was used to compute the stationary distribution of the chain and compared to the Bayesian results.

Section 4.6 introduces the idea of a transition graph which is a representation of a Markov chain. The R package igraph is employed to implement such graphs and provide one with additional information about the behavior of the process. The section includes a discussion of Bayesian inferences for irreducible chains, that is those where all the states communicate, that is there is only one class. Bayesian inferences are demonstrated with the three-by-three irreducible chain with transition matrix (4.70). Specifically, the entries of the third row of the chain are estimated with the Bayesian paradigm in the usual way with multinomial observations generated for the third row and the results reported in Table 4.14.

It is well known that there are two types of states in a Markov chain, transient and recurrent, such states are defined in section 4.6.3. Example of a chain with both states is the one with three states and transition matrix (4.71). It is easy to show that 1 and 2 are recurrent, but that 3 is transient. Realizations generated via the R function Markov illustrate that 3 is transient and that 1 is recurrent. For the Bayesian analysis, tests of hypotheses about the third row of the transition matrix are carried out. The social class example (4.61) with three states is irreducible and employed to illustrate the average return time to a particular state. The goal for the Bayesian is to estimate those average return times, and BUGS code 4.6 is executed for the posterior analysis with the results reported in Table 4.8.

Section 4.7 explains the Bayesian approach to making inferences about the period of state of a Markov chain. The example has transition matrix (4.7) where it is known that each state has period 2. The problem for the investigator is to test the hypothesis of period say for example state 1 is period 2. This is a very interesting example of Bayesian inference. The posterior analysis is reported in Table 4.10.

Time reversibility is the subject of section 4.8 and is an interesting property of those chains that exhibit it. Such chains demonstrate the same behavior whether looking into the future or going backwards to the past. The concept is defined and two examples are explored: one where it is known there is no

TABLE 4.14

Initial Value 1 with 200 Transitions

---
1 2 1 2 1 1 2 1 2 1 2 1 2 1 2 1 2 1 1 2 1 1 2 1 2 1 2 1 2 1 2 1 2 1 2 1 1 2 1
1 1 2 1 2 1 2 1 1 1 1 1 1 1 1 2 1 1 1 2 1 2 1 1 1 2 1 2 1 2 1 2 1 1 2 1 2
1 2 1 2 1 1 2 1 2 1 2 1 2 1 2 1 1 2 1 2 1 1 1 2 1 1 2 1 2 1 2 1 1 2 1 2 1
2 1 1 1 2 1 2 1 2 1 1 2 1 1 1 1 2 1 2 1 1 2 1 2 1 2 1 2 1 2 1 2 1 2 1 1 2
1 2 1 2 1 2 1 2 1 2 1 1 2 1 1 2 1 2 1 2 1 1 2 1 1 2 1 1 1 2 1 2 1 1 2 1 2
1 1 1 2 1 2 1 2 1 2 1 1 2 1 1 2 1 2 1
---

time reversibility and the other where there is time reversibility. When time reversibility is present for a three-state chain, there are three conditions that must be satisfied. Therefore, the Bayesian approach is to test the hypothesis that the chain is time reversible. One assumes the chain is irreducible and uses the Bayesian approach to testing hypotheses, see section 2.5.3 of Chapter 2. Using the stationary distribution of the chain is essential and BUGS code 4.9 implements the analysis and the posterior analysis reported in Table 4.13.

Lastly, the chapter concludes with the Bayesian approach to estimating the absorbing states of a Markov chain. The basic idea of absorbing states is well-illustrated with the gambler's ruin problem, where there are three communicating classes: {1} the gambler has lost all, {N} the gambler has won the pot, and the rest {2,3,...,N − 1}. The two absorbing states are 1 and N, where N = 5 and k = 2 (the initial capital), and the Bayesian analysis consists of estimating the probability the gambler will lose and estimate the average duration of the game. Also presented is a brief description of the current coronavirus considered as a stochastic time series.

Bayesian inference for Markov chains is an active area of interest and what follows are several references that are applicable to the presentation given here. When using Jeffreys' prior for the inference of a Markov chain, Assodou and Essebbar [8] provide an interesting perspective. With regard to time reversible chains, see Diaconis and Rolles [9] and if your interest is a general account of Bayesian inference for Markov chains, refer to Eichelsbacher and Ganesh [10] as well as the book by Insua, Ruggeri, and Wiper [11]. Also of interest is the relation between Markov chains and associated decision problems, and Martin [12] details the relationship. The empirical Bayes approach to inference is not considered in this book; however, it is adopted by Meshkani and Billard [13] who explain the subtleties of that method. Lastly Welton and Ades [14] deal with the important topic of using partially observed data to estimate the transition probabilities of a Markov chain. For a more complete list of Bayesian inference for Markov chains, see Insua, Ruggeri, and Wiper.

4.12 Exercises

1. Write a two page essay summarizing Chapter 4.
2. Refer to the one-step transition matrix (4.4), the Diaconis example of a biased coin.
   a. To what extent is the coin biased?
   b. Using the markov function of R, generate 200 observations with initial value heads.

TABLE 4.15

Posterior Distribution of P_{01}

Parameter	Mean	SD	Error	2 1/2	Median	97 1/2
P_{01}	.5769	.06797	.000385	.4423	.5766	.7066

    c. Using the transition counts generated in b, give the usual estimates of P_{11} and P_{12}.

3. Refer to the transition matrix (4.10), the transition matrix for the random walk on a cycle. Using the matrixpower function of R, confirm the entries of the matrix P^6, the six-state transition matrix corresponding to (4.21).

4. Use the R function rmultinom to generate cell counts for the first row of the transition matrix P (4.12) with n = 50. Using this as the sample information, the cell counts in the first row will follow a multinomial distribution, and assuming an improper prior distribution for the first row entries of P, what is the Bayesian posterior distribution of P_{01}? Execute the Bayesian analysis with 35,000 observations for the simulation with a burn in of 5,000. Your results should be similar to those reported in Table 4.15.

5. Refer to the transition probability matrix (4.23)

    a. Use the R code 4.2 and verify the entries of P^{17} and P^{18}.

    b. What is the long-term risk of the forest fire index with five states?

6. Duplicate the five multinomial realizations appearing in Table 4.2 of the first row of the transition matrix (4.23) using a total count of 100.

7. For the forest fire index example, consider the test of the hypothesis
    H_0: P_{11} = .755, P_{12} = , 118, P_{13} = .172, P_{14} = .109, P_{15} = .026 based on equations (4.36)–(4.41), show that the posterior probability of the null hypothesis is P_0 = .1845.

8. Refer to the probability transition matrix (4.51), the social mobility example, and using R code 4.3, verify the stationary distribution as π = (.0623, .6234, .3141). In the long term, what is the probability a person will be in the middle class?

9. a. Using the first realization for the social mobility example (Table 4.5), and assuming an improper prior distribution for the first row of the transition probability matrix P (4.51), show the posterior distribution of the first row is Dirichlet (98, 84, 18).

    b. Based on the third realization reported in Table 4.5, show posterior distribution of the first row is Dirichlet (86, 106, 8).

    c. What are the implications for having two different Dirichlet distributions for the posterior distribution of the first row of P?

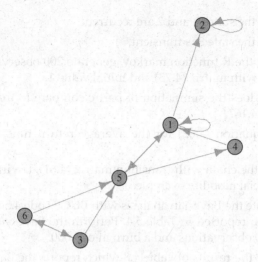

FIGURE 4.1
Partitioning of Six States

10. Refer to the social mobility example with transition matrix P (4.51). Based on BC 4.3 and generating 40,000 observations for the simulation with a burn in of 5,000, execute a Bayesian analysis for the stationary distribution of the chain. Refer to Table 4.4. Your results should be similar.

11. Using R code 4.4, verify the transition graph Figure 4.1. You will need to download the package "igraph" to the R platform.

12. Based on the transition graph 4.4, explain why the chain is irreducible.

13. Based on the first multinomial realization (Table 4.5) of the third row of the chain and assuming an improper prior distribution for the third for the parameters:

    a. Show the posterior distribution probabilities of the third row are as follows:

        i. $P_{31} \sim beta(1,102)$, $P_{32} \sim beta(31,72)$, $P_{33} \sim beta(71,32)$.

        ii. Verify the posterior analysis of Table (4.6).

        iii. What is the 95% credible interval for P_{31}?

        iv. Plot the posterior density of P_{31}.

        v. Based on the density of P_{31}, is the distribution symmetric?

14. Verify the transition graph Figure 4.1, which is based on transition probability matrix (4.62).

15. Refer to the Markov chain with transition probability matrix (4.67).

    a. Show the states 1 and 2 are recurrent.

    b. Show the state 3 is transient.

    c. Using the R function markov, generate 200 observations from the chain with matrix (4.73) and initial value 1.

    d. How does the simulation of part c compare to that appearing in Table 4.16?

16. Verify equation (4.62) for the average return time to a particular state.

17. Refer to the chain with transition matrix (4.61), the irreducible chain of the social mobility example.

    a. Execute the Bayesian analysis with BUGS code 4.5 using the information reported in Table 5.4. Perform the Bayesian analysis with 35,000 observations and a burn in of 5,000.

    b. Verify the results of Table 4.8 which reports the Bayesian analysis for the first return times for each of the three states (n lower, middle, and higher social class).

    c. Are the results of Table 4.8 reasonable? Explain in detail and justify your answer.

    d. Explain why R code 4.5 computes the average return time to the states of a Markov chain.

    e. Compare the Bayesian estimate of the average return time

    f. (reported in Table 4.8) to that computed by R code 4.8.

18. Refer to the transition probability matrix (4.76).

    a. Show that state 1 has period 2.

    b. Using the igraph package with R code 4.6, generate the transition graph of the chain (4.76). Your results should look like Figure 4.2.

    c. Does the graph show each state has period 2? Why?

19. Based on the entries of the estimated transition matrices of P (4.80), namely P^2(4.70) and P^4(4.72), is the period of each state of P is of period 2?

20. Verify the Bayesian analysis reported in Table 4.8 of the 1-1 element of the two-step transition matrix P^2. Do the results imply that each state of the chain is of period 2? Explain your answer in detail.

21. Time reversibility of a Markov chain is defined by (4.75). Does the Bayesian analysis reported in Table 4.10 support the conjecture that the chain is time reversible?

22. Using BC 4.7, execute the Bayesian analysis with 35,000 observations for the simulation with a burn in of 5,000 and verify the posterior analysis of Table 4.9.

TABLE 4.16

Initial Value 3: 200 Transitions

3 3 2 1 2 1 1 2 1 2 1 2 1 2 1 1 1 1 2 1 1 1 2 1 2 1 1 1 1 2 1 1 1 2 1 2 1
2 1 2 1 1 2 1 1 2 1 2 1 2 1 2 1 1 2 1 1 1 2 1 2 1 2 1 2 1 1 2 1 2 1 2 1 2
1 2 1 2 1 2 1 2 1 2 1 2 1 1 2 1 2 1 2 1 1 1 1 2 1 1 2 1 2 1 2 1 1 2 1 2 1
2 1 1 1 2 1 2 1 2 1 1 1 2 1 2 1 2 1 2 1 2 1 2 1 2 1 1 1 2 1 1 2 1 2 1 2 1
2 1 1 2 1 2 1 2 1 1 2 1 2 1 2 1 2 1 2 1 2 1 2 1 2 1 1 2 1 2 1 1 2 1 2 1 1
2 1 2 1 1 1 2 1 1 1 1 1 2 1 1 2

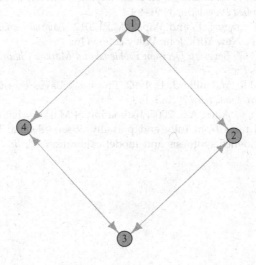

FIGURE 4.2
Transitions Among

23. Refer to section 4.9 and the stochastic epidemic: perform a Bayesian analysis with 35,000 for the simulation with 5,000 initial values. Use BC 4.7 for the Bayesian analysis. Your results should be similar to Table 4.13.

References

1. Markov, A.A. 1906. Rasprostranenie zakona bol'shih chisel na velichiny, zavi-syaschie drug ot druga. *Izvestiya Fiziko-matematicheskogo obschestva pri Kazanskom universitete, 2-ya seriya* 15: 135–156.
2. Diaconis, P. 2007. Dynamical bias in coin tossing, *SIAM Review*, 49(2):211–235.
3. Dobrow, R.P. 2016. *Introduction to Stochastic Processes with R*. New York, John Wiley & Sons Inc.

4. Martell, D.L. 1999. A Markov chain model of day to day changes In the Canadian Forest Fire Weather Index. *International Journal of Wildland Fire*, 9(4):265–273.
5. Ross, S.1996. *Stochastic Processes*. New York, John Wiley & Sons Inc.
6. DeGroot, M.H. 1970. *Optimal Statistical Decisions*. New York. McGraw Hill.
7. Bailey, N.T.J. 1964. *The Elements of Stochastic Processes*. New York, John Wiley & Sons Inc.
8. Assodou, S. and Essebbar, B. 2003. A Bayesian model for Markov Chains via Jeffreys' prior. *Communications in Statistics: Theory and Methods* 32:2163–2184.
9. Diaconis, P. and Rolles, S. 2006. Bayesian analysis for reversible Markov chains. *Annals of Statistics* 34:1270–1292.
10. Eichelsbacher, P. and Ganesh, A. 2002. Bayesian inference for Markov chains. *Journal of Applied Probability* 39:91–99.
11. Insua, D.R., Ruggeri, F. and Wiper, M.P. 2012. *Bayesian analysis of Stochastic Process Models*. New York, John Wiley & Sons Inc.
12. Martin, J.J. 1967. *Bayesian Decision Problems and Markov Chain*. New York, John Wiley & Sons Inc.
13. Meshkani, M.R. and Billard, L. 1992. Empirical Bayes estimators for a finite Markov chain. *Biometrika* 79:185–193.
14. Welton, N.J. and Ades, A.E. 2005. Estimation of Markov chain transition probabilities and rates from fully and partially observed data: Uncertainty propogation, evidence synthesis and model calibration. *Medical Decision Making* 25:633–645.

5

Biological Examples Modeled by Discrete Markov Chains

5.1 Introduction

Bayesian inferential techniques will be employed to gain a deeper understanding of the mechanism of various biological phenomena. Several examples will illustrate the Bayesian approach to making inferences: (1) the general birth and death process, (2) the logistic growth process, (3) a simple model for an epidemic, (4) the chain binomial model, (5) Greenwood and the Reed–Frost versions of the epidemic models, and (6) Stochastic epidemic models.

Bayesian inferences will include determining the posterior distribution of the relevant parameters, testing hypotheses about those parameters, and determining the Bayesian predictive distribution of future observations. Such Bayesian procedures will closely follow those presented in Chapter 4, and will comprise generating simulations from the chain, displaying the associated transition graph for the chain of each example, and employing the appropriate R code and WinBUGS code for the analysis. It is important to note that the biological examples included here serve as an introduction to elementary biological examples, leading up to more sophisticated examples of the coronavirus pandemic.

5.2 Birth and Death Process

A general birth and death process is formulated as a discrete time Markov chain. We consider a finite population of maximum size N and a chain $\{X(n), n = 0,1,2,..\}$ with state space $\{0, 1, 2, \ldots , N\}$, where $X(n)$ is the size of the population at time n. The birth and death probabilities b_i and d_i depend on the size of population where

$$P_{ij} = \Pr\{X(n+1) = j \mid X(n) = i\}$$
$$= b_i, j = i+1,$$
$$= d_i, j = i-1, \tag{5.1}$$
$$= 1-(b_i + d_i), j = 1,$$
$$= 0, otherwise$$

and i = 1,2, , $P_{00} = 1$, $P_{0j} = 0$, $j \neq 0$. Also, note that $P_{N,N+1} = b_N = 0$, therefore the N + 1 by N + 1 transition matrix is given by

$$P = \begin{pmatrix} 1,0,0,0,0,\ldots\ldots,,,,,,,,,,,,,,,,,,,,,,,,,,,,,,,,,,,,,,,0 \\ d_1,1-(d_1+b_1),b_1,0,0,0,0,0,0,0,\ldots,,0 \\ 0,d_2,1-(d_2+b_2),b_2,0,0,0,0,0,0,\ldots,0 \\ \vdots \\ 0,0,0,\ldots\ldots\ldots,0,d_{N-1},1-(d_{N-1}+b_{N-1}),b_{N-1} \\ 0,0,\ldots\ldots\ldots\ldots\ldots\ldots\ldots\ldots\ldots,0,d_N,1-d_N \end{pmatrix}. \tag{5.2}$$

Thus the population increases by one, decreases by one, or remains the same. There are two communicating classes where {0} and {1, 2, ..., N}, where 0 is an absorbing state and the remaining are transient. In addition, it can be shown that there is a unique stationary distribution.

As an example of a birth and death process let N=10 and $b_i = bi$, i = 1, 2, .., 9, $d_i = di$, i = 1, 2, ..., 10, where b and d are constants.

Three cases are considered: (a) b = .02 < .03 = d, (b) b = .025 = d, and (c) b = .03 > .02 = d.

For the first case the transition matrix is given by equation (5.3).

$$P = \begin{pmatrix} 1,0,0,0,0,0,0,0,0,0,0 \\ .03,.95,.02,0,0,0,0,0,0,0,0 \\ 0,.06,.9,.04,0,0,0,0,0,0,0 \\ 0,0,.09,.85,.06,0,0,0,0,0,0 \\ 0,0,0,.12,.8,.08,0,0,0,0,0 \\ 0,0,0,0,.15,.75,.10,0,0,0,0 \\ 0,0,0,0,0,.18,.70,.12,0,0,0 \\ 0,0,0,0,0,0,.21,.65,.14,0,0 \\ 0,0,0,0,0,0,0,.24,.60,.16,0 \\ 0,0,0,0,0,0,0,0,.27,.55,.18 \\ 0,0,0,0,0,0,0,0,0,.30,.70 \end{pmatrix} \tag{5.3}$$

Recall the following R code Markov function that generates observations from the chain with transition matrix P.

RC 5.1

```
markov <- function(init,mat,n,labels) {
+ if (missing(labels)) labels <- 1:length(init)
+ simlist <- numeric(n+1)
+ states <- 1:length(init)
+ simlist[1] <- sample(states,1,prob=init)
+ for (i in 2:(n+1))
+ {simlist[i] <- sample(states,1,prob=mat[simlist[i-1],])}
+ labels[simlist]
+}
```

The first simulation has initial value 2 and the process is absorbed by the state 1.

```
> init<-c(0,1,0,0,0,0,0,0,0,0,0)
> markov(init,p,100)

2 2 2 2 2 2 2 2 2 2 2 2 3 3 3 3 3 3 3 3 3 3 3 3 3 3 2 2 2 2 2 2
2 2 2 2 2 2
2 2 2 2 2 2 2 2 2 2 2 2 2 2 2 2 2 1 1 1 1 1 1 1 1 1 1 1 1 1 1 1
1 1 1 1 1 1
1 1 1 1 1 1 1 1 1 1 1 1 1 1 1 1 1 1 1 1 1 1 1 1 1 1 1 1 1 1 1 1
```

The second simulation begins with the state 3 and stays in the state 2 for the remaining observations.

```
> init<-c(0,0,1,0,0,0,0,0,0,0,0)
>init<-c(0,0,1,0,0,0,0,0,0,0,0)
>markov(init,p,100)

3 3 3 3 4 4 3 3 3 3 3 3 3 3 3 3 3 3 3 3 3 3 3 3 3 3 3 3 3 3 3 3
3 3 3 3 3 3 3 3 3 3 3 3 3 3 3 3 3 3 3 3 3 3 3 3 3 2 2 2 2 2 2 2 2 2
2 2 2 2 2 2 2 2 2 2 2
2 2 2 2 2 2 2 2 2 2 2 2 2 2 2 2 2 2 2 2 2 2 2 2 2 2 2 2 2 2 2 2 2.
```

The student should experiment with the markov R function with additional simulations using different initial values. Also of interest is the R function stationary, which when applied to the transition P gives the stationary distribution π reported in Table 5.1.

```
stationary <- function(P) {
+ x = eigen(t(mat))$vectors[,1]
+ as.double(x/sum(x))
+ }
>
> stationary(P)
```

TABLE 5.1

Stationary Distribution Birth
and Death Process

π_0	0.001782713
π_1	0.009306754
π_2	0.032048848
π_3	0.032048848
π_4	0.217523222
π_5	0.481424409
π_6	0.120759090
π_7	0.033324661
π_8	0.009965581
π_9	0.003265024
π_{10}	0.001287085

Our last goal for this example of a birth and death process is to estimate the birth and death rates using a Bayesian approach, whereby multinomial realizations will be generated form the first three components of the second row of P, namely (.03,.95,.02) which are the values assigned to the vector $(d_1, 1 - (b_1 + d_1), b_1)$. The R code

```
p<-c(.03,.95,.02)
> rmultinom(5,100,p)
```

generates the following five realizations of size 100 depicted in Table 5.2.

Based on the fifth realization, the usual estimates of the death and birth rates d_1 and b_1 are .02 and .07, respectively, compared to the values of .03 and .02, respectively, used to generate those realizations. Also apparent is the variation demonstrated between the five realizations. Recall the Bayesian analysis is based on assuming the realizations have a multinomial distribution and an improper prior assigned to the unknown parameters d_1 and b_1, that the prior density is

$$g\left(b_1, d_1\right) \propto 1 / b_1 d_1, 0 < b_1 < 1, 0 < d_1 < 1. \tag{5.4}$$

TABLE.5.2

Five Realizations for Birth and Death Process

	R1	R2	R3	R4	R5
d_1	5	1	1	1	2
$1 - (d_1 + b_1)$	93	96	97	96	91
b_1	2	3	2	3	7

Based on the fifth realization and the prior density (5.3), the posterior density of b_1 is beta (7,93) and that d_1 beta (2,98) and the complete Bayesian analysis is executed with BUGS code 5.1.

BC 5.1

```
model;
{
d1~dbeta(7,93)
b1~dbeta(2,98)
}
```

I executed the analysis with 70,000 observations for the simulation and a burn in of 5,000.

The actual value the birth rate is .02, and the posterior mean is .02006 with a 95% credible interval of (.0023,.0552), but the actual value of the death rate is .03 and is estimated with the posterior median of .0672 with a 95% credible interval (.0287,.1269). Note that also the credible interval for d_1 does include .03. Both posterior distributions appear to be skewed to the right. See the posterior density of b_1 shown in Figure 5.13.

The last aspect of Bayesian inference for the birth and death process is to derive the predictive distribution of the multinomial distribution used to generate realizations, Table 5.4, for the counts of the birth and death process (5.1) with transition matrix (5.2).

In general, the predictive density of the future transition counts (m_1, m_2, m_3) of the first three components of the first row of P (5.3);

$$
\int\int\int [m!/m_1!m_2!m_3!]\left[\Gamma\left(\sum_{j=1}^{j=3}m_j+\alpha_j\right)/\prod_{j=1}^{j=3}\Gamma(m_j+\alpha_j)\right]
$$

$$
\times\prod_{j=1}^{j=3}P_j^{m_j+n_j+\alpha_j-1}dP_1dP_2dP_3
$$

$$
=\left[m!/\prod_{j=1}^{j=3}m_j!\right]\left[\Gamma\left(\sum_{j=1}^{j=3}(n_j+\alpha_j)\right)\right]/\left[\prod_{j=1}^{j=3}\Gamma(n_j+\alpha_j)\right]
$$

$$
\times\left[\prod_{j=1}^{j=3}\Gamma(n_j+m_j+\alpha_j)/\Gamma\left(\sum_{j=1}^{j=3}(n_j+m_j+\alpha_j)\right)\right]
$$

(5.5)

where the posterior density of (P_{11}, P_{12}, P_{13}) is Dirichlet $(n_1+\alpha_1, n_2+\alpha_2, n_3+\alpha_3)$, and the corresponding prior density is Dirichlet $(\alpha_1, \alpha_2, \alpha_3)$. Note by letting the alpha hyper parameters be zero, one is in effect assuming an improper prior for the three transition parameters, which simplifies the predictive density to

TABLE 5.3

Posterior Analysis for Birth and Death Process. Fifth Realization

Parameter	Mean	SD	Error	2 1/2	Median	97 1/2
b_1	.02006	.01402	.0000821	.002347	.01696	.05521
d_1	.07009	.02538	.000142	.02875	.06727	.1269

TABLE 5.4

Multinomial Realizations for Birth and Death Process

Population Size	d	1-d-b	b	n_1	n_2	n_3
1	.03	.95	.02	2	97	21
2	.06	.90	.04	8	86	6
3	.09	.85	.06	7	91	2
4	.12	.8	.08	15	81	4
5	.15	.75	.10	11	76	13
6	.18	.7	.12	17	66	17
7	.21	.65	.14	22	64	14
8	.24	.6	.16	23	59	18
9	.27	.55	.18	27	57	16
10	.30	.70		28	72	

$$g(m_1,m_2,m_3) = A / B \qquad (5.6)$$

where

$$A = [m!/ m_1! m_2! m_3!]\Gamma(100)\Gamma(2+m_1)\Gamma(91+m_2)\Gamma(7+m_3)$$

and

$$B = \Gamma(2)\Gamma(91)\Gamma(7)\Gamma(100+m_1+m_2+m_3).$$

Recall that the cell count m_1 corresponds to the death rate d_1, m_2 to $1 - (d_1 + b_1)$, and m_3 to b_1. For example, it can be shown that

$$g(2,3,5) = .000008392 \qquad (5.7)$$

Of special interest is the expected time to extinction of the birth and death process. According to Dobrow [1,p118], the average time to extinction of the birth and death process $\{X(n), n = 0,1,2,\ldots\}$ with

$$X(0) = m \geq 1, b_0 = 0 = d_0, b_i > 0, i = 1,2,\ldots,N-1$$

and $d_i > 0, i = 1, 2, \ldots, N$ is given by

$$
\begin{aligned}
\mu_m &= 1/d_1 + \sum_{i=2}^{i=N} (b_1\ldots b_{i-1}/d_1\ldots d_i), m = 1 \\
&= \mu_1 + \sum_{s-1}^{s=m-1} [d_1\ldots d_s/b_1\ldots b_s][\sum_{i=s+1}^{i=N} [b_1\ldots b_{i-1}/d_1\ldots d_i], m = 2,\ldots,N
\end{aligned}
$$

(5.8)

Using formula (5.28), it can be shown that the average time to extinction is $\mu_1 = 54.7933$ time points. Note this estimate does not have a standard error attached, and this problem can be avoided using Bayesian inferential techniques. Is this value reasonable? Remember that if the population size is one, one would need a death for extinction, but the probability of a death is .03, a small chance that that extinction is imminent. Also, recall the probability the population size remains at one with probability .95 at each time point.

The Bayesian approach will generate multinomial data using the transition matrix P of equation (5.2). I generated a multinomial realization of size 100 for the transition counts corresponding to the 10 population sizes which correspond to the various birth and death rates listed in columns 2 and 4. For example, corresponding to the population of size 5 with death rate .15 and birth rate .10, the multinomial realization of size 100 is (11,76,13). Thus, the usual estimate of the death rate is .11 compared to the actual value of .15. Of course, we would expect the estimated rates to differ from the actual.

Assuming an improper prior density of the birth and death rates, the posterior distribution of the transition probabilities (the birth and death rates) of each will be beta. For example, the posterior distribution of d_2 is beta (8,92), which has a posterior mean of .08. I executed the posterior analysis with BUGS code 5.2 with 70,000 observations for the simulation and a burn in of 5,000.

BC 5.2

```
model;
{

d1~dbeta(2,98)
b1~dbeta(1,99)
d2~dbeta(8,92)
b2~dbeta(6,94)
d3~dbeta(7,93)
b3~dbeta(2,98)
d4~dbeta(15,85)
b4~dbeta(4,96)
```

```
d5~dbeta(11,89)
b5~dbeta(13,87)
d6~dbeta(17,83)
b6~dbeta(17,83)
d7~dbeta(22,78)
b7~dbeta(14,86)
d8~dbeta(23,77)
b8~dbeta(18,82)
d9~dbeta(27,73)
b9~dbeta(16,84)

d10~dbeta(28,72)

b12<-b1*b2
b13<-b12*b3
b14<-b13*b4
b15<-b14*b5
b16<-b15*b6
b17<-b16*b7
b18<-b17*b8
b19<-b18*b9

d12<-d1*d2
d13<-d12*d3
d14<-d13*d4
d15<-d14*d5
d16<-d15*d6
d17<-d16*d7
d18<-d17*d8
d19<-d18*d9
d110<-d19*d10

mu1<- (1/d1)+(b1/d12)+(b12/d13)+(b13/d14)+(b14/d15)+(b15/d16)+
(b16/d17)+(b17/d18)+(b18/d19)+(b19/d110)

}
```

The Bayesian analysis is reported in Table 5.5.

The posterior distribution of μ_1 is extremely skewed to the right. Refer to formula (5.8) for μ_1 which shows that the numerator and denominator of the terms are extremely small sometimes in very large values for the simulation. Because of the asymmetry of the posterior distributions, I recommend the

TABLE 5.5

Birth and Death Process

Parameter	Mean	SD	Error	2 1/2	Median	97 1/2
μ_1	134.4	465	1.702	21.53	76.55	574.4

median of 76.55 time points as the estimate of the time to extinction. This implies that on the average it will take 77 time points to reach a population size of 0, starting with a population of size 1. This is because the probability of a death is only .03. Note one is assuming the time between events so that in small time intervals at most one event will occur.

5.3 The Logistic Growth Process

The logistic growth process is a variation of the birth and death process that satisfies

$$b_i - d_i = ri(1 - i/K), i = 0,1,2,\ldots,N, N > K \tag{5.9}$$

where r is the intrinsic growth rate, K is the carrying capacity, b_i is the birth rate when the population is of size i, and d_i the corresponding death rate. The process is observed at various time points, such that the time between time points is sufficiently small so that $\{d_i + b_i\} \leq 1$. It can be seen that the behavior of the process various according to the size of the population. Note that when I = 0 or I = K (the carrying capacity) the birth and death rates are the same. Two cases are considered:

$$b_i = r(i - i^2/2K), d_i = ri^2/2K, i = 0,1,2,\ldots,2K$$
$$b_i = ri, i = 0,1,2,\ldots,N-1; d_i = ri^2/K, i = 0,1,2,\ldots,N \tag{5.10}$$

For the first case, the maximum population size is N = 2K, and the birth probability increases when the population size < K and decreases for population sizes > K, but the death rate is always increasing. On the other hand, for the second case, both the birth and death probabilities increase with the population size. Refer to Allen [2, pp. 123–127] for additional details about the logistic growth process.

For the Bayesian analysis interest is restricted to the second case with N=20, K=10, r=.004, and $b_i = ri$, $d_i = ri^2/K$. The one-step 21-by-21 transition matrix for the second case is given by P below. The analysis consists of generating multinomial realizations of size 1000 for the non-zero entries of each row of P. In this way the sample information is available, then this is combined with the prior information for the unknown parameters (the transition parameters of the transition matrix, of which there are three for each row of P). As before an improper prior distribution is assigned, which when combined with the realizations of Table 5.4 results in Dirichlet distributions for the transition rows of P.

$$P = \begin{pmatrix} 1,0,0,0,0,0,0,0,0,0,0 \\ .03,.95,.02,0,0,0,0,0,0,0,0 \\ 0,.06,.9,.04,0,0,0,0,0,0,0 \\ 0,0,.09,.85,.06,0,0,0,0,0,0 \\ 0,0,0,.12,.8,.08,0,0,0,0,0 \\ 0,0,0,0,.15,.75,.10,0,0,0,0 \\ 0,0,0,0,0,.18,.70,.12,0,0,0 \\ 0,0,0,0,0,0,.21,.65,.14,0,0 \\ 0,0,0,0,0,0,0,.24,.60,.16,0 \\ 0,0,0,0,0,0,0,0,.27,.55,.18 \\ 0,0,0,0,0,0,0,0,0,.30,.70 \end{pmatrix} \tag{5.11}$$

TABLE 5.6

Multinomial Realizations for the Logistic Growth Model

Population Size	d	1-b-d	b	n_1	n_2	n_3
1	.0004	.9956	.004	1	992	7
2	.0016	.9904	.008	1	996	3
3	.0036	.9844	.012	5	988	7
4	.0064	.9776	.016	4	977	19
5	.01	.9700	.020	9	964	27
6	.0144	.9616	.024	15	961	24
7	.0196	.9524	.028	18	952	30
8	.0256	.9242	.032	26	943	31
9	.0324	.9316	.036	29	935	36
10	.04	.92	.04	48	912	40
11	.0484	.9076	.044	41	914	41
12	.0576	.8944	.048	62	888	50
13	.0676	.8804	.052	74	880	46
14	.0784	.8656	.056	63	882	55
15	.09	.85	.06	84	859	57
16	.1024	.8336	.064	93	841	66
17	.1156	.8164	.068	109	824	67
18	.1296	.7984	.072	132	801	67
19	.1444	.7790	.076	139	781	80
20	.16	.84		154	846	

The first column of Table 5.6 designates the population size, and the second, third, and fourth rows are the transition probabilities (the death and birth rates) of the transition matrix of the logistic growth model, while the last three columns of Table 5.6 are the corresponding multinomial realizations.

Each realization is based on a sample of size 1000 and the realizations provide sample information for the Bayesian analysis.

For example, corresponding to a population size 10, the death and birth rates are each .04 and the corresponding multinomial realization is (48,912,40), giving .48 and .40 as the usual estimates of the death and birth rates, respectively, when the population is of size 10. I chose 1000 for the realization size because the birth and death rates are very small. I wanted to avoid a transition count of zero. Note that the last row of Table 5.6 does not have an entry (corresponding to the population of size 20, the maximum size), since a birth is impossible, but a death can occur with probability .16.

Using formula (5.8), the goal of the Bayesian analysis is to estimate the time to extinction assuming a population of size 1.

BC 5.3

```
model;
{
d1~dbeta(1,999)
d2~dbeta(1,999)
d3~dbeta(5,995)
d4~dbeta(4,996)
d5~dbeta(9,991)
d6~dbeta(15,985)
d7~dbeta(18,982)
d8~dbeta (26,974)
d9~dbeta(29,971)
d10~dbeta(48,952)
d11~dbeta(41,959)
d12~dbeta(62,938)
d13~dbeta(74,926)
d14~dbeta(63,937)
d15~dbeta(84,916)
d16~dbeta(93,917)
d17~dmodelbeta(109,891)
d18~dbeta(132,868)
d19~dbeta(139,861)
d20~dbeta(154,846)
b1~dbeta(7,993)
b2~dbeta(3,997)
b3~dbeta(7,993)
b4~dbeta(19,981)
b5~dbeta(27,973)
b6~dbeta(24,976)
b7~dbeta(30,970)
b8~dbeta(31,969)
b9~dbeta(36,964)
```

```
b10~dbeta(40,960)
b11~dbeta(41,959)
b12~dbeta(50,950)
b13~dbeta(46,954)
b14~dbeta(55,945)
b15~dbeta(57,943)
b16~dbeta(66,936)
b17~dbeta(67,933)
b18~dbeta(67,933)
b19~dbeta(80,920)
d.12<-d1*d2
d.13<-d.12*d3
d.14<-d.13*d4
d.15<-d.14*d5
d.16<-d.15*d6
d.17<-d.16*d7
d.18<-d.17*d8
d.19<-d.18*d9
d.110<-d.19*d10
d.111<-d.110*d11
d.112<-d.111*d12
d.113<-d.112*d13
d.114<-d.113*d14
d.115<-d.114*d15
d.116<-d.115*d16
d.117<-d.116*d17
d.118<-d.117*d18
d.119<-d.118*d19
d.120<-d.119*d20

b.12<-b1*b2
b.13<-b.12*b3
b.14<-b.13*b4
b.15<-b.14*b5
b.16<-b.15*b6
b.17<-b.16*b7
b.18<-b.17*b8
b.19<-b.18*b9
b.110<-b.19*b10

b.111<-b.110*b11
b.112<-b.111*b12
b.113<-b.112*b13
b.114<-b.113*b14
b.115<-b.114*b15
b.116<-b.115*b16
b.117<-b.116*b17
b.118<-b.117*b18
b.119<-b.118*b19

mu1<-1/d1+b1/d.12+b.12/d.13+b.13/d.14+b.13/d.14+b.14/d.15+
b.15/d.16+b.16/d.17+b.17/d.18+b.18/d.19+b.19/d.110+b.110/d.111
```

TABLE 5.7

Posterior Analysis of Logistic Growth Model

Parameter	Mean	SD	Error	2 1/2	Median	97 ½
b_1	.00699	.00263	.000008	.0028	.0066	.0130
b_2	.0030	.0017	.000005	.00062	.0026	.0071
b_3	.0069	.0026	.000007	.0028	.0066	.0130
d_1	.0009	.0009	.000003	.000025	.0006	.0036
d_2	.0010	.00099	.000003	.00002	.0006	.0036
d_3	.0049	.00223	.000006	.00163	.0046	.0102
μ_1	$5.37*10^7$	$3.4*10^9$	$1.04*10^7$	24200	919400	$1.2*10^8$

```
+b.111/d.112+b.112/d.113+b.113/d.114+b.114/d.115+b.115/d.116
+b.116/d.117+b.117/d.118+b.118/d.119+b.119/d.120

}
```

I used 55,000 observations for the simulation with a burn in of 5,000 and the results are reported in Table 5.7.

The posterior distribution of three death and birth rates is portrayed in Table 5.7, while the posterior median to the time to extinction is 919,400 time units. When the population is size 1, note that the probability of a death is .0004, thus it is not surprising that the median time to extinction is extremely large. The student will be asked to enlarge the posterior analysis to the parameter μ_{10}, the average time to extinction, assuming the population is size 10.

5.4 Epidemic Processes

5.4.1 Introduction

This section deals with using Markov chains to model the evolution of an epidemic and then explores the use of Bayesian techniques to provide inferences for the unknown transition probabilities (which contain the basic parameters that describe the epidemic) of the process. First to be discussed is an explanation of the basic principles of an epidemic, which is the biological foundation of an epidemic. Next, a deterministic version of a simple epidemic is presented, which lays rudiments of the stochastic version of an epidemic model. Of primary importance in the study of epidemics is to determine the average duration of the epidemic. Various versions that generalize the simple epidemic are the chain binomial models which include the Greenwood model and the Reed–Frost model. The relationship between the epidemic model and the previously discussed birth and death process is elucidated.

The model is referred to as the SIS model because susceptible individuals (S) becomes infected (I) but do not develop immunity after they recover. This is designated by $S \to I \to S$, because the infected individuals can again become infected. No latent period is included in the simple epidemic model; thus, people that become infected can pass the disease to others. Also assumed is no vertical transmission of the disease, that is the infection cannot be passed on to the mother's offspring. Thus, the offspring immediately become susceptible. Because the number of births and deaths are the same, the total population size is $N = S + I$. Suppose the interval between time n and time n+1 is small enough so that at most one event occurs. Therefore, the following can occur: (1) a susceptible person becomes infected, (2) a susceptible person give birth (and a corresponding death of either a susceptible or infected individual), or (3) an infected person recovers. Suppose the probability of a susceptible individual becoming infected is $\beta I/N$, where β is the number of contacts made by one infectious individual that results in one infection during the interval $(n, n+1)$; thus, only $\beta S/N$ of these contacts may result in a new infection, and the total number of new infections by the whole class of infected individuals is $\beta SI/N$. Suppose susceptible and infected persons are born or die with probability b, and that infected individuals recover with probability γ.

5.4.2 Deterministic Model

Let $I(n)$ and $S(n)$ denote the number of infected and number of susceptible individuals at time n respectively, where the dynamics of the chain follow the system of difference equations:

$$S(n+1) = S(n) - \beta S(n)I(n)/N + I(n)(b+\gamma)$$
$$I(n+1) = \beta S(n)I(n)/N + I(n)(1-b-\gamma) \tag{5.12}$$

where, $n = 0, 1, 2, \ldots, S(0) > 0, I(0) > 0, S(n) + I(n) = N$.

These equations are interpreted as follows: The number of new susceptible individuals at time n + 1 is the number of individuals that did not become infected $S(n)[1 - \beta I(n)/N]$, plus the number of infected individuals that recovered, namely $\gamma I(n)$, and plus the offspring (newborns) from the infected group $bI(n)$. Since the total population size is constant, the number of offspring from the susceptible class is the same as the number of susceptible people that die, namely, $bS(n)$. The restrictions on the unknown parameters is $0 < \beta \le 1, 0 < b + \gamma \le 1$.

In the second equation of (1.32), $S(n)$ is replaced by $N - I(n)$ giving

$$I(n+1) = I(n)\left[\beta(N-I(n))/N\right] + 1 - b - \gamma$$
$$= I(n)\left[1 + \beta - b - \gamma - \beta I(n)/N\right] \tag{5.13}$$

There are two equilibrium solutions, that is where

$$I(n+1) = I(n) = E \tag{5.14}$$

which are $E = 0$ and $E = N[1 - (b + \gamma)/\beta]$.

The equilibrium point is a function of the reproduction number

$$R_0 = \beta/(b+\gamma), \tag{5.15}$$

which has an interesting meaning in epidemiology: It is when the whole population is susceptible and one infectious person is introduced into the population, R_0 is the average number β of successful contacts during the period of infectivity $1/(b+\gamma)$ that will result in a new infected person. Note that if $R_0 > 1$, then one infected individual produces more than one new infection and if $R_0 < 1$, then one infectious individual produces less than one new infection.

5.4.3 Stochastic Model

Assume the facts about the simple model in the deterministic case, but where $I(n)$ is random variable denoting the number of infected individuals at time n, where the population is of size $N = I(n) + S(n)$, and $S(n)$ is a random variable denoting the number of susceptible people at time n, n = 0,1,2,... . Now assume that the time interval from n to n + 1 is small enough so that there is at most one change over that time period. For the Bayesian analysis focus will be on the number of infected people

$I(n)$ with state space $\{0, 1, 2, ..., N\}$, which has two classes: $\{0\}$ and $\{1, 2, ..., N\}$, where state 0 is absorbing, denoting that the infection dies out. The transition matrix is defined by the following three equations:

$$\begin{aligned}
P_{i,i+1} &= \Pr\left[I(n+1) = i+1 \mid I(n) = i\right] = \beta i(N-i)/N = \lambda_i \\
P_{i,i-1} &= \Pr\left[I(n-1) = i-1 \mid I(n) = i\right] = (b+\gamma)i,
\end{aligned} \tag{5.16}$$

and

$$P_{i,i} = \Pr\left[I(n+1) = i \mid I(n) = i\right] = 1 - \lambda_i - (b+\gamma)i.$$

Thus, the one-step transition matrix of the number of infected people is

$$P = \begin{pmatrix}
1, 0, \dots\dots\dots\dots\dots\dots\dots\dots\dots\dots\dots\dots\dots, 0 \\
b+\gamma, 1-b-\gamma-\lambda_1, \lambda_1, 0, \dots\dots\dots\dots, 0 \\
0, 2(b+\gamma), 1-2(b+\gamma)-\lambda_2, 0, \dots\dots\dots, 0 \\
\vdots \\
0, \dots\dots\dots\dots, 0, N(b+\gamma), 1-N(b+\gamma)
\end{pmatrix}, \tag{5.17}$$

The goal as a Bayesian is to make inferences about the unknown parameters: the birth rate b, β the number of contacts, and γ the number of infected people that recover. I will begin with estimating the parameters b, γ, and β using as data transition counts for the first three entries of the second row of P, where the transition counts will be realizations generated via the multinomial distribution.

Consider the multinomial distribution with parameter p = (.005,.9851,.0099), then using the R function rmultinom, the following realization was generated with transition counts $(n_{10}, n_{11}, n_{12}) = (3,993,4)$ corresponding to the transition probabilities

$$P_{10} = b + \gamma,$$
$$P_{11} = 1 - \lambda_1 - (b + \gamma),$$
$$P_{12} = \lambda_1 = \beta(N-1)/N, \tag{5.18}$$
$$N = 100,$$
$$b = \gamma = .0025,$$

and

$$\beta = .01.$$

Therefore, the transition probabilities are estimated as $P_{10}^- = .003$, $P_{11}^- = .973$, and $P_{12}^- = .004$. Thus, using (5.9), the estimates for the parameters of the epidemic are .0040404 for β and .0015 for b and γ. What are the Bayesian estimates?

Assume the prior distribution for the transition probabilities is the improper prior

$$\zeta(P_{10}, P_{11}, P_{12}) = \sum_{j=0}^{j=2} P_{1j}^{-1}, \tag{5.19}$$

where

$$\sum_{j=0}^{j=1} P_{1j} = 1, 0 < P_{1j} < 1, \text{ and } j = 1, 2, 3.$$

It can be shown the posterior distribution of the transition probabilities is Dirichlet with parameter $(n_{10}, n_{11}, n_{12}) = (3,993,4)$, thus the marginal posterior distribution of P_{10} is beta(3,997), of P_{11} is beta(993,7), and that of P_{12} beta(4,996).

The Bayesian analysis is executed with BUGS code 5.8 with 35,000 observations for the simulation and a burn in of 5,000. The step command g2 gives the posterior probability that $R_0 > 1$.

BC 5.4

```
model;
{
p10~dbeta(3,997)
p11~dbeta(993,7)
p12~dbeta(4,996)
bplusgamma<-p10
N<-100
beta<-p12*N/(N-1)
b<-bplusgamma/2
R0<-beta/bplusgamma
g1<-step(R0-.5)
g2<-step(R0-1)
}
```

As a result of the simulation, the Bayesian analysis for the simple epidemic model is reported in Table 5.8.

Note that the posterior probability that $R_0 > 1$ is .663, that is in symbols $g_2 = \Pr[R_0 > 1 \mid data] = .663$. The estimates of the other parameters P_{10}, P_{11}, and P_{12} are similar to the usual estimates given above. Recall that the transition probabilities $P_{10} = .005$, $P_{11} = .9851$, $P_{12} = .0099$ were used to generate the multinomial realization $(n_{10}, n_{11}, n_{12}) = (3,993,4)$ for the Bayesian analysis, and these values for the transition probabilities should be compared to the posterior means $(.0029, .993, .0039)$ of Table 5.8. It appears that the posterior means are quite close to these values. See Broemeling [3,*ch5*] for additional information about stochastic models for epidemics.

For additional information about the stochastic epidemic model refer to Allen and Burgin [4], Daley and Gani [5], and Jacquez and Simon [6].

TABLE 5.8

Posterior Distribution of Epidemic Model

Parameter	Mean	SD	Error	2 1/2	Median	97 1/2
R_0	2.029	2.655	.0097	.2935	1.389	7.538
b	.00149	.000859	.0000032	.00031	.00133	.00361
$b+\gamma$	.002986	.001718	.0000064	.00062	.00267	.00722
P_{10}	.002986	.001718	.0000064	.00062	.00267	.00722
P_{11}	.993	.00262	.0000096	.987	.9933	.9972
P_{12}	.00399	.001992	.0000083	.0011	.00366	.00879
β	.004037	.002003	.0000112	.00113	.003705	.00886
g2	.663	.4727	.002646	0	1	0

5.4.4 Chain Binomial Epidemic Models

The following description of chain binomial models relies heavily on Allen [2,pp. 137–143]. Let S(n) and I(n) denote discrete random variables for the number of susceptible and infected people at time n respectively, where the time interval between time n and n + 1 is the latent period, that is the time until individuals become infectious, for n = 0,1,2,... Thus, the number of infected individuals I(n) represents newly infected individuals who were latent during the time period n − 1 to n, and these people are infectious. They will contact susceptible individuals at time n, who consequently could become infected at time n + 1. The infected I(n) individuals are removed or recovered in the next time interval from n to n + 1. Births and deaths do not occur and the newly infected individuals at time n + 1 and those susceptible at that time represent all those who were susceptible at time n, thus

$$S(n+1)+I(n+1)=S(n) \tag{5.20}$$

The epidemic terminates when I(n)=0 for some n. The above explanation for chain binomial models is somewhat simplified and the reader is referred to Daley and Gani [5] for additional information about the subject. Let α be the probability of a contact between an infected and susceptible individual, and suppose β is the chance that the contact results in the susceptible person become infected, therefore, the probability that a susceptible person does not become infected is

$$p = 1 - \alpha\beta. \tag{5.21}$$

In view of (5.21), 1-p is the probability of a contact not resulting in an infection, and as will be revealed, p is an important parameter in both versions of the chain binomial model.

There are two versions of the chain binomial model: (a) The Greenwood and (b) the Reed–Frost.

First the Greenwood model is investigated. At time n + 1 there are S(n + 1) susceptible people among which S(n + 1) contacts were not successful and the number of contacts that were successful is I(n+1) = S(n + 1) − S(n). This implies that the probability of a one-step transition from S(n + 1) to S(n) is

$$P_{S(n),S(n+1)} = \binom{s(n)}{s(n+1)} \left[p^{i(n)} \right]^{s(n+1)} \left[1 - p^{i(n)} \right]^{s(n)-s(n+1)}. \tag{5.22}$$

where s(n + 1) = 0,1,2,..,s(n), and $0 < p < 1$. Note this determines the s(0)-by-s(0) transition matrix of the Greenwood model (1.41) for an epidemic, which is to be initiated with I(0) >0 infectious people. Note that the state process for the chain {S(n), n = 1,2,,,,}, where S(0) is positive. A realization of the process is depicted by {s(0), s(1),...,s(t)} where the number of infected people at time t is zero that is, $I(t) = 0$, which is equivalent to $S(t-1) = S(t)$. The duration of the epidemic is t and the size of the epidemic is the number of susceptible people who became infected during the duration or $S(0) - S(t)$. This type of epidemic is of the chain binomial type because the distribution of $S(n+1)$ is binomial with parameters $s(n)$ and p. From (5.13), the $(s(0)+1)$ by $(s(0)+1)$ is

$$P = \begin{pmatrix} 1,0,0,\dots\dots\dots\dots\dots\dots\dots\dots\dots\dots\dots\dots\dots\dots\dots\dots\dots,0 \\ (1-p),p,0,\dots\dots\dots\dots\dots\dots\dots\dots\dots\dots\dots\dots\dots\dots,0 \\ (1-p)^2,2p(1-p),p^2,0,\dots\dots\dots\dots\dots\dots\dots\dots\dots,0 \\ \vdots \\ (1-p)^{s(0)},\binom{s(0)}{1}p(1-p)^{s(0)-1},\binom{s(0)}{2}p^2(1-p)^{S(0)-2},\dots\dots,p^{s(0)} \end{pmatrix}. \quad (5.23)$$

- Now let $s(0) = 3$, the four-by-four matrix P reduces to

$$P = \begin{pmatrix} 1,0,\dots\dots\dots\dots\dots\dots\dots\dots\dots,0 \\ 1-p,p,0,\dots\dots\dots\dots\dots\dots\dots,0 \\ (1-p)^2,2p(1-p),p^2,\dots\dots\dots\dots,0 \\ (1-p)^3,3p(1-p)^2,3p^2(1-p),p^3 \end{pmatrix} \quad (5.24)$$

Now let $\beta = .05$, the probability that a susceptible person is infected after contact with an infected person, and suppose the probability of a contact between a susceptible individual and an infected individual is $p = .025$, which is the probability a susceptible person is infected. Substitute .025 for p in (5.15) to give as the transition matrix

$$P = \begin{pmatrix} 1,0,0,0 \\ .02500,.97500,0,0 \\ .000625,.04875.95060,0 \\ .0000156,.001821,.07129,.92685 \end{pmatrix} \quad (5.25)$$

In terms of α and β, the transition matrix is

$$P = \begin{pmatrix} 1,0,0,0 \\ \alpha\beta,1-\alpha\beta,0,0 \\ \alpha^2\beta^2,2(1-\alpha\beta)\alpha\beta,(1-\alpha\beta)^2,0 \\ \alpha^3\beta^3,3(1-\alpha\beta)\alpha^2\beta^2,3\alpha^2\beta^2(1-\alpha\beta),(1-\alpha\beta)^3 \end{pmatrix} \quad (5.26)$$

There are two classes {0} and {1,2,3} where the latter states are transient and the first is absorbing. Does it have a limiting distribution?

The following R code generates realizations from the Greenwood process using the transition matrix P (5.16).

RC 5.2

```
markov <- function(init,mat,n,labels) {
+ if (missing(labels)) labels <- 1:length(init)
+ simlist <- numeric(n+1)
+ states <- 1:length(init)
+ simlist[1] <- sample(states,1,prob=init)
+ for (i in 2:(n+1))
+ {simlist[i] <- sample(states,1,prob=mat[simlist[i-1],])}
+ labels[simlist]
+}
> p<-matrix(c(1,0,0,0,
.02493,.9751,0,0,
.001567,.04672,.9517,0,
.000156,.004232,.004232,.9298),nrow=4,ncol=4,byrow=TRUE)
```

A realization of size 25 is generated by the markov function
    markov(init,p,25) with starting value the state 1:

```
init<-c(0,1,0,0)
1,1,1,1,1,1,1,1,1,1,1,1,1,1,1,1,1,1,1,1,1,1,1,1,1,1.
```

With starting value 2:

```
init<-c(0,0,1,0)
2,2,2,2,2,2,2,2,2,2,2,2,2,2,2, 1,1,1,1,1,1,1, 0,0,0,0.
```

With initial value 3:

```
init<-c(0,0,0,1)
3,3,3,3,3,3,3,3,3,3,3,3,3,3,3,3,3,3,3,3,3,3,3,3,3,3,
```

and starting value 0:

```
init<-c(1,0,0,0)
0,0,0,0,0,0,0,0,0,0,0,0,0,0,0,0,0,0,0,0,0,0,0,0,0,0.
```

Do these simulations demonstrate the transient behavior of the states 1,2, and 3 and that 0 is an absorbing state?

For the Bayesian analysis, I used multinomial realizations of size 500 for each row of P (5.16) which generates the transition count matrix Q (5.46). The transition counts will serve as the sample information for Bayesian estimation of p (the second entry of the second row of P), the fundamental unknown parameter of the process with transition matric P (5.16).

$$Q = \begin{pmatrix} 500,0,0,0 \\ 10,490,0,0 \\ 1,17,482,0 \\ 1,2,2,495 \end{pmatrix}. \tag{5.27}$$

Assuming a uniform prior for p, the posterior density of p is beta (491,11), with posterior mean $491/502 = .978087649$. A more compete analysis is executed with BUGS code 5.5.

BC 5.5

```
model;
{
p~dbeta(491,11)
p10<-1-p
p11<-p
p20<-pow(1-p,2)
p21<-2*p*(1-p)
p22<-pow(p,2)
p30<-pow(1-p,3)
p31<-3*p*pow(1-p,2)
p32<-3*pow(p,2)*(1-p)
p33<-pow(p,3)
p3219<-p32*p21*p10
q310<-3*p*pow(1-p,2)*(1-p*p)
s3210<-6*pow(p,3)*pow(1-p,3)
}
```

The Bayesian simulation is for the transition probabilities of the transition matrix P (5.16), whose entries are in terms of the fundamental parameter p. For example, note that p30 of the code is the first entry P_{30} of the last row of (5.16). The posterior analysis is executed with 45,000 observations for the simulation and 5,000 for the burn in. The Bayesian analysis shown in Table 5.9 is quite complete, in which the relevant posterior information is shown for all the entries of the transition matrix.

Thus the fundamental parameter p (the probability that a susceptible person does not become infected) is estimated with the posterior mean as .9781

TABLE 5.9

Posterior Analysis for Greenwood Model

Parameter	Mean	SD	Error	2 1/2	Median	97 1/2
P	.9781	.00648	.000037	.9637	.9787	.989
P_{10}	.0219	.00648	.000037	.01104	.02132	.03631
P_{11}	.9781	.00648	.000037	.9637	.9787	.989
P_{20}	.000522	.000314	.000001	.000122	.000454	.001318
P_{21}	.0428	.01236	.000071	.02184	.04172	.06998
P_{22}	.9567	.01267	.000073	.9287	.9578	.978
P_{30}	.000013	.000012	.0000000	.000001	.000009	.000047
P_{31}	.00152	.000906	.0000052	.000361	.001334	.003812
P_{32}	.0626	.0176	.000101	.0324	.06125	.1012
P_{33}	.9358	.0185	.000107	.895	.9374	.9672
P_{3210}	.000074	.000068	.0000003	.000007	.000054	.00026
s_{3210}	.000074	.000068	.0000003	.000007	.000054	.00026

with a 95% credible interval (.9637,.989). Based on the posterior medians, the transition matrix P (5.43) is estimated as

$$\tilde{P} = \begin{pmatrix} 1,0,0,0 \\ .0212,.9787,0,0 \\ .000454,.04172,.9578,0 \\ .000009..001334,.06125,.937 \end{pmatrix}. \tag{5.28}$$

of the last row of the table which shows the posterior distribution of the sample path $\{s(0), s(1), s(2), s(3)\} = \{3,2,1,0\}$ to extinction of the epidemic is estimated as .000074 with the posterior mean and a 95% credible interval (.000007,.00026). Thus, the posterior probability that the epidemic ends after 4 times units along that particular path is extremely small.

Up to this point, Bayesian inference has focused on estimation of the fundamental parameter p, the probability a susceptible person does not become infected, now the focus will be on predicting future transition counts for the Greenwood model. That is starting with a given number of susceptible and infected individuals, what is the Bayesian predictive mass function for the future number of infected persons?

Recall that given $S(n) = s(n)$, the distribution of $I(n + 1)$ is binomial with parameters $s(n)$ and $(1 - p)s(n)$, thus, given $s(n)$ susceptible people at time n, the average number of infections is

$$E\left[I(n+1)\mid S(n) = s(n)\right] = (1-p)s(n), \tag{5.29}$$

where $(1 - p)$ is the probability a susceptible person will be infected.

The predictive mass function of $I(n + 1)$ is easily determined. The conditional mass function of $I(n + 1)$ given $S(n) = s(n)$ is binomial with parameters $s(n)$ and $(1 - p)s(n))$ which is averaged with respect to p over the posterior distribution of p (which is beta with parameters 490 and 11). Recall that of the number of susceptible people, that on the average, $(1 - p)$ will become infected.

A slight variation of the Greenwood model is the Reed–Frost version of a chain binomial epidemic. It is very similar to the Greenwood model but with a slightly different transition matrix

$$P_{S(n),S(n+1)} = \binom{s(n)}{s(n+1)} \left[p^{i(n)} \right]^{s(n+1)} \left[1 - p^{i(n)} \right]^{s(n)-s(n+1)} .s \qquad (5.30)$$

where i(n) is the number of infected people at time n and the number infected at time n is $I(n) = S(n-1) - S(n)$ for $n = 1,2,\dots$ The primary difference between the Greenwood version (1.41) and the Reed–Frost is that the probability p of a susceptible individual being infected depends on the number of infected, namely the probability $p^{i(n)}$. Let us evaluate the posterior probability of the path $\{s(0),s(1),s(2),s(3)\} = \{3,2,1,0\}$, which has probability

$$P_{32}P_{21}P_{10} = 3p^2(1-p)2p(1-p)p(1-p) = 6p^3(1-p)^3$$
$$= 6(.975)^3(.025)^3 = 6(.926859)(.000015625) = .000086893$$

With the Bayesian approach, refer to BUGS CODE 5.9, the statement s_{3210}, and the last row of Table 5.9, which is identical to the next to last row which in turn corresponds to the posterior probability of the same sample path. The posterior distribution of the two probabilities P_{3210} and s_{3210} are the same, as they should be. Since the number of infections, $E[I(n + 1) | S(n) = s(n)] = (1 - p)s(n)$, the transition probabilities of the Reed–Frost model (5.21) are the same as those for the Greenwood model (1.43). For the two models to differ, $i(n)>1$, for some n.

Now consider the sample path $\{s(0),s(10,s(2),s(3)\}=\{3,1,0,0\}$ which occurs with probability

$$P_{31}P_{10} = 3p(1-p)^2(1-p^2) = 3(.975)(.275)^2(.049375) = .0109219$$

It is left for the student to do the Bayesian analysis to estimate $P_{31}P_{10}$. Refer to BUGS Code 5.8 and the bugs statement s3210<-6*pow(p,3)*pow(1-p,3) which is the probability of the sample path $\{3,1,0,0\}$ assuming the Reed–Frost model.

5.5 Duration and Size

Let T denote the duration of an epidemic, and let W denote the size of the epidemic or the total number of susceptible individuals who become infected. Consider the sample path $\{s_0, s_1, \ldots, s_{t-1}, s_t\}$, $T = t$ and $W = s_0 - s_t$. For a given number of initial susceptible and infected individuals, $s_0 > 0$ and $i_0 > 0$, the maximum value of T is $s_0 + 1$, where $T \in \{0, 1, \ldots, s_0 + 1\}$, and the maximum value of W is s_0, where $W \in \{0, 1, \ldots, s_0\}$. The epidemic may end in one-time step if there are no infections initially, that is when $T = 1$ and $W = 0$ or after $s_0 + 1$ time points when one individual contacts the infection at each time step, that is when $T = s_0 + 1$ and $W = s_0$. Note also that T and W are random variables with distributions that can be determined from the probabilities of the various sample paths.

Consider the example given by Allen [2, pp. 141–142]. This example specifies the probability distribution of T, the duration of the epidemic, assuming the Greenwood model with initially three susceptible and one individual infected, denoted by $s_0 = 3$ and $i_0 = 1$, therefore

$$\begin{aligned} \Pr[T = 1] &= p^3 \\ \Pr[T = 2] &= (1-p)^3 + 3p^2(1-p)^2 + 3p^4(1-p) \\ \Pr[T = 3] &= 3p(1+p)(1-p)^3 + 6p^4(1-p)^2, \end{aligned} \tag{5.31}$$

and

$$\Pr[T = 4] = 6p^3(1-p)^3.$$

Note that p is the probability of a contact not resulting in an infection.

We now present another derivation of the distribution of T and W, assuming the Greenwood model described in section 5. Our presentation is based on that of Daley and Gani [5]. Consider the transition matrix of the Greenwood model (5.13).

$$P = \begin{pmatrix} 1, 0, 0, \ldots\ldots\ldots\ldots\ldots\ldots\ldots\ldots\ldots\ldots\ldots\ldots\ldots\ldots\ldots\ldots\ldots\ldots\ldots, 0 \\ (1-p), p, 0, \ldots\ldots\ldots\ldots\ldots\ldots\ldots\ldots\ldots\ldots\ldots\ldots\ldots\ldots\ldots\ldots\ldots, 0 \\ (1-p)^2, 2p(1-p), p^2, 0, \ldots\ldots\ldots\ldots\ldots\ldots\ldots\ldots\ldots\ldots\ldots, 0 \\ \vdots \\ (1-p)^{s(0)}, \binom{s(0)}{1} p(1-p)^{s(0)-1}, \binom{s(0)}{2} p^2 (1-p)^{S(0)-2}, \ldots\ldots, p^{s(0)} \end{pmatrix} \tag{5.32}$$

Now partition the transition P given below into two matrices as $P = U + D$, where U is a strictly lower triangular matrix with zeros down the diagonal, namely

$$U = \begin{pmatrix} 0,0,0,\dots\dots\dots\dots\dots\dots\dots\dots\dots\dots\dots\dots\dots\dots\dots,0 \\ 1-p,0,0,0,\dots\dots\dots\dots\dots\dots\dots\dots\dots\dots\dots\dots\dots,0 \\ (1-p)^2,2p(1-p),0,\dots\dots\dots\dots\dots\dots\dots\dots\dots,0 \\ \vdots \\ (1-p)^{s_0},\binom{s_0}{1}p(1-p)^{s_0-1},\binom{s_0}{2}p^2(1-p)^{s_0-2},\dots,0 \end{pmatrix} \tag{5.33}$$

and D is the diagonal matrix $D = diag\,(1,p,p^2,\dots,p^{s}_0)$.

The matrix U represents the transitions that do not return to the same state in one step with probability p_{ij} for $i \ne j$, and D represents those transitions that do return to the same in one time unit with probability p_{ii}. When $s_t = s_{t-1}$ or $p^{(n)}_{s_t,s_t} > 0$, there is a positive probability that the epidemic ends at time n. The elements of the matrix U^{n-1} represent the probability of transitions between i and j in n-1 time units, namely $p^{(n-1)}_{ij}$, where $i \to j$, $i \ne j$. Now let $p(n) = [p_0(n),p_1(n),\dots,p_{s_0}(n)]^t$ denote the probability distribution for the state of susceptible individuals at time n, then $U^{n-1}p(0)$ represents the probability $p(n-1)$ given that the epidemic has not ended at time $n-1$. Multiplying by D gives $DU^{n-1}p(n-1)$ represents the probability that the epidemic has terminated at time n, denoted by $Pr[T = n]$. Let $E = (1,1,1,\dots,1)$ be a row vector of ones, then

$$Pr[T = n] = EDU^{n-1}p(0).$$

Since the epidemic can end at states 0, 1, ..., s_0, the probability generating function of T, the duration of the epidemic is represented by the equation

$$\sum_{n=1}^{s_0+1} DU^{n-1}p(0)t^n = \sum_{n=1}^{s_0+1} Pr[T = n]t^n.$$

In a similar fashion, the probability generating function of W, the size of the epidemic, can be derived as was shown by Daley and Gani [5]. For the Greenwood model, let

$$U(t) = \begin{pmatrix} 0,0,0,\dots\dots\dots\dots\dots\dots\dots\dots\dots\dots\dots\dots\dots,0 \\ (1-p)t,0,0,\dots\dots\dots\dots\dots\dots\dots\dots\dots\dots,0 \\ [(1-p)t]^2,2p(1-p)t,0,\dots\dots\dots\dots,0 \\ \vdots \\ [(1-p)t]^{s_0},\binom{s_0}{1}p[(1-p)t]^{s_0-1},\dots,0 \end{pmatrix} \tag{5.34}$$

Note that the previous matrix U is U(1) and the elements $p_{ij}(t)$ of $U(t)$ are $p_{ij}(t) = p_{ij}t^{i-j}$. The elements of U(t) $p_{ij}(t)$, $i \neq j$ represent generating elements for the probability if the epidemic has not ended in one-step transitions. Since the number of susceptible individuals has gone from I to j, the size of the epidemic is i – j. In addition, the elements of $U^2(t)$ are $p_{ij}^2(t) = p_{ij}^2 t^{i-j}$. If in two consecutive times, the number of susceptible individuals has gone from I to j, then the size of the epidemic is i – j. Therefore, $EDU^{n-1}(t)p(0)$ is the generating function of the size of the epidemic when it terminates in n time steps. Because the epidemic can end in 1,2,…, $s_0 + 1$ time points, the probability generating function of W is

$$\sum_{n=1}^{s_0+1} EDU(t)^{n-1} p(0) = \sum_{k=0}^{s_0} pr[W = k]t^k. \qquad (5.35)$$

Based on this, it can be shown that if $s_0 = 3$ and $i_0 = 1$, then

$$\begin{aligned}
\Pr[W = 0] &= p^3 \\
\Pr[W = 1] &= 3p^4(1-p) \\
\Pr[W = 2] &= 3p^2(1+2p^2)(1-p)^2 \\
\Pr[W = 3] &= (1-p)^3(1+3p+3p^2+6p^3).
\end{aligned} \qquad (5.36)$$

5.6 Example of an Epidemic with the Greenwood and Reed–Frost Models

Table 5.10 is taken from Allen [2,p139] and displays possible sample paths, duration, and size for the Greenwood and Reed–Frost models. Assume initially there are three susceptible individuals and one with infection.

5.7 The Covid-19 Pandemic. Statistical Concepts and Perspectives

With the world in the grip of a pandemic of coronavirus disease, newspapers, TV news broadcasts, websites, and social media are flooded with numbers. There are daily reports of cases, treatments, and deaths plus the following analysis to digest; however, a lot of the reports discus concepts for example

TABLE 5.10

Sample Paths with Three Susceptible and One Infection

Sample Path	Duration T	Size W	Greenwood	Reed–Frost
3,3	1	0	p^3	p^3
3,2,2	2	1	$3(1-p)p^4$	$3(1-p)p^4$
3,2,1,1	3	2	$6(1-p)^2p^4$	$6(1-p)^2p^4$
3,1,1	2	2	$3(1-p)^2p^2$	$3(1-p)^2p^3$
3,2,1,0,0	4	3	$6(1-p)^3p^3$	$6(1-p)^3p^3$
3,2,0,0	3	3	$3(1-p)^3p^2$	$3(1-p)^3p^2$
3,1,0,0	3	3	$3(1-p)^3p$	$3(1-p)^3p(1+p)$
3,0,0	2	3	$(1-p)^3$	$(1-p)^3$

From Allen, page 139 Table 3.2

SIR models, that is those report the number of susceptible individuals, the number infected, and the number removed from the population of interest. Also discussed are fatality ratios, transmission rates, as well as reproduction numbers. Some of these ideas will not be familiar to the reader.

That is to say, it can all be unfamiliar and overwhelming. The present issue of *Significance* is committed to explaining statistical ideas and concepts, which will help readers to understand what is going on and to make sense of the information that confronts them as well as to put it in the appropriate context. Contributors to this issue of Significance responded to the call to describe the statistical analysis of COVID-19, and what is to follow should benefit the reader. As one past contributor recently summarized the situation as probably the most relevant, statistically speaking, global crisis ever. Many statisticians are doing important work to understand the spread of the virus and measure its virulence. In tandem, others are fighting the spread of false information, which can have a negative impact on the public health.

For additional information see Volume 17 of the June 2020 issue of *Significance*.

5.8 Comments and Conclusions

This chapter presents the birth and death process and several models for epidemics that deal with deterministic and stochastic versions.

The birth and death process is defined by $\{X(n), n = 0, 1, 2, \ldots\}$, where $X(n)$ is the size of the population at time n, and is the next subject to be presented. The transition matrix is a function of the birth and death rates which give the probabilities of a birth and death, respectively, at each time point. The birth and death rates depend on the present size of the population, and the process is illustrated with a birth and death rates $b_i = bi$ and $d_i = di$, where i is the present size of the population and b=.02 and d=.03. Since the basic death rate is more than that of the birth rate, one would expect the population to become extinct. Of interest for the Bayesian is to estimate the time to extinction. The logistic growth process is a special case of the birth and death process and fundamental parameter of the process are estimated via Bayesian methods using multinomial realizations for the data and an improper prior distribution for the birth and death rates.

Much of the chapter is devoted to Bayesian inferences for several versions of an epidemic. In the simplest case at a given time point there are two types individuals, infected or susceptible, in a fixed population of individuals. Also infected individuals can again become susceptible. A more realistic version of the epidemic process is presented as an exercise at the end of the chapter. First to be described is the deterministic process which includes definitions of the basic parameters. In the stochastic version of the epidemic, the one-step transition matrix is defined in terms of the number of the number of infected people in the population. β, b, and γ are the fundamental parameters of the process and their meaning is made clear in the following explanation: Suppose the interval between time n and time n+1 is small enough so that at most one event occurs. Therefore the following can occur: (1) a susceptible person becomes infected, (2) a susceptible person give birth (and a corresponding death of either a susceptible or infected individual), or (3) an infected person recovers. Suppose the probability of a susceptible individual becoming infected is $\beta I/N$, where β is the number of contacts made by one infectious individual that results in one infection during the interval $(n, n + 1)$, thus only $\beta S/N$ of these contacts may result in a new infection, and the total number of new infections by the whole class of infected individuals is $\beta SI/N$. Suppose susceptible and infected persons are born or die with probability b, and that infected individuals recover with probability γ. The transition matrix of the process is determined by the three parameters β, b, and γ. The Bayesian posterior analysis is executed, where the sample information is data generated by multinomial realizations and an improper prior used for prior information. Another version of the epidemic model is presented and is called the chain binomial model because the transition probabilities are computed according to the binomial distribution. For this model the parameters are α, β and p, where α is the probability a susceptible person comes in contact with an infected person, β is the probability the contact results in an infection, and the probability a susceptible person is not infected. There are two versions of the chain binomial model: (1) Greenwood and (2) Reed–Frost. For the Greenwood model the transition matrix is given by the binomial distribution where the probability of success is given by p, whereas for the Reed–Frost model the probability of success is given by $p^{i(n)}$, where i(n) is the number of infected at time n and the I(n) process satisfies $S(n) + I(n) = S(n-1)$ for n=1,2,...

For additional information about epidemics see Allen [2] and Anderson and May [7]. Fundamental contributions to the stochastic theory of epidemics were made by Greenwood [8].

5.9 Exercises

1. Refer to the transition probability matrix for the birth and death process given by (5.3), where d_i and b_i are the death and birth rates when the population is size i. Assume the birth and death rates are given by $b_i = bi$ and $d_i = di$, where b = .02 and d = .03. Thus, the birth rate is increasing at 2 percent per for an increase of one in the population size, while the death rate is increasing at a rate of 3 percent.

   a. Refer to R Code 5.1 and generate 100 observations for the birth and death process using the R function Markov with initial value 1 person.

   b. Using the R function stationary, determine the stationary distribution of this birth and death process.

   c. Generate five multinomial realizations of size 10 for the birth and death process using the probability vector p<-c(.03,.95,.02). See Table 5.2.

   d. Assume an improper prior distribution for the birth and death rates b_1 and d_1, the birth and death rates when the population consists of only one individual. Use the fifth multinomial realization for the sample information and execute BUGS code 5.1 with 45,000 observations for the simulation and 5,000 for the burn in. Your results should be similar to those presented in Table 5.3.

   e. What is the 95% credible interval for d_1.

   f. Are the posterior distributions for these birth and death rates skewed?

   g. Demonstrate their skewness by plotting the posterior density of the birth and death rates.

2. Refer to the time of extinction of the birth and death given by (5.8).

   a. Generate multinomial realizations of size 100 of the 10 birth and death processes presented in Table 5.4.

b.   Assume an improper prior for the birth and death rates. Execute a Bayesian analysis using BC 5.5 for estimating the 10 birth and death rates b and d (where $b_i = bi$ and $d_i = di$, i = 1,2,...,10) and time to extinction. Use 35,000 observations for the simulation and 4,000 for the burn in.

c.   What are the posterior characteristics for the 10 average times to extinction?

d.   What are the 95% credible intervals for d_3 and b_3 ?

e.   The posterior median of μ_1 is 76.55. Does this seem reasonable to you?

3. a.   Read Section 5.4 and describe the SIS epidemic model.

b.   Carefully explain the difference equation (5.3) for the evolution of an epidemic. What is the solution to the difference equation?

c.   Define the parameters β, b, and γ of the deterministic version

d.   Describe the transition matrix as defined by (5.8).

e.   Refer to equation (5.9) which determines the transition probability matrix for the special case N = 100, $\gamma = b = .0025$, $\beta = .01$.

f.   Generate multinomial realizations of size 1000 using the probability vector p < −c(.005,.9851,.0099). This should result in the transition count (3,993,4) for the transition counts corresponding to the second row of the transition matrix (5.9).

g.   Assume an improper prior distribution (5.10) corresponding to the first three entries of the second row of the transition count vector (3,993,4). The latter serves as data for the Bayesian analysis for estimating the parameters, $(b + \gamma)$, b, β, P_{10}, P_{11}, P_{12}. Execute BC 5.6 for the posterior analysis with 35,000 observations for the simulation, and 5,000 for burn in. The results should be similar to those presented in Table 5.8.

h.   What is the posterior mean and median of b? Is this skewed? The posterior mean of b is .00149. Is this reasonable? Why?

4. a.   Refer to section 5.4.3 and describe the purpose of the parameters α, β, and $1 − \alpha\beta$.

b.   Verify that the matrix P (5.13) is the one-step probability transition matrix of the Greenwood model.

c.   Show that (5.15) reduces to the matrix (5.15) when s(0) = 3.

d. As a special case let $\alpha = .5$, $\beta = .05$ and verify the probability transition matrix is (5.16).

e. What states are transient for the special case?

f. Using the R function markov, generate 25 observations for the epidemic with initial value 2.

g. For each row of the transition matrix (5.13), generate multinomial realizations of size 500. The result should be similar to the matrix Q (5.18).

h. Assuming a uniform prior distribution for the parameter p, and show the posterior distribution of p is beta (491,11).

i. In order to estimate p and the other entries of the transition matrix (5.16), execute BC 5.5 with 35,000 observations for the simulation and 5,000 for the burn in. Your results should be similar to those presented in Table 5.9.

j. What is the 95% credible interval for p? Is this a reasonable value? Explain why?

5. The SIR model is an abbreviation for susceptible people, infected, and removed individuals during the course of an epidemic. A person is susceptible if they have not had the disease infected if currently have the disease, and removed if they have had the disease and have since recovered (and are now immune) or have died. Time is measured in discrete steps and at each step each individual can infect susceptible individuals or can recover/die, at which point the infected is removed. Therefore, this version of an epidemic is more realistic than the previous model. Suppose S(t), I(t), and R(t) denote the number of susceptible individuals, infected, and removed at time t, where at each time point each infected has a probability α of infecting each susceptible (this assumes each person has an equal chance of contacting all susceptible persons). At the end of each step, after having had a chance to infect people, each infected person has probability β of being removed. The initial conditions are $S(0) = N$, $I(0) = 1$, $R(0) = 0$, where the total population is of size $N + 1$ and remains fixed (is not random), that is, $S(t) + I(t) + R(t) = N + 1$, for all $t = 0,1,2,\ldots$

Note at each time point the chance a person remains uninfected is $(1 - \alpha)^{I(t)}$, that is each infected must fail to pass on the infection to the susceptible individuals. Because each infected has a probability β of being removed,

$$R(t+1) \sim R(t) + bin\big(I(t),\beta\big). \tag{5.37}$$

Also,

$$S(t+1)\, \text{given}\, S(t)\, \text{is binomial} \left[S(t), (1-\alpha)^{I(t)} \right] \qquad (5.38)$$

In addition, that if S(t+1) and R(t+1) are known, then

$$I(t+1) = N + 1 - S(t+1) - R(t+1). \qquad (5.39)$$

The following R code stipulates the instructions for simulating the SIR epidemic if one knows the inputs $a = \alpha$, $b = \beta$, N the total population size, and T the number of time points the epidemic is followed.

R CODE for SIR model

```
SIR<-function(a,b,N,T){+ S<-rep(0,T+1)+ I<-rep(0,T+1)+
R<-rep(0,T+1)+ S[1]<-N+ I[1]<-1+ R[1]<-0+ for ( i in 1:T){+
S[i+1]<-rbinom(1,S[i],(1-a)^I[i])+ R[i+1]<-
R[i]+rbinom(1,I[i],b)+ I[i+1]<-N+1-R[i+1]-S[i+1]+ }+ return(ma
trix(c(S,I,R),ncol=3))+ }> a<-.001> b<-.1> N<-1000> T<-100
```

An epidemic will be simulated with the following inputs:

a = .001, b = .1, N = 1000, and T = 100. Thus an infected person has a probability .001 of infecting a susceptible, while the probability is .1, that an infected is removed. Table 5.11 portrays a SIR simulation with the above inputs. I used 100 time points but the table displays the first 14 time points. It is interesting to observe that by time 14, there are already 638 infected individuals and 322 have been removed. The student should simulate the epidemic for all 100 time points.

Now the interesting aspect of this exercise is to make Bayesian inferences for the α and β parameters of the SIR model, given the data in Table 5.12. Does the information in this table allow one to estimate α and β with reliable values? In order to estimate these two parameters, the following BUGS CODE SIR will be used to execute the posterior analysis. In the code, alphamean is the mean of the 13 alphas and betameans is the mean of the 13 betas. Assuming an improper prior for the alphas and gams their corresponding posterior distribution is beta. The Bayesian analysis is executed with 70,000 observations for the simulation and 5,000 for the burn in.

BC SIR

```
model;

{

beta4~dbeta(2,16)
beta5~dbeta(2,32)
beta6~dbeta(8,45)
```

```
beta7~dbeta(5,97)
beta8~dbeta(11,177)
beta9~dbeta(33,308)
beta10~dbeta(52,452)
beta11~dbeta(61,570)
beta12~dbeta(69,621)
meanbeta<-(beta4+beta5+beta6+beta7+beta8+beta9+beta10+beta11+b
eta12)/9

gam1~dbeta(998,2)
gam2~dbeta(994,4)
gam3~dbeta(982,12)
gam4~dbeta(964,18)
gam5~dbeta(933,31)
gam6~dbeta(886,47)
gam7~dbeta(795,91)
gam8~dbeta(631,164)
gam9~dbeta(435,196)
gam10~dbeta(256,179)
gam11~dbeta(136,120)
gam12~dbeta(67,69)
gam13~dbeta(41,26)

alpha1<-1-gam1
alpha2<-1-pow(gam2,1/2)
alpha3<-1-pow(gam3,1/3)
alpha4<-1-pow(gam4,1/4)
alpha5<-1-pow(gam5,1/5)
alpha6<-1-pow(gam6,1/6)
alpha7<-1-pow(gam7,1/7)
alpha8<-1-pow(gam8,1/8)
alpha9<-1-pow(gam9,1/9)
alpha10<-1-pow(gam10,1/10)
alpha11<-1-pow(gam11,1/11)
alpha12<-1-pow(gam12,1/12)
alpha13<-1-pow(gam13,1/13)

meanalpha<-(alpha1+alpha2+alpha3+alpha4+alpha5+alpha6+alpha7+a
lpha8+alpha9+alpha10+alpha11+alpha12+alpha13)/13
}
```

a. Using BUGS CODE SIR with 70,000 observations for the simulation with a burn in of 5,000 execute the Bayesian analysis appearing in Table 5.12.

b. What does the posterior distribution for $\bar{\alpha}$ appearing in Table 5.12 imply about $\alpha =.001$ used to generate the epidemic data given in Table 5.18.

c. What does the posterior distribution of $\bar{\beta}$ imply about $\bar{\beta} =.1$, the value used to generate the epidemic given in Table 5.11?

TABLE 5.11

Simulation of SIR Epidemic

Time	S	I	R
1	1000	1	0
2	998	3	0
3	994	7	0
4	982	18	1
5	964	34	3
6	933	63	5
7	886	102	13
8	795	188	18
9	631	341	29
10	435	504	62
11	256	631	114
12	136	690	175
13	67	690	244
14	41	638	322

TABLE 5.12

Bayesian Analysis for SIR Model

Parameter	Mean	SD	Error	2 1/2	Median	97 1/2
$\bar{\alpha}$	.02421	.000985	.0000038	.02235	.02419	.0262
$\bar{\beta}$	.0916	.01139	.0000413	.07213	.0906	.1167

Note that $\bar{\alpha}$ is the posterior mean of the average of the 13 alphas, and $\bar{\beta}$ is the posterior mean of the mean of the 9 betas calculated with BC SIR. The posterior mean for α, which should be compared to the value of $\alpha = .001$ to generate the data for the epidemic. In a similar way, the posterior mean of β should be compared to $\beta = .1$ the value used to generate the epidemic data of Table 5.18.

References

1. Dobrow, R.P. 2016. *Introduction to Stochastic Processes with R*. New York, John Wiley & Sons Inc.
2. Allen, J.S.L. 2011. *An Introduction to Stochastic Processes with Applications to Biology, Second Edition*. Boca Raton, CRC Press, Taylor & Francis.
3. Broemeling, L.D. 2018. *Bayesian Inference for Stochastic Processes*. Boca Raton, CRC Press, Taylor and Francis.
4. Allen, L.J.S. and Burgin, A. 2000. Comparison of deterministic and stochastic SIS and SIR models in discrete time, *Math. Biosci.*, 163:1–33.
5. Daley, D.J. and Gani, J. 1999. *Epidemic Modeling: An Introduction. Cambridge Studies in Mathematical Biology* 15. Cambridge UK, Cambridge University Press.

6. Jacquez, J.A. and Simon, P.C. 1993. The Stochastic SI model with recruitment and deaths. Comparison with the closed SIS model. *Math. Biosciences*, 117, 77–125.
7. Anderson, R.M. and May, R.M. 1992. *Infectious Diseases in Humans: Dynamics and Control*. Oxford UK, Oxford University Press.
8. Greenwood, M. 1931. On the statistical measure of infectiousness. *J. Hyg.*, 31:336–351.

6

Inferences for Markov Chains in Continuous Time

6.1 Introduction

Our main goal is to present Bayesian inferences for processes in continuous time in this chapter. The material presented in this chapter lays the foundation for the study of epidemics taking place in continuous time. Recall that Chapter 4 played a similar role in laying the foundation for Chapter 5 that presented the epidemic process in discrete time. As in earlier chapters, Bayesian ways to estimate parameters, test hypotheses about those parameters, and predicting future observations will be developed. There are many examples of Markov chains in continuous times and the best known is the Poisson process.

The definition of the Poisson process begins Chapter 6, which is followed by a description of the arrival and inter-arrival times, then various generalizations are considered such as the nonhomogeneous Poisson processes, which include compound processes and processes that contain covariates. Of course, R is employed to generate realizations from the several examples of homogeneous and nonhomogeneous Poisson processes.

Of course, infectious diseases evolve continuously through time and of special interest is the present pandemic of the covid-19 virus.

6.2 The Poisson Process

The Poisson process is a counting process, a collection $\{N(t), t \geq 0\}$ of nonnegative integers where if $0 \leq s \leq t, N(s) \leq N(t)$.

Note that a counting process is indexed by a continuum, the set of positive numbers, and with a state space consisting of the non-negative integers. Now to be described are three equivalent definitions of the Poisson process. For additional information, see Dobrow [1, pp. 224–229].

Definition (a)

A Poisson process with parameter λ is a counting process $\{N(t), t \geq 0\}$ such that

1. $N(0) = 0$,
2. For all $t > 0$, $N(t)$ has a Poisson distribution with parameter λt,
3. The process has stationary increments, that is, for all time $s, t > 0$, $N(t + s) - N(s)$ has the same distribution as $N(t)$, thus,

$$\Pr\left[N(t+s) - N(s)\right] = \Pr\left[N(t) = 0\right] = e^{-\lambda t}\left(\lambda t\right)^{k}/k! \tag{6.1}$$

4. The process has independent increments, that is, for $0 \leq q < r \leq s < t$, $N(t) - N(s)$ and $N(r) - N(q)$ are independent.

Consequently, the distribution of the number of events depends only on the length of the interval. It should be noted that the mean and variance of the process are $E[N(t)] = Var[N(t)] = \lambda t$ for all $t > 0$. The next definition of a Poisson process is given in terms of the arrival times of the events. The arrival times are the times the event occur while the inter-arrival times are the times between consecutive events. It will be shown that the inter-arrival times are independent and have identical exponential distributions.

Definition (b)

For a Poisson process with parameter λ let Y be the time of the first arrival after time 0, then

$$P[Y > 0] = P\left[N(t) = 0\right] = e^{-\lambda t}, \quad t > 0 \tag{6.2}$$

Y is distributed exponential with parameter λ (with mean $1/\lambda$). Therefore, it is true that the inter-arrival times between all of the following events (after the first) follow the same exponential distribution. This is so because after the first event, the succeeding events start the process all over again.

Let $Y_1, Y_2, \ldots$ be a sequence of i.i.d. exponential random variables with parameter λ and let

$$N(t) = \max\left\{n : Y_1 + Y_2 + \cdots + Y_n \leq t\right\}$$

where $N(0) = 0$, then $\{N(t), t > 0\}$ is a Poisson process with parameter λ.

The arrival time for the n-th event is

$$S_n = Y_1 + Y_2 + \cdots + Y_n$$

Thus, the inter-arrival time between the event k-1 and the event k

$$Y_k = S_k - S_{k-1}, k = 1, 2, \ldots$$

It can be shown that the distribution of $S_n \sim Gamma(n, \lambda)$ with density

$$f(s) = \lambda^n s^{n-1} \exp{-\lambda s} / (n-1)! \quad s > 0, \tag{6.3}$$

with moments

$$E(S_n) = n/\lambda$$

and

$$Var(S_n) = n/\lambda^2.$$

Definition (c)

A Poisson process with parameter λ is a counting process $\{N(t), t \geq 0\}$ satisfying the following properties.

1. $N(0) = 0$
2. The process has stationary and independent increments.
3. $P[N(t) = 0] = 1 - \lambda h + o(h)$

$$P\big[N(t) = 1\big] = \lambda h + o(h) \tag{6.4}$$

4. $P[N(t) > 1] = o(h)$
   whereas $h \to 0$, then $o(h)/h \to 0$.

The restrictions 3–5 insure that it is impossible for infinite number of arrivals in a finite interval and that for very small intervals there may occur at most one event. It is left to reader in exercise 1 to show that the three definitions for a Poisson processes are equivalent. See Dobrow [1, pp. 234–235]. The beginning sections have laid the foundation for the Poisson process, and the following section will introduce Bayesian inferential techniques for the parameter λ.

6.3 Bayesian Inferences for λ

This section begins with R code for simulating the arrival times of a Poisson process with parameter $\lambda = 1/2$ over the time interval (0,40].

R Code 6.1

```
> t<-40
> lamda<-1/2
> N<-rpois(1,lamda*t)
> unifs<-runif(N,0,t)
> arrivals<-sort(unifs)
> arrivals
2.976133, 3.248414, 4.721712, 13.677706, 18.775247, 20.919774,
24.250771, 26.427624, 29.565929, 33.931659, 36.650545,
39.282970.
```

Thus the first event arrives at time 2.976133, the second at time 3.248414, and the last the 12-th is at time unit 39.28297, consequently $N(39.28) = 12$.

Consider the following fact about the minimum n of independent. exponential random variables $Y_1, Y_2, ..., Y_n$ with parameters $\lambda_1, \lambda_2, ..., \lambda_n$ respectively. Let $M = \min(Y_1, Y_2, ... Y_n)$ t and $t > 0$, then

$$P[M > t] = \exp{-t(\lambda_1 + \lambda_2 + \cdots + \lambda_n)} \tag{6.5}$$

For $k = 1, 2, ..., n$

$$P[M = Y_k] = \lambda_k / (\lambda_1 + \lambda_2 + \cdots + \lambda_n) \tag{6.6}$$

The first assertion above implies that M has an exponential distribution with parameter $\lambda_1 + \lambda_2 + \cdots + \lambda_n$.

6.4 Thinning and Superposition

The thinning of a Poisson event (arrival) can be one of several types, each occurring with some nonzero probability. The initial process has a given rate λ, but the subsequent thinned processes have rates smaller than λ induced by the thinning probabilities of the component processes. A good example of this is the birth of humans, where the overall birth rate is say λ, and the birth rates for males and females are say $p\lambda$ and $(1-p)\lambda$ respectively, where p is the probability of a male birth.

If the overall birth process follows a Poisson process, it can be shown that the male births follow a Poisson process, as do the females, and that both component processes have stationary and independent increments.

More generally, suppose $\{N(t), t > 0\}$ is a Poisson process with parameter λ, and assume each arrival (independent of previous arrivals) is marked by a type k event with probability p_k such that $\sum_{k=1}^{k=n} p_k = 1$, thus, there are n-thinned processes. Now let $\{N^k(t), t > 0\}$, be the type-k component process, then it can be shown that it is a Poisson process with parameter λp_k, where the n processes are independent. See Dobrow [1, pp. 238–240] for additional details.

Returning to the birth Poisson process discussed earlier, according to the United Nations Population Division, the probability of a male birth is $p = .519$ and assume that births at a large municipal hospital is a Poisson process occurring at $\lambda = 2$ births per hour. Consider the following three problems:

(a) On a 8-hour shift, what is the expectation and standard deviation of the number of female births.

(b) Find the probability that only girls were born between 2 and 5 p.m.

(c) Assume the three babies were born at the hospital yesterday. Find the probability that two are female.

Suppose that $\{N(t), t > 0\}$, $\{M(t) > 0\}$ and $\{F(t), t > 0\}$ denote the overall, male and female processes respectively and consider the first problem (a) above. It is obvious that the females form a Poisson process with parameter $\lambda(1 - p) = 2(1 - .519) = .962$ births per hour. Therefore, the mean of the number of female births over an 8-hour process is

$$E\left[F(\delta)\right] = \delta(2)(.481) = 7.696 = Var\left[F(\delta)\right], \tag{6.7}$$

The average number of female births over an 8-hour period.
Now consider the second question (b), namely

$$P\left[M(3) = 0, F(3) > 0\right] = P\left[M(3) = 0\right] P\left[F(3) > 0\right]$$
$$= \exp\left[-2(.519)4\right]\left[1 - \exp\left(-2(.481)3\right)\right] = .042$$

Lastly for the third problem (c), the desired probability is

$$\binom{3}{2}(.481)^2(.519) = .3602. \tag{6.8}$$

The solution to problems (a), (b), and (c) are based on the "true" values of λ and p; however, in practice these true values are not available. Instead what is available are observations from the three processes $\{N(t), t > 0\}$, $\{M(t) > 0\}$, an $\{F(t), t > 0\}$. From the overall process one can estimate λ, and from that for males one can estimate $p\lambda$, and consequently p. The following R code generates observations for the overall births over a 8-hour period with a birth rate of λ per hour and generates male birth with $2(.519) = 1.038$ births per hour.

R Code 6.2

```
> t<-8
> lamda<-2
> N<-rpois(1,lamda*t)
> unifs<-runif(N,0,t)
> births<-sort(unifs)
> arrivals
1.263526, 1.414724, 1.593349, 2.248500, 2.329316, 2.597407,
2.653645, 2.861839, 3.654373, 3.881924, 4.310339, 4.450808,
5.0
5.008346, 5.085663, 5.315546, 6.850246, 7.320440, 7.524868.
```

R Code 6.3

```
> t<-8
> lamda<-1.038
> N<-rpois(1,lamda*t)
> unifs<-runif(N,0,t)
> malebirths<-sort(unifs)
> malebirths
1.284937, 1.861346, 2.364378, 2.823737, 3.577798, 4.628334,
5.542943, 6.022781, 6.304477, 6.743645, 6.779419.
```

There are 18 overall births with 11 male births over the 8-hour period, which implies a maximum likelihood estimate of $18/8 = 2.25$ births per hour for the overall birth rate, while that for the male birth rate the estimate is $11/8 = 1.375$, and consequently the maximum likelihood estimate of p is $1.375/2.25 = .611$. The overall rate of 2.25 should be compared to 2, the value used to generate the data with R code 6.2. In the same way, the male birth rate estimate of .611 should be compared to the "true" value of .519.

What is the Bayesian approach to estimating the overall and male birth rates over an 8-hour period? First, consider estimating the overall birth rate λ, using the conditional distribution of the waiting time S_{18}, given λ as the likelihood function. When this is combined with the improper prior density (6.10), the posterior distribution of λ is gamma$(18, S_{18})$, where $S_{18} = 7.524868$. In a similar fashion, it can be shown that the posterior distribution of $\gamma = p\lambda$ is gamma $(11, 6.779419)$.

TABLE 6.1

Bayesian Analysis for Overall and Male Birth Rates

Parameter	Mean	SD	Error	2 1/2	Median	97 1/2
γ	1.62	.4909	.00248	.8064	1.571	2.72
λ	2.388	.5622	.00288	1.425	2.344	3.603
p	.7182	.2866	.00142	.3043	.6711	1.414

BUGS CODE 6.1

```
model;
{ lamda~dgamma(18,7.5248)
  gam~dgamma(11,6.7794)
 p<-gam/lamda
}
```

BUG CODE 6.1 is executed with 70,000 observations for the simulation with a burn in of 5,000, and the Bayesian analysis is reported in Table 6.1.

The posterior distributions for p and γ are skewed; thus, I recommend the posterior median as the estimate of the parameter. For example, the posterior median of γ is 1.572 which should be compared to $\gamma = p\lambda = 1.038$, the "true" value" of that parameter. In the same manner, the posterior median of λ is 2.343 should be compared to the "true" value of $\lambda = 2$. Also the "true" value of p is .519, which should be compared to the posterior median of .672. These so-called true values are the values used to generate the realizations from the relevant Poisson process via R Code 6.2 and 6.3. One can see the uncertainty of posterior estimates induced by the sample realizations.

6.5 Spatial Poisson Process

The spatial Poisson process is a generalization of the one-dimensional process studied in Section 6.4 to two or higher dimensions, and there are many examples: models of location of trees in a forest, the distribution of galaxies in the universe, and clusters of disease epidemics. Let the dimension $d > 1$ and the subset $A \subset R^d$ Suppose the random variable $N(A)$ counts the number of points in the subset A and denote $|A|$ as the size of A in one dimension $|A|$ would be a length and in two an area, etc.), then the spatial Poisson process $\{N(A), A \subset R^d\}$ is defined as follows.

a. For each set A $\{N(A), A \subset R^d\}$ is a spatial process with parameter $\lambda |A|$,
b. Whenever A and B are disjoint sets, $N(A)$ and $N(B)$ are independent random variables.

Note how properties *a* and *b* generalize the Poisson process to higher dimensions, where *a* is the generalization of stationary increments and *b* a generalization of independent increments.

Consider the following problem, in two dimensions with parameter $\lambda = 1/3$, then what is the probability that a circle of radius 2 centered at (3,4) contains 5 points?

Let C denote the circle, where $|C| = \pi r^2 = 4\pi$, then

$$P\left[N(C)=5\right]=e^{-\lambda|C|}\left(\lambda|C|\right)^5/5!=e^{-(1/3)(4\pi)}\left(4\pi/3\right)^5/5!=.1629.$$

Recall how the uniform distribution arises with a Poisson process in one dimension, and one see it generalizes to the spatial case. Suppose $N(A) = n$, then the locations of the points in A are uniformly distributed in A. In order to simulate a spatial Poisson process, first simulate a Poisson process with parameter $\lambda \mid A|$, then generate *n* points uniformly distributed in A. The following R code, RC 6.4, generates a realization from a Poisson process with parameter $\lambda = 100$ on the unit square. The circle C inside the square is centered at (.7,.7) with radius *r* = .2. The simulation was repeated 100,000 times counting the number of points in the circle at each location. Figure 6.1 depicts one realization of the simulation and Tables 6.2 and 6.3 list the *x* and *y* coordinates of the points appearing in the square.

TABLE 6.2

Abscissa for Spatial Poisson

0.69947304,	0.752098439,	0.123763154,	0.296506146,	0.928317846,
0.429585261,	0.488405587,	0.697309565,	0.993607834,	0.532608426,
0.756079691,	0.826716592,	0.034607809,	0.730601819,	0.118687329,
0.852127976,	0.263830818,	0.793649223,	0.745337202,	0.176954050,
0.452190885,	0.038280711,	0.734769342,	0.901897682,	0.042760698,
0.493274997,	0.367916513,	0,81977386,	0.624886743,	0.867079208,
0.960224926,	0.725773072,	0.225712035,	0.818893997,	0.884597214,
0.577080285,	0.572040944,	0.08996827,	0.195316027,	0.189498151,
0.095972550,	0.038441649,	0.061324936,	0.307401637,	0.999510041,
0.257187202,	0.707372153,	0.477685743,	0.993814115,	0.213965860,
0.147804266,	0.045082209,	0.166208690,	0.188101258,	0.264188643,
0.613630638,	0.003161575,	0.810800111,	0.563908210,	0.989670485,
0.676237988,	0415593890,	0.545226286,	0.565639704,	0.723113632,
0.205693715,	0.291846363,	0.833905545,	0.222310579,	0.627019410,
0.918520986,	0.233912573,	0933558643,	0.943388963,	0.647354387,
0.455108665,	0.251903168,	0.511865139		

TABLE 6.3

Ordinates

0.26124186, 0.44396077, 0.72392878, 0.49111736, 0.89497749,
0.99227313,] 0.56237175, 0.86285194, 0.77451082, 0.03185146,
0.71030768, 0.43206807, 0.83520226, 0.65923869, 0.80783829,
0.99454636, 0.19521338, 0.92224793, 0.16692210, 0.65440660,
0.13786445, 0.17622265, 0.47331905, 0.78017173, 0.66753798,
0.90558875, 0.70708760, 0.22333211, 0.61457419, 0.72894909,
0.70386713, 0.44872583, 0.95518757, 0.40273958, 0.82697592,
0.59400583, 0.76483304, 0.18288699, 0.30049257, 0.27454940,
0.44961878, 0.08830324, 0.35170958, 0.43822516, 0.81478120,
0.13588946, 0.82128662, 0.01149270, 0.68743833, 0.57614086,
0.20674913, 0.80565632, 0.94538263, 0.70551711, 0.58287165,
0.42483037, 0.90379620, 0.53658911, 0.16208827, 0.06086748,
0.47875291 0.64352514, 0.75371784, 0.16645801, 0.53436726,
0.31414601, 0.30729664, 0.33627592, 0.36142669, 0.81547725,
0.66096427, 0.71732857, 0.67960241, 0.57335401, 0.41865694,
0.47824777, 0.10624367, 0.69410526

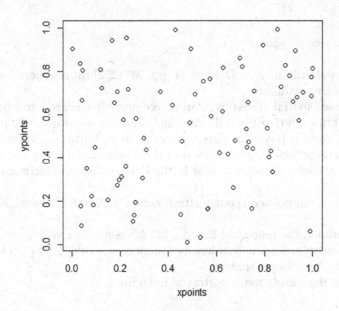

FIGURE 6.1
One realization of the simulation.

RC 6.4

```
lamda<-100
> squarearea<-1
> trials<-100000
> simlist<-numeric(trials)

> for( i in 1:trials){
+ N<-rpois(1,lamda*squarearea)
+ xpoints<-runif(N,0,1)
+ ypoints<-runif(N,0,1)
+ ct<-sum((xpoints-0.7)^2+(ypoints-0.7)^2<=0.2^2)
+ simlist[i]<-ct}
> mean(simlist)
[1] 12.56054
> var(simlist)
[1] 12.58442
> xpoints

> ypoints

> lamda*pi*(0.2)^2
[1] 12.56637
> plot(xpoints,ypoints)
```

The reader should refer to Dobrow [1, pp. 249–252] for additional information about this simulation.

Of course, spatial statistics is an active area of research and for additional details refer to Bivand, Pebesma, and Gomez-Rubio [2, pp. 249–252], and from a Bayesian perspective, to Blangiardo and Camdelli [3}. The R package "spatstat" is very useful for additional ideas about simulation of spatial processes similar to the Poisson. See the technical report from UCLA.

http://scc.stat.ucla.edu/page_attachments/0000/0094/spatial_R_1_09S.pdf.

For example, the following R code, RC 6.5 is another way to simulate a spatial Poisson process with intensity function $f(x,y) = 50(x^2 + y^2)$. One must employ the R package "spatstat."

A plot of the simulation is portrayed in Figure 6.2.

pp1

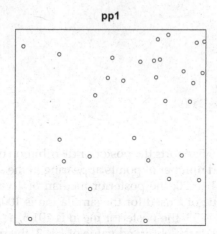

FIGURE 6.2
Spatial Poisson process with intensity $f(x, y) = 50(x^2 + y^2)$.

RC 6.5

```
pp1<-rpoispp(function(x,y) {50*(x^2+y^2) )})
plot(pp1)
```

From a Bayesian viewpoint, how would one estimate the parameter λ of a spatial Poisson process with parameter λ with probability mass function

$$\Pr\left[N(A) = k\right] = (\lambda | |A| |)^k \exp(-\lambda | |A| |) / k!, \tag{6.9}$$

where A is a subset of R^n and the known $|A|$ is the "size" of A?

If one combines the improper prior density

$$g(\lambda) = 1 / \lambda, \lambda > 0 \tag{6.10}$$

with the likelihood function (6.9), then via Bayes theorem, the posterior distribution of λ is gamma with parameters k (the observed number of points appearing in the subset A) and the size of A, namely $|A|$. Recall the previous simulation where $\lambda = 100$ and A is the circle centered at $(.7,.7)$ with radius A, thus, $|A| = \pi r^2 = .12566$

I used Bugs Code 6.2 for the Bayesian estimation of λ with 45,000 observations for the simulation and a burn-in of 5,000. Referring to Table 6.4, the number of points in A is varied from 1 to 20.

TABLE 6.4

Number of Points in Target Circle C

Counts	0–4	5–9	10–14	15–19	20–24	25–29
	522	19,200	50,028	24,975	3,135	106

BC 6.2

```
model;
{
for ( k in 1:20){
delta[k]~dgamma(k,.125)}
}
```

The following Table 6.5 reports the posterior distribution of λ for various values of k, the observed number of points appearing in the subset A.

As k varies from 1 to 20, the posterior median of λ varies from 5.544 to 157.5. Recall the value of λ used for the simulation is 100, thus if in fact the observed value of k is 13, the posterior mean is 101.6, a "good" estimate of λ. On the other hand, if the observed value of k is 3, the posterior median is 21.3, somewhat far away from the "true" value $\lambda = 100$. This shows how the sample variation effects the posterior median on the observed number of points in the circle. Remember when $\lambda = 100$ and, the above spatial Poisson process has parameter$|A| = .1256$ per unit area.

TABLE 6.5

Posterior Distribution of the Poisson Rate Parameter

k	Mean	SD	Error	2 1/2	Median	97 1/2
1	8	8.028	.04148	.202	5.544	29.65
2	16.09	11.45	.05355	1.954	13.44	45.06
3	23.93	13.85	.06663	4.884	21.3	57.77
4	31.98	15.98	.07236	8.732	29.35	70.13
5	39.92	17.86	.09785	12.95	37.27	82.21
6	48.01	19.64	.09033	17.51	45.37	93.82
7	55.96	21.22	.1043	22.52	53.23	104.6
8	63.94	22.51	.1128	27.74	61.44	115.1
9	72.12	23.97	.135	33.16	69.41	126.4
10	79.89	25.12	.1241	38.66	77.31	136.4
11	88.08	26.44	.135	44.56	85.43	147.1
12	95.98	27.82	.1291	49.54	93.19	157.8
13	104.1	28.91	.133	55.07	101.6	167.7
14	112.2	29.9	.1393	61.64	109.6	177.6
15	120.2	31.1	.1507	67.41	117.4	188.8
16	127.8	31.9	.1634	73.3	125.1	198
17	135.9	33.08	.1586	78.86	133.4	207.8
18	143.9	33.81	.1684	85.08	141.2	216.7
19	151.8	34.81	.1787	91.46	149.2	227
20	160.1	35.77	.1647	96.98	157.5	236.8

The last stage for Bayesian inferences for spatial Poisson processes is to test the hypothesis

$$H : \lambda = 100 \quad \text{versus} \quad A : \lambda \neq 100 \tag{6.11}$$

Recall the case discussed previously where simulations were generated from a spatial Poisson process with $\lambda = 100$. See Figure 6.2 for a graph of the simulations, Table 6.4 for the counts of the number of points in the target circle of radius .2, and finally the estimation of λ depicted in Table 6.5. All this information is needed to implement the Bayesian test of H versus A.

The posterior probability of the null hypothesis is

$$p_0 = \pi_0 g\left(k| \lambda = 100\right) / \left[\pi_0 g\left(k| \lambda = 100\right) + \pi_1 g_1\left(k\right)\right], \tag{6.12}$$

where

$$g\left(k| \lambda = 100\right) = \left[\left(100 \,|\, A \,|\right)^k \exp\left(-100 \,|\, A \,|\right)\right] / k!, \tag{6.13}$$

$$g_1(k) = \int_0^\infty \zeta_1(\lambda) g\left(k| \lambda\right) d\lambda, \tag{6.14}$$

$$g\left(k| \lambda\right) = \left[\left(\lambda |\, A |\right)^k \exp\left(-\lambda |\, A |\right)\right] / k!, \tag{6.15}$$

and

$$\zeta_1(\lambda) = \beta^\alpha \lambda^{\alpha-1} e^{-\lambda\beta} / \Gamma\left(\alpha\right)$$

is the prior density of λ under the alternative hypothesis ($\lambda \neq 100$). Thus one must choose the hyper parameters α and β. If one chooses an improper prior for λ, namely $\zeta_1(\lambda) = 1/\lambda$, can show

$$g_1(k) = 1/k. \tag{6.16}$$

When $k = 13$, it can be shown that

$$g\left(13| \lambda = 100\right) = .109127284 \tag{6.17}$$

and

$$g_1(13) = .076923072, \tag{6.18}$$

thus

$$p_0 = .5865, \tag{6.19}$$

which implies that the null hypothesis is indeed plausible. In the exercises, the reader will be asked to compute p_0 for values of $k = 1, 2, \ldots, 20$.

This concludes the presentation of Bayesian methods for estimating the parameter of a spatial Poisson process.

6.6 Concomitant Poisson Processes

Three versions of concomitant Poisson processes are considered: (a) independence, (b) complete similarity, and (c) partial similarity.

Suppose k Poisson processes $N_i(t)$ with parameters λ_i, $i = 1, 2, ..., k$, where n_i events are observed over the interval $(0, t_i]$. The processes could be related. For example, consider the case where the different processes correspond to different intersections in a large city where for the i-th intersection, $N_i(t)$ counts the number of accidents at intersection i and the average number of accidents per day (over a 24 hour period) is denoted by λ_i. If enough is known about the network of intersections, such as their proximity to each other and their location to busy businesses etc. In large cities traffic communication centers continuously monitor the accidents at each intersection in the networks. Thus, there are k homogeneous Poisson processes, and we present Bayesian inferences about the parameters λ_i for the cases, namely of independence and complete and partial similarity between the k processes.

6.7 Nonhomogeneous Processes

6.7.1 The Intensity Function

To understand the nonhomogeneous Poisson process, one must understand the concept of its intensity function, which is defined as

$$\lambda(t) = \lim P\left(N(t, t + \Delta t) \geq 1\right) / \Delta t \tag{6.20}$$

where the limit is as $\Delta t \to 0$, and $N(t)$ has a Poisson distribution. It can be shown that

$$P[N(s, t) = n] = \left[\left(\int_s^t \lambda(x)dx\right)^n \exp\left(-\int_s^t \lambda(x)dx\right)\right] / n!. \tag{6.21}$$

Also note that the mean value function of the process is

$$E\left[N(t)=m(t)\right]=\int_0^t \lambda(x)dx, \quad t>0. \tag{6.22}$$

Consequently,

$$E[N(s,t)=m(s,t)=\int_s^t \lambda(x)dx, s\langle t,s,t\rangle 0 \tag{6.23}$$

and if m is differentiable, it follows from (6.62) that

$$dm(t)/dt = \lambda(t). \tag{6.24}$$

Since the intensity function and the mean value function can vary over time, in general the nonhomogeneous Poisson process does not have stationary increments; however, it does have independent increments and the superposition, the sum of independent Poisson process has a Poison distribution, the valid coloring theorem, when the events occur with a set of multinomial probabilities are valid.

The goal of this section is to develop Bayesian inferences for the parameters of the mean value function or equivalently the intensity function. Of special interest is the intensity function

$$\lambda(t) = M\beta t^{\beta-1} \tag{6.25}$$

where M and β are unknown positive parameters.

Note if $M = 1$ and $\beta = 1$, the Poisson process is homogenous but the intensity function is quite flexible in that it can represent increasing, decreasing, convex, and concave properties.

Corresponding to $\lambda(t)$ is the mean value function

$$m(t) = \int_0^t \lambda(x)dx = \int_0^t M\beta t^{\beta-1} = Mt^\beta, \quad t>0. \tag{6.26}$$

Consider observations taken at times $t_1 < t_2 < \ldots < t_k$ with corresponding counts
$N(t_i) = n_i, i = 1, 2, \ldots, k$, then

$$P\left[N(t_i)=n_i\right]=\left\{\left[m(t_i)\right]^{n_i}\exp\left(-m(t_i)\right)\right\}/n_i! \tag{6.27}$$

Now use the mean value function (6.27), then (6.28) reduces to

$$P\left[N(t_i)=n_i\right]=M^{n_i}t_i^{\beta n_i}\exp\left(-Mt_i^\beta\right)/n_i! \tag{6.28}$$

See Ntzoufras [4] for making Bayesian inferences for the parameters of nonstandard distributions, such as the nonhomogenous Poisson process (6.28) with the power law intensity function. Ntzoufras [4, p. 275] shows how one can provide Bayesian inferences using an approximation to the likelihood function. This approach to approximating the likelihood function will be demonstrated in the next section.

6.7.2 Choosing the Intensity Function

An example involving reliability will illustrate how one can choose the appropriate intensity function. At different times, many systems are subject to reliability decay or growth, and the intensity function is chosen on the basis of exploratory data analysis and prior information about the study at hand. To choose the intensity function and hence the corresponding mean value function, it is helpful to assess whether the expected number of failures over time becomes infinite or remains at some asymptotic level. If the mean value function remains finite as time increases, then Cox–Lewis [5] nonhomogeneous Poisson process with mean value function

$$m(t) = M\left(1 - e^{-\beta t}\right) / \beta \tag{6.29}$$

is a possible alternative; however, as stated by Insua, Ruggeri, and Wiper [6], if the mean value function becomes unbounded as time increases, a possible alternative is the Musa–Iannino–Okumoto [7] mean value function

$$M(t) = M \log(t + \beta). \tag{6.30}$$

As mentioned earlier, a very flexible intensity function is the power law

$$\lambda(t) = M \beta t^{\beta - 1} \tag{6.31}$$

which includes a variety of behavior, including constant, growth, or decaying reliability. For example, when $\beta = 1$, the reliability is constant, and if $\beta > 1$ reliability decays, and finally when $0 < \beta < 1$, there is reliability growth.

When $0 < \beta < 1$, the nonhomogeneous Poisson process is useful in detecting software bugs assuming new bugs are not introduced during testing. For our purpose, an example described by Insua, Ruggeri, and Wiper [6] is adopted. The intensity function exhibits a bathtub behavior for the reliability, which is modeled as a change point with three stages. The change points y_1 and y_2 with three intervals $I_1 = (0, y_1]$, $I_2 = (y_1, y_2]$, and $I_3 = (y_2, y]$ with the same parameter M, but different $\beta_1, \beta_2,$ and β_3. Assume there are n observations $T_1, T_2, \ldots,$

T_n in the interval $(0, y]$ where n_i are in interval i for $i = 1, 2, 3$. The likelihood function is

$$l(M, \beta_1, \beta_2, \beta_3, data) = l_1(M, \beta_1) l_2(M, \beta_2) l_3(M, \beta_3), \tag{6.32}$$

where

$$l_1(M, | \beta_1, | data) = M^{n_1} \beta_1^{m_1} \prod_{i=1}^{i=n_1} T_i^{\beta_1 - 1} \exp\left(-M y_1^{\beta_1}\right), \tag{6.33}$$

$$l_2(M, | \beta_2, | data) = M^{n_2} \beta_2^{n_2} \prod_{i=n_1+1}^{i=n_2} T_i^{\beta_2 - 1} \exp\left(-M y_1^{\left(y_2^{\beta_2} - y_1^{\beta_2}\right)}\right), \tag{6.34}$$

and

$$l_3(M, | \beta_3, | data) = M^{n_3} \beta_3^{n_3} \prod_{i=n_1+n_2+1}^{i=n_3} T_i^{\beta_3 - 1} \exp\left(-M y_1^{\left(y^{\beta_3} - y_3^{\beta_3}\right)}\right) \tag{6.35}$$

As an example, the following data points are generated according to the posterior distributions given by (6.32) through (6.35) using the following code.

RC 6.6

```
M<-1
> beta<-.4
> t<-30
> N<-rpois(1,lamda)
> unifs<-runif(N,0,t)
> arrivals<-sort(unifs)
> arrivals
```

When the mean value function is

$$m(t) = t^{.4}, 20 < t < 30, \tag{6.36}$$

there are only two events with arrival times at

20.54698, 22.14968.

RC 6.7

```
> t<-20
> M<-1
> beta<-1
> lamda<-M*t**beta
> N<-rpois(1,lamda)
> unifs<-runif(N,0,t)
> arrivals<-sort(unifs)
> arrivals
```

When the mean value function is

$$m(t) = t^\cdot, 10 < t < 20 \qquad (6.37)$$

there are 11 events with arrival times

```
11.127021,  11.570835,  12.520865,  12.714158,  13.288865,
15.761193  16.741561,  16.948549,  17.125616,  18.301101,
18.812169.
```

RC 6.8

```
> t<-10
> M<-1
> beta<-2
> lamda<-M*t**beta
> N<-rpois(1,lamda)
> unifs<-runif(N,0,t)
> arrivals<-sort(unifs)
> arrivals
```

When the mean value function is n b

$$m(t) = t^2, 0 < t < 10, \qquad (6.38)$$

there are 94 events with arrival times

```
0.01929614,  0.16683374,  0.30868937,  0.45783466,  0.45783841,
0.60971629,  0.69073963,  0.72312287,  0.73048354,  0.78726970,
0.87282923,  1.11631418,  1.19893630,  1.24930384,  1.29853977,
```

1.86708471, 1.99640772, 2.09816973, 2.31948325, 2.31964980,
2.31978450, 2.32668238, 2.38249653, 2.39276180, 2.40731530,
2.51792069, 2.69428169, 2.86724672, 2.93153171, 2.95547242,
3.09350756, 3.11019411, 3.41164040,3.48050033, 3.51716059,
3.52967131, 3.66419103, 3.70468339, 3.73201358, 3.76651419,
3.77171997, 3.80131188, 3.83412594, 4.27709175, 4.32951888,
4.33360442, 4.45838177, 4.46452007, 4.67891457, 4.72167716,
4.81387984, 5.00014701, 5.24055764,5.30405366, 5.45888764,
5.49390880, 5.52179333, 5.66381047, 6.16508507, 6.24032858,
6.2442796, 6.29753330, 6.30779498, 6.31612410, 6.41120937,
6.41448096, 6.43383395, 6.77219317, 6.84154629, 6.90076633,
6.92867827, 6.93095933, 7.10138919, 7.26750958, 7.27311966,
7.33515741, 7.50370963, 7.52847685, 7.67226142, 7.6930181,
7.73796714, 7.78828417, 8.08008341, 8.42653468,
8.42955573,8.43619858 8.50564013 8.70426517 8.74478266
8.80415160,] 9.0581363, 9.27984186, 9.28731328, 9.35034508,
9.51775680, 9.74506902, 9.96410355, 9.98975439.

Thus, this is the bath tub sort of intensity function with three stages over the three intervals (0,10],(11,20], and (21,30], where there are 94 observations in the first, 11 in the second, and 2 in the third. See

See Ntzoufras [4] for making Bayesian inferences for the parameters of nonstandard distributions given by the likelihood function (6.70). Bayesian estimation for M, β_1, β_2, and β_3 is based on BC 6.10 with code that closely follows Equations (6.32)–(6.35) (Table 6.6).

I executed the analysis with 45,000 observations for the simulation and 5,000 for the burn in.

TABLE 6.6

Posterior Distribution for the Bathtub Mean Value Function

Parameter	Mean	SD	Error	2 1/2	Median	97 1/2
M	3.309	7.196	.0101	.00000	.231	27.33
β_1	.4991	.7065	.001028	.000493	.2277	2.5
β_2	1.001	.9969	.001381	.02528	.6952	3.696
β_3	1.999	1.411	.00197	.2431	1.681	5.554

BC 6.3

```
model;
{
am<-1
bm<-1
n<-108
#see (6.70)
M~dgamma(c1,c2)
c1<-n+am
c2<- bm+pow(10,beta1)+
pow(20,beta2)-pow(10,beta2)+pow(30,beta3)-pow(20,beta3)
# the prior distributions for the regression coefficients
beta1~dgamma(.5,1)
beta2~dgamma(1,1)
beta3~dgamma(2,1)
a1<-1
b1<-1
n1<-94
# see (6.71)
# this is the log likelihood function M and beta1
for ( i in 1:95){
l1[i]<-(a1+n1-1)*log(beta1)-b1*beta1-M*pow(10,beta1)+beta1*log
(T[i])}
n2<-11
a2<-1
b2<-1
# see (6.72)
# this is the log likelihood function for M and beta2
for( i in 96:107){
l2[i]<-(a2+n2-1)*log(beta2)-b2*beta2-M*(pow(20,beta2)-pow(10,b
eta2))+beta2*log(T[i])}
a3<-1
b3<-1
# see (6.73)
# this is the likelihood function for M and beta3
for ( i in 108:110){
l3[i]<-(a3+n-n1-n2-1)*log(beta3)-b3*beta3-M*(pow(30,beta3)-pow
(20,beta3))+beta3*log(T[i])}
}
```

```
list(T= c(0.01929614, 0.16683374, 0.30868937, 0.45783466,
0.45783841, 0.60971629, 0.69073963, 0.72312287, 0.73048354,
0.78726970, 0.87282923, 1.11631418, 1.19893630, 1.24930384,
1.29853977, 1.86708471, 1.99640772, 2.09816973, 2.31948325,
2.31964980, 2.31978450, 2.32668238, 2.38249653, 2.39276180,
2.40731530, 2.51792069, 2.69428169, 2.86724672, 2.93153171,
2.95547242, 3.09350756, 3.11019411, 3.41164040,3.48050033,
3.51716059, 3.52967131, 3.66419103, 3.70468339, 3.73201358,
3.76651419, 3.77171997, 3.80131188, 3.83412594, 4.27709175,
4.32951888, 4.33360442, 4.45838177, 4.46452007, 4.67891457,
4.72167716, 4.81387984, 5.00014701, 5.24055764,5.30405366,
5.45888764, 5.49390880, 5.52179333, 5.66381047, 6.16508507,
6.24032858,
6.2442796, 6.29753330, 6.30779498, 6.31612410, 6.41120937,
6.41448096, 6.43383395, 6.77219317, 6.84154629, 6.90076633,
6.92867827, 6.93095933, 7.10138919, 7.26750958, 7.27311966,
7.33515741, 7.50370963, 7.52847685, 7.67226142, 7.6930181,
7.73796714, 7.78828417, 8.08008341, 8.42653468,
8.42955573,8.43619858, 8.50564013, 8.70426517, 8.74478266,
8.80415160, 9.0581363, 9.27984186, 9.28731328, 9.35034508,
9.51775680, 9.74506902, 9.96410355, 9.98975439, 11.127021,
11.570835, 12.520865, 12.714158, 13.288865, 15.761193,
16.741561, 16.948549, 17.125616, 18.301101, 18.812169,
20.54698, 22.14968))
list(beta1=.2, beta2=1,beta3=3,M=1)
```

Recall that the "true" values for β_1, β_2, and β_3 are .5, 1, and 2 respectively and that of M is 1. The posterior means are very close to these values, but the posterior mean of M is 3.309 and the posterior median is .231. Also note that the posterior distributions for β_1, β_2, β_3 are skewed to the right. As an exercise, the student will be asked to study the sensitivity of the posterior distributions to their priors. The following example is similar to that above for the washtub shaped mean value function, but instead the mean value function is the reverse to that of the washtub shape.

This section on nonhomogeneous Poisson processes is concluded with an example presented by Dobrow [1, p. 253] in the form of a problem. Students arrive at a cafeteria for lunch according to a Poisson process, where the rate of arrival varies in a linear way from 100 to 200 students over the time interval from 11:00 AM to noon, but the rate stays constant over the next two hours (from noon to 2:00 PM), then decreases linearly decreasing to 100 from 2:00 to 3:00 PM. Find the probability that there are at least 400 people in the cafeteria between 11:30 AM and 1:30 PM. The intensity function is given by

$$\lambda(t) = 100 + 100t, 0 < t < 1,$$
$$= 200, \quad 1 < t < 3, \qquad\qquad (6.39)$$
$$= 500 - 100t, 3 < t < 4.$$

It is easy to see that the answer to the question is as follows: The mean value function is

$$E\big[N(2.5) - N(0.5)\big] = \int_{.5}^{1}(100 + 100t)\,dt + \int_{1}^{2.5}200t\,dt = 387.5 \qquad (6.40)$$

Thus,

$$P\big[N(2.5) - N(.5) \geq 400\big] = 1 - \sum_{k=0}^{k=399}(387.5)^k \exp(-387.5)/k! = .269.$$

Our approach will take more of a statistical approach by generating observations from the nonhomogeneous Poisson process with intensity function (6.77), then based on that information estimate the expected value of the process and consequently estimate the required probability.

The following is the R code for generating the inter-arrival times for the process with intensity function (6.39) over the range $0 < t < 1$.

RC 6.9

```
t<-1
> lamda<-200*t
> N<-rpois(1,lamda)
> unifs<-runif(N,0,t)
> arrivals<-sort(unifs)
> arrivals
```

There are 129 arrivals corresponding to the intensity function $\lambda(t) = 100 + 100t, 0 < t < 1$.

```
0.002514378,  0.019175922,  0.021953457,  0.024550520,  0.031322105,
0.035207160,  0.042003951,  0.066021339,  0.069204332,  0.070603115,
0.074403316,  0.078209166,  0.081210360,  0.089738117,  0.108841185,
0.113504869,  0.118042807,  0.120448525,  0.127535137,  0.148708492,
0.155505013,  0.160686959,  0.165564084,  0.171232042,  0.185665243,
0.194464218,  0.202340639,  0.212150896,  0.216791938,  0.229751281,
0.233844860,  0.237426403,  0.240561157,  0.257191631,  0.259427338,
```

0.261023988, 0.261239244, 0.264757474, 0.264951792, 0.265082411,
0.276758405, 0.280244587, 0.311615852, 0.324892686, 0.341942644,
0.347802898, 0.350671225, 0.359282152, 0.372455910, 0.375604996,
0.391797577, 0.395026651, 0.398594826, 0.406915699, 0.417825938,
0.421420146, 0.435862032, 0.436892793, 0.445679733, 0.469381181,
0.478037560, 0.479947491, 0.485462589, 0.494364918, 0.495973951,
0.510708708, 0.516524876, 0.522994348, 0.555194473, 0.565705654,
0.590331443, 0.595593126, 0.606269287, 0.625587527, 0.629214609,
0.633505706, 0.639148909, 0.639599133, 0.646117045, 0.656630432,
0.660690608, 0.676695661, 0.679830155, 0.684899308, 0.684988749,
0.699697015, 0.706919646, 0.716615237, 0.727993494, 0.738322579,
0.739148218, 0.739186125, 0.742365563, 0.745413160, 0.747257771,
0.750100336, 0.755538156, 0.757015456, 0.757025317, 0.759269100,
0.779462443, 0.780866463, 0.781078923, 0.782396013, 0.783245994,
0.784139053, 0.786832943, 0.796762091, 0.801637811, 0.808890634,
0.822337339, 0.823737507, 0.831439372, 0.848291475, 0.874408497,
0.874706832, 0.883884702, 0.888856504, 0.913807917, 0.916263616,
0.916435269, 0.935536873, 0.937345495, 0.937769405, 0.950301845,
0.959554330, 0.966411747, 0.982074249, 0.990829274

When the intensity function is $\lambda(t) = 200t$, there are 375 arrivals

1.013929345, 1.017299016, 1.020494032, 1.023492119, 1.029293662,
1.032535843, 1.034444443, 1.037337014, 1.044150100, 1.047903597,
1.048080343, 1.048804146, 1.055148176, 1.058901393, 1.062717973,
1.064533587, 1.069731262, 1.073189439, 1.081210021, 1.084091396,
1.099257308, 1.102238394, 1.111405018, 1.113974762, 1.115141771,
1.119604075, 1.122310411, 1.128649801, 1.129954257, 1.131515992,
1.134076646, 1.139261891, 1.140393564, 1.140692617, 1.145096267,
1.150237783, 1.163802895, 1.164433796, 1.165833532, 1.165907854,
1.176382628, 1.181937235, 1.182783321, 1.184585128, 1.196833924,
1.215449107, 1.227184298, 1.229106881, 1.242416283, 1.252645860,
1.252659581, 1.256543911, 1.258500341, 1.263674010, 1.269127304,
1.283127524, 1.286516622, 1.289281019, 1.290950422, 1.298855664,
1.300081327, 1.311437985, 1.329287803, 1.333032885, 1.337514530,
1.339356022, 1.340879801, 1.340931009, 1.341674382, 1.352022462,
1.357608653, 1.370389704, 1.373695941, 1.377188421, 1.403674372,
1.412190809, 1.416503148, 1.416678626, 1.418442181, 1.422087779,
1.424918116, 1.429967697, 1.444163951, 1.447379901, 1.452092366,

1.455721355, 1.458417613, 1.481371435, 1.485535010, 1.500044102,
1.500944988, 1.508367766, 1.516415729, 1.517187150, 1.521979619,
1.547682925, 1.566067752, 1.572167292, 1.577183020, 1.582464693,
1.590667617, 1.591216097, 1.593355230, 1.603135045, 1.615538036,
1.618061811, 1.626994546, 1.628422921, 1.630330539, 1.632926330,
1.635977235, 1.637666293, 1.645006708, 1.647880308, 1.648163049,
1.648172640, 1.652674647, 1.653589362, 1.656538000, 1.657236307,
1.661943821, 1.669053135, 1.699143140, 1.708281809, 1.709955084,
1.713104594, 1.714725234, 1.719333043, 1.724069923, 1.731021449,
1.735625281, 1.744656268, 1.746371425, 1.752927465, 1.753558599,
1.758681826, 1.759282306, 1.762545862, 1.767443548, 1.769469178,
1.773373658, 1.774687876, 1.778749374, 1.788461942, 1.790885404,
1.792485123, 1.795371861, 1.818204767, 1.827249561, 1.827614513,
1.834176804, 1.837328507, 1.839253480, 1.844222442, 1.847155063,
1.849525522, 1.850213237, 1.872098574, 1.873283888, 1.878129812,
1.889259991, 1.891425377, 1.892338493, 1.894636884, 1.894837229,
1.897565121, 1.907123635, 1.908636525, 1.910457973, 1.923362812,
1.924344287, 1.930150185, 1.949453704, 1.949761146, 1.953641534,
1.963653137, 1.963705628, 1.965964503, 1.977688008, 1.980482935,
1.985755443, 1.993329713, 1.999674787, 2.004291961, 2.007671704,
2.012298288, 2.017793437, 2.017909379, 2.028398239, 2.031657952,
2.033711193, 2.033917471, 2.047056607, 2.050281285, 2.052463886,
2.053530491, 2.054419905, 2.054703643, 2.059919972, 2.063083232,
2.063497233, 2.069296796, 2.070229900, 2.074059980, 2.078603481,
2.079287798, 2.083572979, 2.084623537, 2.093311061, 2.095123729,
2.101438373, 2.101883553, 2.109193094, 2.119495949, 2.130416757,
2.136031440, 2.136091095, 2.139714617, 2.140818849, 2.140982116,
2.143215024, 2.143642017, 2.147456241, 2.151059430, 2.159486218,
2.165581206, 2.171049164, 2.173861756, 2.174151290, 2.176017579,
2.180252875, 2.181935899, 2.184849538, 2.200547223, 2.208170009,
2.212822450, 2.213719575, 2.220661806, 2.239305554, 2.241199394,
2.243685161, 2.251112889, 2.254011817, 2.258543056, 2.275763491,
2.279060312, 2.285134647, 2.288586070, 2.289982291, 2.294147501,
2.296366955, 2.298688979, 2.301678425, 2.307905431, 2.321390142,
2.321833524, 2.323235367, 2.325190695, 2.336485252, 2.345230376,
2.363177724, 2.364178989, 2.365743879, 2.372871519, 2.373774794,
2.375236578, 2.375773515, 2.376371675, 2.391577682, 2.400035776,
2.411478949, 2.424025024, 2.427385656, 2.432976392, 2.434047745,
2.442873146, 2.446176723, 2.472320898, 2.483721139, 2.486104882,

2.490810028, 2.495618162, 2.510926709, 2.511234161, 2.513839507,
2.519147823, 2.520375510, 2.526825013, 2.527719625, 2.527960403,
2.528866718, 2.530859574, 2.531298494, 2.535594637, 2.542282276,
2.547550235, 2.551692040, 2.555513599, 2.568842423, 2.570009794,
2.573882751, 2.578535879, 2.583370734, 2.591475289, 2.592686206,
2.599859480, 2.611279551, 2.619419517, 2.620431709, 2.623434798,
2.623813957, 2.627428332, 2.629607411, 2.641245481, 2.654289036,
2.655992781, 2.669850807, 2.676764303, 2.678075310, 2.688720737,
2.698684317, 2.703161751, 2.717440890, 2.719578907, 2.724078030,
2.728939681, 2.735276548, 2.735783146, 2.745158123, 2.745165184,
2.746823335, 2.760853430, 2.761141808, 2.761796885, 2.769162985,
2.769795155, 2.777490208, 2.783952558, 2.786193984, 2.792533542,
2.793089024, 2.798631219, 2.800673852, 2.802583046, 2.805103524,
2.821825363, 2.832271894, 2.836535176, 2.837648671, 2.846627899,
2.850492782, 2.855327041, 2.878247633, 2.882553231, 2.883212790,
2.889528822, 2.892304451, 2.911982264, 2.913785207, 2.923520705,
2.926015311, 2.939286368, 2.943335389, 2.945615221, 2.946840695,
2.956556404, 2.958435072, 2.970019833, 2.970869889, 2.978547289,
2.979987915, 2.987539444, 2.989231064, 2.995278765, 2.996926318

When the intensity function is $m(t) = 500t - 50t^2$ there are 292 events,

3.0394055042, 3.0395649960, 3.0497750333, 3.0515539590,
3.0534064593, 3.0550988168, 3.0603179419, 3.0611753678,
3.0638260543, 3.0684684142, 3.0690515153, 3.0701252520,
3.0710977903, 3.0761675294, 3.0789520564, 3.0870140810,
3.0901728366, 3.0940281730, 3.1025335584, 3.1041963296,
3.1046456881, 3.106,436313, 3.1156511167, 3.1157595599,
3.1171774771, 3.1178429807, 3.1203698972, 3.1262418255,
3.1303598192, 3.1336451545, 3.1356885713, 3.1359373592,
3.1372633446, 3.1387056960, 3.1472093416, 3.1476380508,
3.1481734151, 3.1515996931, 3.1557536889, 3.1578143174,
3.1655712742, 3.1660238905, 3.1675412720, 3.1700455686,
3.1709044836, 3.1710038716, 3.1710768277, 3.1807788387,
3.1844945773, 3.1865160577, 3.1982697193, 3.1989803519,
3.2010379033, 3.2034131940, 3.2041366743, 3.2121709464,
3.2217008546, 3.2264809981, 3.2292034011, 3.2307586530,
3.2316791369, 3.2357311882, 3.2366268234, 3.2477117376,
3.2505444707, 3.2612449862, 3.2624498317, 3.2690377990,

```
3.2699324042,  3.2726698127,  3.2808823753,  3.2881072043,
3.2917402433,  3.2969507733,  3.3015268594,  3.3015537094,
3.3063119072,  3.3096362194,  3.3164327303,  3.3168281792,
3.3212339133,  3.3241597982,  3.3273486616,  3.3274049992,
3.3323849887,  3.3333767094,  3.3339362908,  3.3363375543,
3.3369981498,  3.3470437285,  3.3504107334,  3.3604161320,
3.3611478573,  3.3624880472,  3.3654973106,  3.3666472705,
3.3799138367,  3.3843323132,  3.3963465840,  3.3980996637,
3.4005952124,  3.4013850382,  3.4036674043,  3.4044647310,
3.4091130989,  3.4127464471,  3.4152737586,  3.4190298095,
3.4272268470,  3.4378765291,  3.4381807251,  3.4381879056,
3.4405560624,  3.4420253634,  3.4503981983,  3.4537759321,
3.4647708368,  3.4727968536,  3.4743528450,  3.4746357612,
3.4767445046,  3.4786015302,  3.4810818359,  3.4830563124,
3.4834156064,  3.4838489853,  3.4844182320,  3.4893770060,
3.4913737085,  3.4926125128,  3.4944544798,  3.4947529892,
3.4955945443,  3.4957072623,  3.5017801821,  3.5019984478,
3.5088554090,  3.5098619508,  3.5190729275,  3.5214515720,
3.5337872561,  3.5338723445,  3.5349942641,  3.5373605257,
3.5374128018,  3.5415375559,  3.5452064471,  3.5490878643,
3.5529638240,  3.5564432358,  3.5567915970,  3.5569886006,
3.5691233557,  3.5804139767,  3.5806436213,  3.5812419420,
3.5821914040,  3.5834934516,  3.5839783000,  3.5847572675,
3.5939939115,  3.5965053625,  3.5973652303,  3.5987382149,
3.5989597440,  3.6125720618,  3.6135758925,  3.6139502143,
3.6165282140,  3.6193393739,  3.6278351685,  3.6300896127,
3.6335888784,  3.6348160263,  3.6383879464,  3.6394935939,
3.6402793005,  3.6429974539,  3.6486793263,  3.6525471816,
3.6569040315,  3.6666116016,  3.6678881897,  3.6687063370,
3.6730838716,  3.6790721621,  3.6885159444,  3.6895445548,
3.6923138006,  3.6925381618,  3.6974107707,  3.7003768077,
3.7019655583,  3.7107408307,  3.7119259490,  3.7147472426,
3.7158508776,  3.7180384109,  3.7188526653,  3.7221041368,
3.7243337510,  3.7297047498,  3.7357104449,  3.7379124304,
3.7393667521,  3.7396834819,  3.7536196075,  3.7553359307,
3.7658056961,  3.7690140931,  3.7693173233,  3.7724120421,
3.7737177517,  3.7764852755,  3.7872026497,  3.7891286425,
3.7931585815,  3.7973917332,  3.7999806516,  3.8075277386,
3.8079434456,  3.8130274843,  3.8147484818,  3.8303364394,
```

```
3.8325500693, 3.8331372524, 3.8335735751, 3.8363890983,
3.8367080148, 3.8419249961, 3.8456002781, 3.8456870727,
3.8456912525, 3.8466627011, 3.8488095850, 3.8496039398,
3.8507244056, 3.8529330473, 3.8531479556, 3.8593404116,
3.8616266381, 3.8682547659, 3.8685721802, 3.8690067939,
3.8702020561, 3.8746858975, 3.8793189283, 3.8806014806,
3.8872348368, 3.8886372708, 3.8891721042, 3.8899864918,
3.8920450564, 3.8939412264, 3.8948968519, 3.8973098779,
3.8977870010, 3.9011845272, 3.9041249128, 3.9141902262,
3.9167675348, 3.9190505901, 3.9190733116, 3.9214201123,
3.9217549330, 3.9334586877, 3.9381146226, 3.9382127598,
3.9390543317, 3.9406094989, 3.9510613997, 3.9525732268,
3.9560717000, 3.9623804362, 3.9641936077, 3.9660449354,
3.9664281784, 3.9665969238, 3.9751119539, 3.9754377482,
3.9763981393, 3.9774438757, 3.9774594707, 3.9805419631,
3.9838282093, 3.9859077316, 3.9871207457, 3.9879421517,
3.9906606367, 3.9927617311, 3.9960442316, 3.9980143020
```

BC 6.4

```
model;
{

for( i in 1:129){

n1[i]~dexp(delta1[i])
lamda1[i]<-beta11*i+beta12*i*i
delta1[i]<-1/lamda1[i]}
beta11~dnorm(100,1)
beta12~dnorm(50,1)

for ( i in 1:375){
n2[i]~dexp(delta2[i])
lamda2[i]<-beta2*i
delta2[i]<-1/lamda2[i]}
beta2~dnorm(200,1)

for( i in 1:292){
n3[i]~dexp(delta3[i])
lamda3[i]<-abs(beta31*i-beta32*i*i)
delta3[i]<-1/lamda3[i]}
beta31~dnorm(500,1)
```

```
beta32~dnorm(-50,1)
E<-beta11/2+3*beta12/8+1.5*beta2
}

list(n1=c(0.002514378, 0.019175922, 0.021953457, 0.024550520,
0.031322105, 0.035207160, 0.042003951, 0.066021339,
0.069204332, 0.070603115, 0.074403316, 0.078209166,
0.081210360, 0.089738117, 0.108841185, 0.113504869,
0.118042807, 0.120448525, 0.127535137, 0.148708492,
0.155505013, 0.160686959, 0.165564084, 0.171232042,
0.185665243, 0.194464218, 0.202340639, 0.212150896,
0.216791938, 0.229751281,
0.233844860, 0.237426403, 0.240561157, 0.257191631,
0.259427338, 0.261023988, 0.261239244, 0.264757474,
0.264951792, 0.265082411, 0.276758405, 0.280244587,
0.311615852, 0.324892686, 0.341942644, 0.347802898,
0.350671225, 0.359282152, 0.372455910, 0.375604996,
0.391797577, 0.395026651, 0.398594826, 0.406915699,
0.417825938, 0.421420146, 0.435862032, 0.436892793,
0.445679733, 0.469381181,
0.478037560, 0.479947491, 0.485462589, 0.494364918,
0.495973951, 0.510708708, 0.516524876, 0.522994348,
0.555194473, 0.565705654, 0.590331443, 0.595593126,
0.606269287, 0.625587527, 0.629214609, 0.633505706,
0.639148909, 0.639599133, 0.646117045, 0.656630432,
0.660690608, 0.676695661, 0.679830155, 0.684899308,
0.684988749, 0.699697015, 0.706919646, 0.716615237,
0.727993494, 0.738322579,
0.739148218, 0.739186125, 0.742365563, 0.745413160,
0.747257771, 0.750100336, 0.755538156, 0.757015456,
0.757025317, 0.759269100, 0.779462443, 0.780866463,
0.781078923, 0.782396013, 0.783245994, 0.784139053,
0.786832943, 0.796762091, 0.801637811, 0.808890634,
0.822337339, 0.823737507, 0.831439372, 0.848291475,
0.874408497, 0.874706832, 0.883884702, 0.888856504,
0.913807917, 0.916263616,
0.916435269, 0.935536873, 0.937345495, 0.937769405,
0.950301845, 0.959554330, 0.966411747, 0.982074249,
0.990829274),
```

```
n2=c(1.013929345, 1.017299016, 1.020494032, 1.023492119,
1.029293662, 1.032535843, 1.034444443, 1.037337014,
1.044150100, 1.047903597, 1.048080343, 1.048804146,
1.055148176, 1.058901393, 1.062717973, 1.064533587,
1.069731262, 1.073189439, 1.081210021, 1.084091396,
1.099257308, 1.102238394, 1.111405018, 1.113974762,
1.115141771,
1.119604075, 1.122310411, 1.128649801, 1.129954257,
1.131515992, 1.134076646, 1.139261891, 1.140393564,
1.140692617, 1.145096267, 1.150237783, 1.163802895,
1.164433796, 1.165833532, 1.165907854, 1.176382628,
1.181937235, 1.182783321, 1.184585128, 1.196833924,
1.215449107, 1.227184298, 1.229106881, 1.242416283,
1.252645860, 1.252659581, 1.256543911, 1.258500341,
1.263674010, 1.269127304,
1.283127524, 1.286516622, 1.289281019, 1.290950422,
1.298855664, 1.300081327, 1.311437985, 1.329287803,
1.333032885, 1.337514530, 1.339356022, 1.340879801,
1.340931009, 1.341674382, 1.352022462, 1.357608653,
1.370389704, 1.373695941, 1.377188421, 1.403674372,
1.412190809, 1.416503148, 1.416678626, 1.418442181,
1.422087779, 1.424918116, 1.429967697, 1.444163951,
1.447379901, 1.452092366,
1.455721355, 1.458417613, 1.481371435, 1.485535010,
1.500044102, 1.500944988, 1.508367766, 1.516415729,
1.517187150, 1.521979619, 1.547682925, 1.566067752,
1.572167292, 1.577183020, 1.582464693, 1.590667617,
1.591216097, 1.593355230, 1.603135045, 1.615538036,
1.618061811, 1.626994546, 1.628422921, 1.630330539,
1.632926330, 1.635977235, 1.637666293, 1.645006708,
1.647880308, 1.648163049,
1.648172640, 1.652674647, 1.653589362, 1.656538000,
1.657236307, 1.661943821, 1.669053135, 1.699143140,
1.708281809, 1.709955084, 1.713104594, 1.714725234,
1.719333043, 1.724069923, 1.731021449, 1.735625281,
1.744656268, 1.746371425, 1.752927465, 1.753558599,
1.758681826, 1.759282306, 1.762545862, 1.767443548,
1.769469178, 1.773373658, 1.774687876, 1.778749374,
1.788461942, 1.790885404,
```

```
1.792485123,  1.795371861,  1.818204767,  1.827249561,
1.827614513,  1.834176804,  1.837328507,  1.839253480,
1.844222442,  1.847155063,  1.849525522,  1.850213237,
1.872098574,  1.873283888,  1.878129812,  1.889259991,
1.891425377,  1.892338493,  1.894636884,  1.894837229,
1.897565121,  1.907123635,  1.908636525,  1.910457973,
1.923362812,  1.924344287,  1.930150185,  1.949453704,
1.949761146,  1.953641534,
1.963653137,  1.963705628,  1.965964503,  1.977688008,
1.980482935,  1.985755443,  1.993329713,  1.999674787,
2.004291961,  2.007671704,  2.012298288,  2.017793437,
2.017909379,  2.028398239,  2.031657952,  2.033711193,
2.033917471,  2.047056607,  2.050281285,  2.052463886,
2.053530491,  2.054419905,  2.054703643,  2.059919972,
2.063083232,  2.063497233,  2.069296796,  2.070229900,
2.074059980,  2.078603481,
2.079287798,  2.083572979,  2.084623537,  2.093311061,
2.095123729,  2.101438373,  2.101883553,  2.109193094,
2.119495949,  2.130416757,  2.136031440,  2.136091095,
2.139714617,  2.140818849,  2.140982116,  2.143215024,
2.143642017,  2.147456241,  2.151059430,  2.159486218,
2.165581206,  2.171049164,  2.173861756,  2.174151290,
2.176017579,  2.180252875,  2.181935899,  2.184849538,
2.200547223,  2.208170009,
2.212822450,  2.213719575,  2.220661806,  2.239305554,
2.241199394,  2.243685161,  2.251112889,  2.254011817,
2.258543056,  2.275763491,  2.279060312,  2.285134647,
2.288586070,  2.289982291,  2.294147501,  2.296366955,
2.298688979,  2.301678425,  2.307905431,  2.321390142,
2.321833524,  2.323235367,  2.325190695,  2.336485252,
2.345230376,  2.363177724,  2.364178989,  2.365743879,
2.372871519,  2.373774794,
2.375236578,  2.375773515,  2.376371675,  2.391577682,
2.400035776,  2.411478949,  2.424025024,  2.427385656,
2.432976392,  2.434047745,  2.442873146,  2.446176723,
2.472320898,  2.483721139,  2.486104882,  2.490810028,
2.495618162,  2.510926709,  2.511234161,  2.513839507,
2.519147823,  2.520375510,  2.526825013,  2.527719625,
2.527960403,  2.528866718,  2.530859574,  2.531298494,
```

2.535594637, 2.542282276,
2.547550235, 2.551692040, 2.555513599, 2.568842423,
2.570009794, 2.573882751, 2.578535879, 2.583370734,
2.591475289, 2.592686206, 2.599859480, 2.611279551,
2.619419517, 2.620431709, 2.623434798, 2.623813957,
2.627428332, 2.629607411, 2.641245481, 2.654289036,
2.655992781, 2.669850807, 2.676764303, 2.678075310,
2.688720737, 2.698684317, 2.703161751, 2.717440890,
2.719578907, 2.724078030,
2.728939681, 2.735276548, 2.735783146, 2.745158123,
2.745165184, 2.746823335, 2.760853430, 2.761141808,
2.761796885, 2.769162985, 2.769795155, 2.777490208,
2.783952558, 2.786193984, 2.792533542, 2.793089024,
2.798631219, 2.800673852, 2.802583046, 2.805103524,
2.821825363, 2.832271894, 2.836535176, 2.837648671,
2.846627899, 2.850492782, 2.855327041, 2.878247633,
2.882553231, 2.883212790,
2.889528822, 2.892304451, 2.911982264, 2.913785207,
2.923520705, 2.926015311, 2.939286368, 2.943335389,
2.945615221, 2.946840695, 2.956556404, 2.958435072,
2.970019833, 2.970869889, 2.978547289, 2.979987915,
2.987539444, 2.989231064, 2.995278765, 2.996926318),

n3=c(3.0394055042, 3.0395649960, 3.0497750333, 3.0515539590,
3.0534064593, 3.0550988168, 3.0603179419, 3.0611753678,
3.0638260543, 3.0684684142, 3.0690515153, 3.0701252520,
3.0710977903, 3.0761675294, 3.0789520564, 3.0870140810,
3.0901728366, 3.0940281730, 3.1025335584, 3.1041963296,
3.1046456881, 3.106,436313, 3.1156511167, 3.1157595599,
3.1171774771, 3.1178429807, 3.1203698972, 3.1262418255,
3.1303598192, 3.1336451545, 3.1356885713, 3.1359373592,
3.1372633446, 3.1387056960, 3.1472093416, 3.1476380508,
3.1481734151, 3.1515996931, 3.1557536889, 3.1578143174,
3.1655712742, 3.1660238905, 3.1675412720, 3.1700455686,
3.1709044836, 3.1710038716, 3.1710768277, 3.1807788387,
3.1844945773, 3.1865160577, 3.1982697193, 3.1989803519,
3.2010379033, 3.2034131940, 3.2041366743, 3.2121709464,
3.2217008546, 3.2264809981, 3.2292034011, 3.2307586530,
 3.2316791369, 3.2357311882, 3.2366268234, 3.2477117376,

```
3.2505444707,  3.2612449862,  3.2624498317,  3.2690377990,
3.2699324042,  3.2726698127,  3.2808823753,  3.2881072043,
3.2917402433,  3.2969507733,  3.3015268594,  3.3015537094,
3.3063119072,  3.3096362194,  3.3164327303,  3.3168281792,
3.3212339133,  3.3241597982,  3.3273486616,  3.3274049992,
3.3323849887,  3.3333767094,  3.3339362908,  3.3363375543,
3.3369981498,  3.3470437285,  3.3504107334,  3.3604161320,
3.3611478573,  3.3624880472,  3.3654973106,  3.3666472705,
3.3799138367,  3.3843323132,  3.3963465840,  3.3980996637,
3.4005952124,  3.4013850382,  3.4036674043,  3.4044647310,
3.4091130989,  3.4127464471,  3.4152737586,  3.4190298095,
3.4272268470,  3.4378765291,  3.4381807251,  3.4381879056,
3.4405560624,  3.4420253634,  3.4503981983,  3.4537759321,
3.4647708368,  3.4727968536,  3.4743528450,  3.4746357612,
3.4767445046,  3.4786015302,  3.4810818359,  3.4830563124,
3.4834156064,  3.4838489853,  3.4844182320,  3.4893770060,
3.4913737085,  3.4926125128,  3.4944544798,  3.4947529892,
3.4955945443,  3.4957072623,  3.5017801821,  3.5019984478,
3.5088554090,  3.5098619508,  3.5190729275,  3.5214515720,
3.5337872561,  3.5338723445,  3.5349942641,  3.5373605257,
3.5374128018,  3.5415375559,  3.5452064471,  3.5490878643,
3.5529638240,  3.5564432358,  3.5567915970,  3.5569886006,
3.5691233557,  3.5804139767,  3.5806436213,  3.5812419420,
3.5821914040,  3.5834934516,  3.5839783000,  3.5847572675,
3.5939939115,  3.5965053625,  3.5973652303,  3.5987382149,
3.5989597440,  3.6125720618,  3.6135758925,  3.6139502143,
3.6165282140,  3.6193393739,  3.6278351685,  3.6300896127,
3.6335888784,  3.6348160263,  3.6383879464,  3.6394935939,
3.6402793005,  3.6429974539,  3.6486793263,  3.6525471816,
3.6569040315,  3.6666116016,  3.6678881897,  3.6687063370,
3.6730838716,  3.6790721621,  3.6885159444,  3.6895445548,
3.6923138006,  3.6925381618,  3.6974107707,  3.7003768077,
3.7019655583,  3.7107408307,  3.7119259490,  3.7147472426,
3.7158508776,  3.7180384109,  3.7188526653,  3.7221041368,
3.7243337510,  3.7297047498,  3.7357104449,  3.7379124304,
3.7393667521,  3.7396834819,  3.7536196075,  3.7553359307,
3.7658056961,  3.7690140931,  3.7693173233,  3.7724120421,
3.7737177517,  3.7764852755,  3.7872026497,  3.7891286425,
3.7931585815,  3.7973917332,  3.7999806516,  3.8075277386,
3.8079434456,  3.8130274843,  3.8147484818,  3.8303364394,
```

```
3.8325500693, 3.8331372524, 3.8335735751, 3.8363890983,
3.8367080148, 3.8419249961, 3.8456002781, 3.8456870727,
3.8456912525, 3.8466627011, 3.8488095850, 3.8496039398,
3.8507244056, 3.8529330473, 3.8531479556, 3.8593404116,
3.8616266381, 3.8682547659, 3.8685721802, 3.8690067939,
3.8702020561, 3.8746858975, 3.8793189283, 3.8806014806,
3.8872348368, 3.8886372708, 3.8891721042, 3.8899864918,
3.8920450564, 3.8939412264, 3.8948968519, 3.8973098779,
3.8977870010, 3.9011845272, 3.9041249128, 3.9141902262,
3.9167675348, 3.9190505901, 3.9190733116, 3.9214201123,
3.9217549330, 3.9334586877, 3.9381146226, 3.9382127598,
3.9390543317, 3.9406094989, 3.9510613997, 3.9525732268,
3.9560717000, 3.9623804362, 3.9641936077, 3.9660449354,
3.9664281784, 3.9665969238, 3.9751119539, 3.9754377482,
3.9763981393, 3.9774438757, 3.9774594707, 3.9805419631,
3.9838282093, 3.9859077316, 3.9871207457, 3.9879421517,
3.9906606367, 3.9927617311, 3.9960442316, 3.9980143020))
list(beta11=100,beta12=50, beta2=200,beta31=500,beta32=-
```

Recall that the value of β_{11} used to generate the arrival times for the first stage is 100 and that for β_{12} is 50, and that the corresponding posterior means are very close to these values. It can also be confirmed that this is also true for the remaining beta parameters. Also recall the expectation

$$E\left[N(2.5) - N(0.5)\right] = \int_{.5}^{1} (100 + 100t)\, dt + \int_{1}^{2.5} 200t\, dt = 387.5$$

However, the posterior mean given by Table 6.7 is 364.9. Why the discrepancy?

TABLE 6.7

Posterior Distribution for Regression Parameters of the Nonhomogeneous Process

Parameter	Mean	SD	Error	2 1/2	Median	97 1/2
β_{11}	99.91	.9997	.01157	97.96	99.9	101.9
β_{12}	47.44	1.031	.01306	45.42	47.44	49.46
β_2	198.1	1.007	.01247	196.1	198.1	200.1
β_{31}	499.9	1.01	.01089	498	499.0	501.9
β_{32}	−44.44	1.064	.01737	−46.54	−44.46	−42.35
E	364.9	1.631	.01614	361.7	364.9	368.2

6.8 General Continuous Time Markov Chains

In this section, Bayesian inferential procedures are presented for continuous time Markov chains more general than the Poisson process. The interarrival times are still an exponential distribution, but the parameter of the exponential distribution depends on state the process currently occupies. Of special interest are homogeneous processes with a finite state space where the system remains for a time with an exponential distribution at each state and upon departing, the state of the system changes with regard to the probabilities that depend solely on the leaving state. The process is completely specified by the initial state, the transition probabilities from the current state to the future state and the parameter of the exponential distribution of the current time the process is in the current state. All phases of inference will be explored which includes estimation, testing hypotheses, and forecasting of future observations (states or inter-arrival times).

Let $\{X(t), t > 0\}$ be a continuous time stochastic process with state space $S = \{1, 2, \ldots, k\}$ such that when the process enters state i, it remains in state i according to the exponential distribution with parameter ν_i (with mean $1/\nu_i$). At the end of this period (being in state i), the process transitions to another state, say $j \neq i$ with transition probability p_{ij} where $\sum_{j=1}^{j=k} p_{ij} = 1$. It should be emphasized that for some j, it is possible that p_{ij} is zero. If one ignores, the time the process occupies the states, the transition probability matrix of the various states is $P = (p_{ij})$ corresponds to what is referred to as the embedded chain. The birth and death process discussed below is an example of a continuous time Markov chain.

In such a process the state space is $S = \{0, 1, \ldots, k\}$ and represents the size of the population. Suppose the process is in state i, then the population can increase by a single birth with rate λ_i and decrease by one unit with a single death occurring at rate μ_i, and the transition matrix is defined as follows.

$$p_{i,i+1} = \lambda_i / (\lambda_i + \mu_i), \quad \text{and} \quad p_{i,i-1} = \mu_i / (\lambda_i + \mu_i). \tag{6.41}$$

Also note that if the population is 0, the size of the population remains zero, and if the population is size k it can only decrease by one death and of course cannot increase by one birth.

Furthermore, in general for a continuous time chains with state space $S = \{1, 2, \ldots, k\}$, when the process is in state i, it remains in state i according to an exponential distribution with parameter $\nu_i > 0$. The jumping intensity from state i to state j is defined by

$$r_{ij} = \nu_i p_{ij}. \tag{6.42}$$

Note that $-v_i = \sum_{j \neq i} r_{ij}$ and the k-th order matrix $R = (r_{ij})$ is called the infinitesimal generator of the process and will be used when computing the equilibrium distribution of the process.

To understand the future behavior of a continuous time chain, the Kolmogorov system of differential equations involving the transition probability function

$$P_{ij}(t) = P\left[X(t+s) = j | X(s) = i\right] = P\left[X(t) = j | X(0) = i\right] \qquad (6.43)$$

is described. Note this follows because the process is homogeneous, that is only the length of the interval is important in determining the transition from i to j.

The formulation of the Kolmogorov equations is explained in Insua, Ruggeri, and Wiper [6] and is closely followed here. Let

$$P_{ij}'(t) = \sum_{k \neq j} r_{kj} P_{ik}(t) - v_j P_{ij}(t) = \sum_k r_{kj} P_{ik}(t) \qquad (6.44)$$

where

$$P'(t) = \left((d/dt)P_{ij}(t)\right).$$

Or in matrix form as

$$P'(t) = RP(t) \qquad (6.45)$$

with

$$I = P(0)$$

where I is the identity matrix and $P(t)$ the matrix of transition probability functions. It is easy to show that the solution to the Kolmogorov system of Equations (6.83) is the exponential form

$$P(t) = \exp(Rt) \qquad (6.46)$$

which according to Moler and Van Loan [8] can be solved for given t using matrix exponentiation.

We now come to the central focus of this section, namely Bayesian inference of continuous time Markov chains. To this end it is assumed that the transition matrix P and the vector v of transition rates are unknown and that P is not a function of v. Assume that the initial state is $x(0)$, which is followed by n transitions times t_i and corresponding observations $x(i)$, $i = 1, 2, \ldots, n$, then the likelihood function is

$$l(P, \mid v, \mid data) = \prod_{i=1}^{i=n} v_{i-1} \exp\left(v_{i-1}\left(t_i - t_{i-1}\right)\right) p_{x(i-1),x(i)}$$

$$= \prod_{i=1}^{i=n} v_i^{n_i} \exp(-v_i t_i) \prod_{i=1}^{i=n} p_{ij}^{n_{ij}} \tag{6.47}$$

where n_{ij} is the number of transitions form state i to j, t_i the time occupying state i (with an exponential distribution with parameter v_i), p_{ij} the probability

of the transition from state i to state j, and $n_{i.} = \sum_{j=1}^{j=k} n_{ij}$ the number of transitions

out of state i. Referring to the likelihood function (6.85), it is understood that state j is $x(j)$, $j = 1, 2, ..., k$. It is obvious from (6.85) that the likelihood function can be written as

$$l(P, \mid v, \mid data) = l_1(v \mid data) l_2(P \mid data). \tag{6.48}$$

Therefore, inferences can be made separately for P and v by first generating transitions n_{ij} from i to j, then generating exponential holding times after the transition to state i. Recall Chapter 4 where RC 4.1 is used to generate transitions according to the transition probability matrix P and to RC 6.10 of this chapter to generate exponential inter-arrival times. Thus starting in state i, one can generate transitions to state j for some of the $j = 1,2,..,k$. If one knows the transition probabilities p_{ij}, $j = 1, 2, ..., k$, one could employ the multinomial distribution to generate the transitions, as was done in Section 4.3 of Chapter 4.

Suppose prior information for the v_i, $i = 1, 2, .., k$ is Gamma (a_i, b_i), then the posterior distribution of v_i is gamma $(n_i + a_i, t_i + b_i)$ with posterior mean $(n_i + a_i)/(t_i + b_i)$. Recall that the posterior mean of the transition time T_i

$$E\left(v_i^{-1} \mid data\right) = \left(t_i + b_i\right)/\left(n_i + a_i - 1\right).$$

Now for the prior distribution of the transition probabilities p_{ij}, because of practical reasons, it is important to remember that some of the p_{ij} are zero, nevertheless that one may employ a Dirichlet distribution for the entries of the row of P; thus, the posterior analysis is demonstrated with an example. Suppose that the probability transition matrix of the embedded chain is

$$P = \begin{pmatrix} p_{11}, 0, p_{13}, p_{14}, 0 \\ 0, p_{22}, 0, p_{24}, 0 \\ 0, 0, p_{33}, p_{34}, p_{35} \\ p_{41}, p_{42}, 0, p_{44}, p_{45} \\ 0, p_{52}, p_{53}, 0, p_{55} \end{pmatrix} \tag{6.49}$$

with permanence rates ν_i, $i = 1, 2, \ldots, 5$, the goal is to provide Bayesian inference for the unknown parameters ν_i, and the non-zero p_{ij} of (6.49). Inferences will be based on the transition counts given by the matrix

$$c = \begin{pmatrix} n_{11}, 0, n_{13}, n_{14}, 0 \\ 0, n_{22}, 0, n_{24}, 0 \\ 0, 0, n_{33}, n_{34}, n_{35} \\ n_{41}, n_{42}, 0, n_{44}, n_{45} \\ 0, n_{52}, n_{53}, 0, n_{55} \end{pmatrix} \tag{6.50}$$

and the observed times t_i occupied in the states i, $i = 1,2,3,4,5$.

Suppose the occupation time distributions T_i are exponential with means 2,7,1,4, and 5 corresponding to exponential parameter values $\nu_1 = 1/2$, $\nu_2 = 1/7$, $\nu_3 = 1$, $\nu_4 = 1/4$, and $\nu_5 = 1/5$. I used the r code rexp(samples, ν_i) with samples =1 to generate the occupation times for the various states and computed $t_1 = 1.3257$, $t_2 = 10.2288$, $t_3 = .11038$, $t_4 = 3.2565$, and $t_5 = 5.65137$. Using the multinomial generator in R, the following transition counts represented by the matrix

$$C = \begin{pmatrix} 1, 0, 17, 2, 0 \\ 0, 10, 0, 20, 0 \\ 0, 0, 7, 4, 4 \\ 10, 7, 0, 7, 6 \\ 0, 6, 8, 0, 16 \end{pmatrix}. \tag{6.51}$$

are computed.

Thus the number of transitions out of the various states are $n_1 = 19$, $n_2 = 20$, $n_3 = 8$, $n_4 = 23$, and $n_5 = 14$. This completes the sample information, therefore, in order to execute the posterior analysis, the prior distributions need to be assigned to the unknown parameters P and ν.

The rows of P are assigned prior Dirichlet distributions as follows (Table 6.8):

TABLE 6.8

Prior Dirichlet Distribution for Rows of P

Row	Parameters
1	(1,0,1,1,0)
2	(0,1,0,1,0)
3	(0,0,1,1,1)
4	(1,1,0,1,1)
5	(0,1,1,0,1)

In addition, the improper prior

$$g(v_i) \propto 1/v_i, i = 1, 2, 3, 4, 5.$$

is assigned to the parameter of the exponential distribution of the occupation times of the various states.

The Bayesian analysis is executed with **BC 6.5** using 45,000 observations for the simulation and 5,000 for the burn in.

BC 6.5

```
Model;

{

nu1~dgamma(19,1.3257)
nu2~dgamma(20,10.2288)
nu3~dgamma(8,.11038)
nu4~dgamma(23,3.2565)
nu5~dgamma(14,5.65132)
p11~dbeta(2,20)
p13~dbeta(17,5)
p14~dbeta(3,19)
p22~dbeta(11,21)
p24~dbeta(21,11)
p33~dbeta(8,10)
p34~dbeta(5,13)
p35~dbeta(5,13)
p41~dbeta(11,23)
p42~dbeta(8,26)
p44~dbeta(8,26)
p45~dbeta(7,25)
p52~dbeta(7,26)
p53~dbeta(9,24)
p55~dbeta(17,16)
mu1<-1/nu1
mu2<-1/nu2
mu3<-1/nu3
mu4<-1/nu4
mu5<-1/nu5
}
```

Table 6.9 reports the Bayesian analysis for the example with five states with five intensity parameters and the probabilities of the transition matrix.

TABLE 6.9

Posterior Distribution for Continuous Markov Chain

Parameter	Mean	SD	Error	2 1/2	Median	97 1/2
μ_1	.07364	.01788	.0000533	.04644	.07099	.1157
μ_2	.538	.1272	.000392	.3442	.519	.838
μ_3	.01573	.006453	.0000213	.007651	.01435	.03184
μ_4	.1481	.03239	.000103	.09786	.1437	.2242
μ_5	.4351	.1255	.000432	.2547	.414	.7382
ν_1	14.34	3.282	.01452	8.67	14.1	21.5
ν_2	1.957	.4385	.001947	1.195	1.927	2.903
ν_3	72.64	25.65	.1173	31.26	69.74	130.5
ν_4	7.058	1.474	.006392	4.468	6.957	10.23
ν_5	2.471	.66087	.00289	1.353	2.409	3.927
p_{11}	-.09073	.06004	.000182	.01151	.07846	.2358
p_{13}	.7732	.08701	.000268	.5831	.7817	.9176
p_{14}	.1362	.07161	.000226	.03036	.1249	.3037
p_{22}	.3435	.08266	.000252	.1927	.3401	.513
p_{24}	.6565	.08262	.000243	.4863	.6597	.8083
p_{33}	.4443	.1141	.000356	.2303	.4424	.6706
p_{34}	.2778	.1025	.000320	.1032	.2696	.498
p_{35}	.2772	.1025	.000325	.1032	.2688	.4976
p_{41}	.3239	.07927	.000251	.1802	.3204	.4883
p_{42}	.2356	.07159	.000231	.111	.2302	.3891
p_{44}	.2351	.07148	.000205	.111	.2299	.398
p_{52}	.2123	.07027	.000215	.093	.2063	.3655
p_{53}	.2727	.07656	.00024	.1372	.268	.4347
p_{55}	.5151	.08579	.000277	.3477	.515	.6817

Most of the posterior distributions are symmetric about the posterior mean, and it appears that the MCMC simulation errors are sufficiently small so that one had confidence in these estimates. The reader should display the posterior densities of the parameters to show that symmetry of the posterior distributions. Chapter 7 will develop in much greater detail the fundamental ideas of continuous time Markov chains which are illustrated with applications in business, biology, and medicine.

6.9 Why Are More Coronavirus Tests Needed Than We Thought Were Needed?

In a misleading statement on April 9 2020, President Donald Trump stated that testing for the presence of the virus would be restricted to individuals who believe they may be infected. However, if testing is limited to those who believe they are infected, one would not be able to understand how deep the disease has infected the population. This would be possible if those who think they are infected did indeed truly representative of the population with respect to the covid-19 infection. Ideally, one would want a random sample of individuals from the appropriate population to infer the fraction of the population that are infected; however, this is very difficult to implement.

The common characteristic of those who believe they are infected is that they show symptoms of infection due to the virus. That is to say, individuals who are undergoing testing are disproportionally showing severe symptoms. This would not be a problem for someone who is infected immediately and shows symptoms, but of course this is unrealistic. There is convincing information that some people develop a mild variant of the disease where the symptoms are not displayed, but do indeed carry the virus without knowing it since they are asymptomatic. Thus, efforts to know the depth of the penetration into the population should include observations of the asymptomatic people.

The estimate of the proportion of the population who are infected can be calculated with the formula

$$P = \left(\# \text{or symptomatic infected} + \# \text{of asymptomatic infected}\right) / \left(\begin{array}{l} \# \text{or symptomatic infected} + \# \text{of asymptomatic infected} \\ + \# \text{not infected} \end{array}\right) \quad (6.52)$$

Thus a random sample of the whole population is required. One must be able to select data from infected people who are showing symptoms, infected people who do not display symptoms, and people who are not infected. As of April 23, leaders in Germany and New York state have begun random testing to measure how widespread is the disease, but there has been resistance from leaders elsewhere. This might be due to ignorance or lack of appreciation of statistical principles – due to a lack of statistical literacy that is all too prevalent in the citizens of most countries. On the other hand, it could be the worry over the limited availability of tests and the aim to devote all these limited tests to those who display symptoms of the novel coronavirus.

Unfortunately, this could inadvertently accelerate the spread of the virus. If a community does not understand the extent of the infection or the contagiousness of the disease, society will not be able to respond in an efficient way in order to slow the progress of the virus. How does one decide what preventive measures are appropriate and necessary? How does one minimize the chance that the disease spreads to a point that the hospitals are overloaded with patients that have the coronavirus? How does one assess progress or if the situation is failing?

Without the evidence that a random sample of the population would provide on is operating in the dark. Operating in this world of ignorance, deaths that could have been prevented will add up and we will continue to take actions that are not effective and cost too much.

Most of the world lacks the ability to test a large number of people and this makes the leaders who appreciate the idea of a random sample hesitant to implement random sampling in the general population. Thus our conclusion is that we need more tests than we think we need.

6.10 Summary

This chapter on continuous time Markov chains begins with three definitions of the Poisson process where the emphasis is on Bayesian inferences for the one parameter λ. R code 6.1 generates arrival times of a Poisson process and these observations are used in the example of Bayesian inferences about λ. All three phases of inferences are displayed including estimation, testing hypotheses, and prediction of future observations. Next to be considered is the concept of the superposition of Poisson processes and the ideas are explained in terms of an example involving major and minor earthquakes in Italy. Included with Bayesian inference is testing the hypothesis, that the rate of occurrence of major earthquakes is the same as that for minor earthquakes.

Next to be presented is a generalization to nonhomogeneous Poisson processes, where the rate of occurrence of events varies over time. An example involving Bayesian estimation of the regression parameters that may affect the rate of occurrence of events is explained in detail. A test of the hypothesis that the regression parameters have no effect is also presented. This chapter is ended with a Bayesian approach to the general continuous time Markov chain, where the parameters of interest are the average occupation of a given state and the transition probabilities of moving from one state to the others.

The reader should be aware of the basic references for continuous time Markov chains, both from a classical and Bayesian perspective. From a non-Bayesian view, see Guttorp [9] and Ross [10], while for a Bayesian flavor refer to Geweke, Marshal, and Zarkin [11], and lastly for those interested in reliability, see Cano, Moguerza, and Rios-Insua [12]. In addition, Insua, Ruggeri, and Wiper [6, pp. 103–108] list more relevant references. As mentioned earlier, this chapter gives the reader the necessary information for the study of epidemics, which will be the main subject of Chapter 7. For additional information about epidemics see Broemeling [14], ch. 7. For information about testing hypotheses from a Bayesian point of view, see Lee [15].

6.11 Exercises

1. Define a Poisson process with parameter λ.

2. Refer to Section 6.2 and show the three definitions (a), (b), and (c) of a Poisson process are equivalent.

3. Show the inter-arrival times of a Poisson process with parameter λ are i.i.d. exponential with mean $1/\lambda$.

4. Use R code 6.1 with t<-40 and lamda<-1/2 to generate the inter-arrival times of a Poisson process with parameter $\lambda = 1/2$. How many inter-arrival times are generated?

5. Show the distribution of the waiting time to the n-th event is gamma with parameters n and $\sum_{i=1}^{i=n} t_i$, where $\sum_{i=1}^{i=n} t_i$ is the waiting time to the n-th event.

6. Assume one has observed n events of a Poisson process with parameter λ and that one employs the improper prior density

$$g(\lambda) \propto 1/\lambda, \lambda > 0$$

   for λ. What is the posterior distribution of λ?

7. Execute BC 6.1 with 45,000 observations for the simulation and a burn in of 5,000 and verify the posterior analysis reported in Table 6.1. What is the 95% credible interval for M? Is the posterior distribution of M symmetric about its mean?

8. Derive the predictive distribution of the waiting time S_{15} given by Equation (6.21).

9. Refer to Section 6.4 and explain the idea behind thinning Poisson processes.

10. Using R code 6.2:

    a. Generate the birth times that follow a Poisson process with $\lambda = 2$ over an 8-hour period.

    b. Generate the birth arrival times of males using R code 6.3 with $\lambda = 1.03$ over an 8-hour period.

    c. Show the posterior distribution of λ of the overall birthrate is gamma with parameters 18 and $S_{18} = 7.524868$.

    d. Show the posterior distribution of $\gamma = p\lambda$ is gamma (11,6.779414).

    e. Verify Table 6.3, the Bayesian analysis for p, λ, and $\gamma = p\lambda$.

11. Refer to Section 6.5 for the spatial Poisson process.

a. Define a spatial Poisson process.

b. Use R code 6.4 with $\lambda = 100$ with a square area of one (the unit square). Using 100,000 trials for generating observations for a spatial process. The goal is to estimate the number of points that fall with a circle of radius $r = .2$ and center $(.7, .7)$. For your answer refer to Table 6.2.

c. By referring to R code 6.4, explain how the plot of Figure 6.1 is conducted.

d. Execute BC 6.2 with 45,000 observations for the simulation and burn in 5,000 and verify the posterior analysis reported in Table 6.5.

12. There are several ways to incorporate covariates in to the Poisson process.

a. Execute BC 6.9 with 35,000 observations for the simulation and a burn in of 5,000. Use your results to verify Table 6.14, the Bayesian analysis for two regression coefficients.

b. Based on the results of Table 6.15, is $\beta_1 = 0$? Explain your answer.

13. a. Execute RC 6.8 using $M = 1$ and beta = 1, generate the arrival times listed below in Table 6.6. The mean value function for this nonhomogeneous Poisson process is $m(t) = 6, 0 < t < 20$.

b. Execute RC 6.8 with the mean value function $m(t) = t^2, 0 < t < 10$, that is use t<1= and M<-1, and beta<-1 as inputs for the code. Your results should be similar to the 94 arrivals times reported below (6.38).

14. a. Execute BC 6.3 with 40,000 observations for the simulation and a burn in of 3,000 and verify Table 6.6.

b. Is the estimate of M reasonable? Explain your answer.

c. Are the estimates of $\beta_1, \beta_2,$ and β_3 reasonable? Explain your answer.

d. What prior distribution is used for $\beta_1, \beta_2, \beta_3,$ and M?

e. Why are the posterior means of these four parameters so close to the "true" values?

15. Refer to Section 6.8.

a. Define a continuous time Markov chain. What is the Markov property of such a process?

b. What is the distribution of the inter-arrival times?

c. What is the parameter of the inter-arrival time when the process leaves state i but has yet to enter a different state j?

d. Describe the transition probability matrix of a continuous time Markov chain.

e. What are the jumping intensities of such a process?

16. a. Explain the solution $P_{ij}(t)$ to the Kolmogorov system of differential Equations (6.44).

    b. Show the solution is given by the exponential form (6.46).

17. Derive the likelihood function (6.47) for the arrival time parameters ν_i, $i = 1, 2, 3, 4, 5$ and the transition probabilities P_{ij}, $i, j = 1, 2, 3, 4, 5$.

18. a. What is the prior distribution of the ν_i, $i = 1, 2, 3, 4, 5$?

    b. Show the posterior distribution of the ν_i, $i = 1, 2, 3, 4, 5$ is $gamma(n_i + a_i, t_i + b_i)$, $i = 1, 2, 3, 4, 5$.

    c. Show the posterior distribution of the rows of the transition probabilities is Dirichlet.

    d. What is the prior distribution of the rows of the transition probabilities?

19. a. Execute BC 6.5 with 41,000 observations for the simulation and a burn in of 2,500.

    b. Verify the Bayesian analysis reported in Table 6.9.

    c. What is the posterior mean of the inter-arrival time when the process leaves state i?

References

1. Dobrow, R.P. (2016). *Introduction to Stochastic Processes with R*, John Wiley & Sons Inc., New York.

2. Bivand, R.S., Pebesma, E.G., and Gomez-Rubio, V. (2013). *Applied Spatial Data Analysis with R*, Springer, New York.

3. Blangiardo, M. and Carmeletti, M. (2015). *Spatial and Spatio-Temperal Bayesian Models with R-INLA*, John Wiley & Sons Inc., New York.

4. Ntzoufras, I. (2009). *Bayesian Modeling Using WinBUGS*, John Wiley & Sons Inc., New York.

5. Cox, D.R. and Lewis, I.A.W. (1966). *Statistical Analysis of Series of Events*. London Muethen.

6. Insua, D.R., Ruggeri, F., and Wiper, M.P. (2012). *Bayesian Analysis of Stochastic Process Models*, John Wiley & Sons Inc., New York.

7. Musa, J.D. and Okumoto, K. (1983). Software reliability models: concepts, classification, comparisons, and practice. In J.K. Skwinzynski (Ed.) *Electronic Systems Effectiveness and Life Cycle Costing, NATO ASI Series*, (395-424), Springer Verlag, Heidelberg.

8. Moler, C. and Van Loan, C. (2003). Nineteen dubious ways to compute the exponential of a matrix, twenty five years later, *Siam Rev.*, 45, 3-49.

9. Guttorp, P. (1995). *Stochastic Modeling of Scientific Data*, Chapman & Hall, Boca Raton, FL.

10. Ross, S.M. (2009). *Introduction to Probability Models*, 10th edition, Academic Press, New York.
11. Geweke, J., Marshal, R., and Zarkin, G. (1986). Mobility indices in continuous time Markov chains, *Econometrica*, 54, 1407-1423.
12. Cano, J., Moguerza, J., and Insua, D.R. (2010). Bayesian reliability, availability, and maintainability analysis for hardware systems described through continuous time Markov chains, *Technometrics*, 52, 324-334.
13. Musa, J.D., Iannio, A., and Okumoto, K. (1987). *Software Reliability Measurement, Prediction, and Application*, McGraw-Hill, New York.
14. Broemeling, L.D. (2018). *Bayesian Inference for Stochastic Processes*, Chapman & Hall/Taylor and Francis Publishers, Boca Raton, FL.
15. Lee, P.M. (1989). *Bayesian Statistics: An Introduction*, 2nd edition, John Wiley & Sons Inc., New York.

7

Bayesian Inference: Biological Processes that Follow a Continuous Time Markov Chain

7.1 Introduction

In Chapter 6, details of the Poisson process, an important case of continuous time Markov chains (CTMC), were presented. In Chapter 7, Bayesian inferences for general CTMC are presented. First to be considered are the important concepts involved in the study of such processes. For example, the ideas of transition rates, holding times, the embedded chain, and transition probabilities are defined and explained. Such concepts are illustrated by using R to compute the transition function and to generate observations from the CTMC. This is followed by a presentation of Bayesian inferences of estimation and testing hypotheses about the unknown parameters of the process. Also developed is the Bayesian predictive distribution for future observations of the CTMC.

As with discrete time chains, the understanding of stationary distributions, absorbing states, mean time to absorption, and time reversibility is an essential part when discussing CTMC.

The chapter is concluded with many examples, including DNA evolution, birth and death processes, and epidemics. The information in this chapter is an introduction to epidemics and infectious diseases and is essential for a more detailed presentation given in Chapters 8 and 9.

7.2 The Foundation of Continuous Time Markov Chains

The reader should refer to Dobrow [1], ch. 7 for an introduction to the essential elements that explain the properties of CTMC and to Insua, Ruggeri, and Wiper [2], ch. 5 for a good account of Bayesian inferential procedures pertaining to CTMC. These references will be closely followed in what is to follow.

For those interested in biological examples of CTMC, see Allen [3], chs. 6, 7 for an in-depth informative approach to the topic. As we have seen, a CTMC behaves like the discrete version except the time between states is distributed as an exponential random variable and events can occur at any time. Thus, there are two sets of parameters that define the CTMC, the parameters of the exponentially distributed inter-arrival times, and the probability transition parameters. As will be seen, the two sets are related by the transition rate parameters.

7.2.1 The Markov Property and Transition Function

Let $\{X(t), t > 0\}$ be a continuous time stochastic process, then it is called a CTMC if

$$
\begin{aligned}
P\big[X(t+s) = j \,|\, X(s) = i \,|\, X(u) = x(u)| \,, 0 \leq u <\big] \\
= P\big[X(t+s) = j \,|\, X(s) = i\big]
\end{aligned}
\tag{7.1}
$$

for all states i, j, and $x(u)$, $0 \leq u < s$. Of course, it is understood that the state space is countable.

Also, a continuous time Markov chain is time homogenous, that is to say

$$
P\big[X(t+s) = j \,|\, X(s) = i\big] = P\big[X(t) = j \,|\, X(0) = i\big] = P_{ij}(t)
\tag{7.2}
$$

Thus, the probabilistic properties of a CTMC over the interval $[s, t + s]$ are the same as over the interval $[0, t]$. Or to express it another way, when the chain visits state i its forward behavior from that time toward the future is the same as if the process started in i at time $t = 0$. Note that the function $P_{ij}(t)$ is called the transition function of the process.

Recall that for a Poisson process the interarrival times are identically exponentially distributed; however, for the CTMC, there is a difference as follows. Let T_i be the holding time of the process, that is, the time the process occupies state i before switching to another state, then it can be shown that T_i has an exponential distribution.

To show T_i is memoryless, consider

$$
\begin{aligned}
P\big[T_i > s+t \,|\, X(0) = i\big] \\
= P\big[T_i > s+t, T_i > s \,|\, X(0) = i\big] \\
= P\big[T_i > s+t \,|\, X(0) = i, T_i > s\big] P\big[T_i > s\big] \\
= P\big[T_i > t \,|\, X(0) = i\big] P\big[T_i > s \,|\, X(0) = i\big]
\end{aligned}
\tag{7.3}
$$

and the last statement of (7.3) shows the process is memoryless. Recall the only continuous distribution which is memoryless is the exponential. The evolution of the process can be described as follows: Starting in state i, the process remains in this state for an exponentially distributed time with parameter q_i (average time in this state is $1/q_i$), then it hits a new state j with probability p_{ij} and remains in state j for a time which has an exponential distribution with mean $1/q_j$, then hits a new state k, $k \neq j$, with probability p_{jk}, etc.

I am assuming that the process does not hit an absorbing state and that the process is not explosive. See Dobrow [1, p. 268–269] for additional information. There is a connection between the transition probabilities p_{ij} and the exponential parameters q_i of the holding times, and this connection is the transition rate of the process.

7.2.2 Transition Rates, Holding Times, and Transition Probabilities

An alternative to describing a CTMC is by transition rates between pairs of states. When the process is in state i, there is a chance that it will change to one of the other possible states, that is, the state i is paired with the state j for all states $j \neq i$. If j can be reached from i, one can associate an alarm that is activated after a time that has an exponential distribution with parameter q_{ij}. When the state i is first occupied, the alarms are all started at the same time, and the first alarm that is activated determines the next state to be occupied. If the alarm (i, j) is first activated and the process moves to state j, a new set of alarms are activated with exponential transition rates $q_{j1}, q_{j2}, \ldots$. Thus, to repeat, the first alarm that is activated determines the next state to be occupied, etc. The q_{ij} are called transition rates and from them, the transition probabilities and holding time parameters can be determined.

Suppose the process starts at i, then the alarms are initiated and the first one that is activated determines the next transition; therefore, the time of the first alarm is the minimum of independent exponential random variable with parameters $q_{i1}, q_{i2}, \ldots$, which is an exponential random variable with parameter $\sum_k q_{ik}$. Thus, the process remains in state i for a holding time which has an exponential distribution with parameter $\sum_k q_{ik} = q_i$. From i the chain moves to state j if the alarm (i, j) is activated first which occurs with probability

$$p_{ij} = q_{ij}/q_i, \tag{7.4}$$

which is the transition probability of moving from state i to state j of the imbedded chain. One sees from (7.4) that the transition probabilities of the chain are completely determined by the transition rates q_{ij}.

As a simple example, consider a four-state chain with the transition rates of the chain are given by

$$(q_1, q_2, q_3, q_4) = (q_{12} + q_{13} + q_{14}, q_{21} + q_{23} + q_{24}, q_{31} + q_{32} + q_{34}, q_{41} + q_{42} + q_{43}) \quad (7.5)$$

Note the imbedded chain has transition matrix

$$P = \begin{pmatrix} 0, q_{12} / q_1, q_{13} / q_1, q_{14} / q_1 \\ q_{21} / q_2, 0, q_{23} / q_2, q_{24} / q_2 \\ q_{31} / q_3, q_{32} / q_3, 0, q_{34} / q_3 \\ q_{41} / q_4, q_{42} / q_4, q_{43} / q_4, 0 \end{pmatrix} \quad (7.6)$$

The transition rates q_{ij} are quite important when studying CTMC. Assume that the continuous time Markov chain has a differentiable transition function $P(t)$, where $p_{ij}(0) = 1$ if $i = j$, otherwise its value is 0.

Note if $X(t) = i$, then the instantaneous transition rate of hitting $j \neq i$ is given by

$$\begin{aligned}
\lim_{h \to 0^+} E\big(\# \text{of transitions to } j \text{ in} (t, t+h] \big) \\
= \lim_{h \to 0^+} P\big[X(t+h) = j \,|\, X(t) = i \big] \\
= \lim_{h \to 0^+} p_{ij}(h)/h \\
= (d/dt) p_{ij}(0) \\
= p'_{ij}(0)
\end{aligned} \quad (7.7)$$

Consider the matrix $Q = P'(0)$, then the off-diagonal elements of Q are the transition rates q_{ij}, that is $q_{ij} = Q_{ij}$, $i \neq j$, and the diagonal entries are $-q_i$, thus, each row of Q has sum 0.

As an example, consider the four-state chain (7.6) where $q_{12} = q_{13} = q_{14} = 1$, $q_{21} = q_{23} = q_{24} = 2$, $q_{31} = q_{32} = q_{34} = 3$, and $q_{41} = q_{42} = q_{43} = 4$, thus $q_1 = 3$, $q_2 = 6$, $q_3 = 9$, and $q_4 = 12$. For this four-state chain, the process remains in state 1 for an average of $1/3$ hours in state 2 for $1/6$ hours, and for state 3, $1/9$ hours, and remains in state 4 for an average of $1/12$ hours. Consequently, the infinitesimal generator matrix is

$$Q = \begin{bmatrix} -3, & 1, & 1, & 1 \\ 2, & -6, & 2, & 2 \\ 3, & 3, & -9, & 3 \\ 4, & 4, & 4, & -12 \end{bmatrix} \quad (7.8)$$

and $\sum_i \pi_i Q_{ij} = 0, \forall j$. Since the transition rates determine the transition probabilities of the imbedded chain, which is the matrix

$$P = \begin{bmatrix} 0, & 1/3, & 1/3, & 1/3 \\ 1/3 & 0, & 1/3, & 1/3 \\ 1/3, & 1/3, & 0, & 1/3 \\ 1/3, & 1/3, & 1/3, & 0 \end{bmatrix}. \tag{7.9}$$

This is a very special transition matrix, because I chose the transition rates in such a way that each transition has the same chance of occurring, namely $1/3$.

7.2.3 The Kolmogorov Forward and Backward Equations and the Matrix Exponential

We now see the role the equation $p_{ij} = q_{ij}/q_i$ plays in determining the transition probability matrix $P(t)$, which is a solution to the forward Kolmogorov equation

$$P'(t) = P(t)Q,$$

where Q is the infinitesimal matrix and $P'(t)$ the derivative matrix with respect to t of the transition probability matrix.

This is also expressed as

$$P'_{ij}(t) = \sum_k p_{ik}(t) q_{kj} = -p_{ij}(t) q_j + \sum_{k \neq j} p_{ik}(t) q_{kj} \tag{7.10}$$

For a proof of (7.10) see Dobrow [1, p. 276]. It is obvious that the solution $P(t)$ to (7.10) is given by the matrix equation

$$P(t) = \exp(tQ), \quad t \geq 0, \tag{7.11}$$

Where, $P(0) = I$.

Also, the solution can be written as

$$P'(t) = (d/dt)e^{tQ} = \sum_{n=0}^{n=\infty} (1/n!)(tQ)^n = I + tQ + t^2 Q^2 / 2 + t^3 Q^3 / 3! + \cdots$$

The next section will use R to express the solution $P(t)$ in matrix form (7.11).

7.2.4 Computing the Transition Function with R

As an example, consider the four-state CTMC, where Q is given by (7.8). The following R code computes the probability transition matrix as the solution (7.11) to the differential equation (the forward Kolmogorov equations) (7.10). Note the package "expm" most be loaded in order to execute the matrix exponential operation.

R Code 7.1

```
>install.packages("expm")
>library(expm)

# Q is the infinitesimal generator matrix

> Q<-matrix(c(-3,1,1,1,
+              2,-6,2,2,
+              3,3,-9,3,
+              4,4,4,-12),ncol=4,nrow=4,byrow=TRUE)
# the following is the command that executes the matrix
exponential
> P<- function (t){expm(t*Q)}
# P(2) is the probability transition matrix at 2
> P(2)
            [,1]        [,2]        [,3]        [,4]
[1,]  0.4800078  0.2399952  0.1599982  0.1199989
[2,]  0.4799903  0.2400060  0.1600023  0.1200014
[3,]  0.4799945  0.2400034  0.1600013  0.1200008
[4,]  0.4799954  0.2400028  0.1600011  0.1200007
# P(0) is the probability transition matrix at t=0.
# this serves as a check since P(0)=I, the identity matrix
> P(0)
      [,1] [,2] [,3] [,4]
[1,]     1    0    0    0
[2,]     0    1    0    0
[3,]     0    0    1    0
[4,]     0    0    0    1
> P(4)
        [,1] [,2] [,3] [,4]
[1,]    0.48 0.24 0.16 0.12
[2,]    0.48 0.24 0.16 0.12
[3,]    0.48 0.24 0.16 0.12
[4,]    0.48 0.24 0.16 0.12
> P(1.2)
            [,1]        [,2]        [,3]        [,4]
[1,]  0.4806526  0.2395971  0.1598456  0.1199047
[2,]  0.4791942  0.2405007  0.1601882  0.1201169
[3,]  0.4795368  0.2402823  0.1601124  0.1200685
[4,]  0.4796187  0.2402339  0.1600914  0.1200561
```

```
>> P(2)
          [,1]         [,2]         [,3]         [,4]
[1,] 0.4800078 0.2399952 0.1599982 0.1199989
[2,] 0.4799903 0.2400060 0.1600023 0.1200014
[3,] 0.4799945 0.2400034 0.1600013 0.1200008
[4,] 0.4799954 0.2400028 0.1600011 0.1200007
> P(0)
       [,1] [,2] [,3] [,4]
[1,]    1    0    0    0
[2,]    0    1    0    0
[3,]    0    0    1    0
[4,]    0    0    0    1
> P(4)
      [,1] [,2] [,3] [,4]
[1,] 0.48 0.24 0.16 0.12
[2,] 0.48 0.24 0.16 0.12
[3,] 0.48 0.24 0.16 0.12
[4,] 0.48 0.24 0.16 0.12
> P(1.2)
          [,1]         [,2]         [,3]         [,4]
[1,] 0.4806526 0.2395971 0.1598456 0.1199047
[2,] 0.4791942 0.2405007 0.1601882 0.1201169
[3,] 0.4795368 0.2402823 0.1601124 0.1200685
[4,] 0.4796187 0.2402339 0.1600914 0.1200561
>
```

For example, when the time is $t = 1.2$ hours, the transition probability matrix is $P(1.2)$, and the probability of changing states from state 1 to 2 over a 1.2-hour interval is .2395, etc.

7.3 Limiting and Stationary Distributions

Limiting and stationary distributions for continuous time Markov chains are determined in much the same way as that for discrete time Markov chains.

Recall the definition of the limiting distribution (as $t \rightarrow \infty$) π of a process as

$$\lim P_{ij}(t) = \pi_j, \qquad (7.12)$$

where π_j is the j-th component of the vector π. The limiting distribution does not have to exist, but if it does it is the stationary distribution of the chain. Of course, the stationary distribution of a CTMC is defined as the vector π that satisfies

$$\pi = \pi P(t), t \geq 0, \qquad (7.13)$$

which is equivalent to

$$\pi_j = \sum_i \pi_i P_{ij}(t), t \geq 0, \tag{7.14}$$

for all states j.

Note the ideas of accessibility, communicating classes, and irreducibility carry over from the discrete case to the continuous. However, note that for CTMC all states are aperiodic. Under what conditions does a CTMC have a stationary distribution?

_____

Basic Limit Theorem

Let $\{X(t), t \geq 0\}$ be a continuous time Markov chain which is irreducible with a finite state space, then the process has a unique stationary distribution, given by the limiting distribution

$\lim_{t \to \infty} P_{ij}(t) = \pi_j$ for all initial states i

or expressed in an equivalent fashion as

$$\lim_{t \to \infty} P(t) = \Pi, \tag{7.15}$$

where each row of Π is the same vector, namely π.

As example, consider the two state CTMC with probability transition matrix

$$P(t) = \left[1/(\lambda + \mu) \right] \begin{pmatrix} \mu + \lambda e^{-(\lambda+\mu)t}, \lambda - \lambda e^{-(\lambda+\mu)t} \\ \mu - \mu e^{-(\lambda+\mu)t}, \lambda + \mu e^{-(\lambda+\mu)t} \end{pmatrix} \tag{7.16}$$

Therefore, in the limit, the matrix reduces to

$$P(t) = \left[1/(\lambda + \mu) \right] \begin{pmatrix} \mu, \lambda \\ \mu, \lambda \end{pmatrix}$$

and the stationary distribution is

$$\pi = \left(\mu/(\lambda + \mu), \lambda/(\lambda + \mu) \right). \tag{7.17}$$

There is a relation between the stationary distribution and the infinitesimal generator matrix Q, given by

$$\pi Q = 0, \tag{7.18}$$

or in scalar terms

$$\sum_i \pi_i Q_{ij} = 0, \forall j$$

The following example is due to Dobrow [1, p. 286–287] with the infinitesimal generator matrix

$$Q = \begin{bmatrix} -2.0, & 1.0, & 1.0 \\ 1/2, & -1, & 1/2 \\ 0, & 1/3, & -1/3 \end{bmatrix}. \tag{7.19}$$

This corresponds to a three-state chain with states eat, play, and sleep.

A newborn baby is in one of three states: eat, play, and sleep. The baby eats on the average for 30 minutes, plays an average one hour, and on the average sleeps approximately three hours. After eating there is a 50-50 chance that he will sleep or play, and after playing a 50-50 chance he will sleep or eat. Lastly after sleeping, the baby will always eat. The corresponding transition matrix of the imbedded chain is

$$P = \begin{bmatrix} 0, & 1/2, & 1/2 \\ 1/2, & 0, & 1/2 \\ 0.0, & 1.0, & 0,0 \end{bmatrix} \tag{7.20}$$

Then using the fact that $q_{ij} = q_i p_{ij}$, the generator matrix is given by (7.19).

Instead of using (7.18), let us find the stationary distribution of this process with R code 7.2. The corresponding code computes the corresponding P matrix, then approximates the limiting distribution P(100).

RC 7.2

```
> Q<-matrix(c(-2,1,1,
+             1/2,-1,1/2,
+             0,1/3,-1/3),nrow=3,byrow=TRUE)
> P<-function(t){expm(t*Q)
+ }
> P(100)
```

	[,1]	[,2]	[,3]
[1,]	0.07142857	0.2857143	0.6428571
[2,]	0.07142857	0.2857143	0.6428571
[3,]	0.07142857	0.2857143	0.6428571

Thus, it is found that the stationary distribution is the vector
π = (.07142, .28571, .64288), therefore, regardless of the initial activity of the baby, in the long run the chance of eating, playing, and sleeping is the same given by the rows of P(100).

7.4 Mean Time to Absorption with R

As with discrete time processes, CTMC can have absorbing states, thus suppose that $\{X(t), t > 0\}$ has states $\{1, 2, ..., k\}$, where one of those states, say a, is absorbing, the all of the other k-1 states are transient. If the chain starts in a transient state, there is a positive probability that the chain will be absorbed.

Suppose the generator matrix is partitioned as

$$(7.21) Q = \begin{bmatrix} 0, & 0^* \\ *, & V \end{bmatrix}$$

where V is the k-1 order submatrix of transient states, then if the chain has initial state i, the mean time to absorption is

$$a_i = \sum_j F_{ij}, \tag{7.22}$$

where F_{ij} is the ij-th element of the fundamental matrix

$$F = V^{-1}. \tag{7.23}$$

Consider the matrix

$$Q = \begin{bmatrix} -(q_{12} + q_{13}), & q_{12}, & q_{13} \\ 0.000000, & -q_{23}, & q_{23} \\ 0,00000, & 0.00, & 0.0 \end{bmatrix}, \tag{7.24}$$

Then according to Bartolomeo [4], the matrix is the generator matrix corresponding to the progression of liver disease among three states: state 1 corresponds to cirrhosis, state 2 liver cancer, and state 3, death. Of course, state

3 is an absorbing state; thus, it is of interest to determine the average time to death, beginning from cirrhosis and from liver cancer.

The fundamental matrix is

$$F = \begin{pmatrix} -(q_{12}+q_{13}), q_{12} \\ 0.000000, -q_{23} \end{pmatrix}^{-1} = \begin{pmatrix} 1/(q_{12}+q_{13}), q_{12}/q_{23}(q_{12}+q_{13}) \\ 0.00000000000000000, 1/q_{23} \end{pmatrix} \quad (7.25)$$

and the mean time to absorption for a person who has cirrhosis is

$$a_1 = \left[1/(q_{12}+q_{13})\right] + \left[q_{12}/q_{23}(q_{12}+q_{13})\right]. \quad (7.26)$$

In a similar way for those with liver cancer, the mean time to death is

$$a_2 = 1/q_{23}. \quad (7.27)$$

For the statistician, one would have to have sample information about the transition rates q_{12}, q_{13}, and q_{13}. Bartolomeo's study estimated these rates as follows: $q_{12} = .0151$, $q_{13} = .0071$, and $q_{23} = .0284$, and these can be substituted into (7.26) and (7.27) for estimates of the mean time to death for those with cirrhosis of the liver and liver cancer, respectively.

Using these estimates, the following R code computes an estimate, using simulation of the average time to death for a patient diagnosed initially with cirrhosis of the liver, where the time unit is months.

RC 7.3

```
> trials<-10000
> simlist<-numeric(trials)
> init<-1
> for ( i in 1:trials){
+ state<-init
+ t<-0
+ while (TRUE){
+ if (state==1){ q12<-rexp(1,0.0151)
+ q13<-rexp(1,.0071)}
+ if (q12<q13) {t<-t+q12
+ state<-2}
+ else{t<-t+q13
+ break}
+ if (state==2){q23<-rexp(1,.0284)
+ t<-t+q23
+ break}
+ }
+ simlist[i]<-t}
> mean(simlist)
[1] 68.37068
```

Therefore, one's estimate of the average time to death for a person initially diagnosed with cirrhosis of the liver is 68.37068 months!

7.5 Time Reversibility

Similar to the discrete case, time reversibility is the last major concept to be defined for CTMC. A continuous time Markov chain with generator matrix Q and stationary distribution π is said to be time reversible if and only if

$$\pi_i q_{ij} = \pi_j q_{ji} \forall i, j. \tag{7.28}$$

Time reversibility is related to the idea of global balance. Let π be the stationary distribution to the CTMC, that is $\pi Q = 0$ is satisfied which in turn implies

$$\sum_{i \neq j} \pi_i q_{ij} = \pi_j q_j, \forall j. \tag{7.29}$$

Note the holding time parameter q_j is the transition rate from j and that π_j is the proportion of the time the process is in state j, thus the right hand side of (7.29) is the long-term rate the process leaves j. Also, it is clear that $\pi_i q_{ij}$ is the long-term rate of transition from i to j, thus the left-hand side of (7.29) is the long-term rate that the process enters state j. This in turn implies that for a stationary process the rates in and out of any state are the same and the equations (7.29) are called the global balance equations. As an example, let

$$P = \begin{pmatrix} 0.0, 1.0, 0.0 \\ 1/3, 0, 2/3 \\ 0.0, 1.0, 0.0 \end{pmatrix} \tag{7.30}$$

be the transition matrix of an embedded chain, where the process remains in state 1 for an average of 5 minutes before moving to state 2, where it remains for a two-minute average before moving to state 3 which is occupied for an average of 4 minutes before moving to state 2. It can easily be shown that the stationary distribution is $\pi = (5/19, 6/19/8/19)$, thus (7.29) implies

$$\left(\pi_1 q_1, \pi_2 q_2, \pi_3 q_3 \right) = \left(1/19, 3/19/2/19 \right). \tag{7.31}$$

Thus, global balance for this example shows that every 19 minutes the process incurs one transition to and from state 1, three transitions to and from state 2, and two transitions to and from state 3.

This concludes the fundamental properties that need to be understood in order to perform Bayesian inferences for CTMC.

7.6 Time Reversibility

For this part of Chapter 7, Bayesian inferences will be performed for a variety of examples, including some from biology, physics, and business.

7.6.1 DNA Evolution

Recall that DNA evolution was presented for the discrete time case in Section 5.7 of Chapter 5, where the chain had four states, namely the four base nucleotides: (1) adenine, (2) guanine, (3), cytocine, and (4) thymine. In the Jukes-Cantor model, the transition rates are all the same with infinitesimal generator matrix

$$Q = \begin{pmatrix} -3r,r,r,r \\ r,-3r,r,r \\ r,r,-3r,r \\ r,r,r,-3r \end{pmatrix} \tag{7.32}$$

where the first row and column correspond to adenine, the second row and column to guanine, the third to cytocine, and the last row and column to thymine. Thus, the corresponding transition matrix is

$$P(t) = \exp(tQ) = (1/4)\begin{pmatrix} 1+3e^{-4rt},1-e^{-4rt},1-e^{-4rt},1-e^{-4rt} \\ 1-e^{-4rt},1+3e^{-4rt},1-e^{-4rt},1-e^{-4rt} \\ 1-e^{-4rt},1-e^{-4rt},1+3e^{-4rt},1-e^{-4rt} \\ 1-e^{-4rt},1-e^{-4rt},1-e^{-4rt},1+3e^{-4rt} \end{pmatrix}. \tag{7.33}$$

Thus, at time t, the probability that the DNA base adenine is replaced by quinine (or to cytosine or to thymine) is $(1/4)(1 - e^{-4rt})$, etc. On the other hand, the probability that adenine at time t is not replaced by another base is $(1/4)(1 + 3e^{-4rt})$.

The statistical problem is to make inferences about the rate r based on observing the evolution at various times.

Based on (7.32), the infinitesimal rates are

$$q_{ij} = r, i \neq j, i, j = 1, 2, 3, 4 \tag{7.34}$$

thus, the holding time exponential parameters are

$$q_i = 3r, i = 1, 2, 3, 4. \tag{7.35}$$

Recall that the transition probabilities are given by

$$p_{ij} = q_{ij} / q_i = r / 3r = 1/3, i \neq j, i, j = 1, 2, 3, 4. \tag{7.36}$$

If one assigns a value to r, one can make inferences about the holding time parameters (7.35) and the transition probabilities (7.36); however, one knows that the transition probabilities are all $1/3$, thus only the holding time exponential parameters will be of interest.

In practice, one would observe the holding times of the various states, then from those observations estimate r. Using WinBUGS, we will assume a value of r then generate the exponential holding times. Consider the holding time for occupying the first state adenine and assume its mean time is 2 time units. The WinBUGS program that follows is based on 50 observations of the holding time for adenine with an average holding time of 2 time units. The main objective is to estimate the average holding time for adenine.

The holding time T_1 for adenine has an exponential distribution with parameter λ, namely

$$f(t_1) = \lambda \exp(-\lambda t_1), t_1 > 0 \tag{7.37}$$

here the mean holding time is

$$E(T_1 | \lambda) = 1 / \lambda = \mu. \tag{7.38}$$

Note let $\lambda = 1/6$ and generate the 50 observations in the list statement of BC 7.1, which corresponds to a mean holding time of 6 time units. Refer to the generator matrix (7.32) for the DNA example where the holding time exponential parameter is 3r, thus I let $3r = 1/6$. It is also assumed that the prior distribution of λ is gamma $(.001, .001)$, a non-informative prior with mean 1 and variance 1000.

BC 7.1 is executed with 45,000 observations for the simulation and a burn in of 5,000. The results of the analysis are reported in Table 7.1.

TABLE 7.1

Posterior Analysis for Holding Time for Adenine

Parameter	Mean	SD	Error	2 1/2	Median	97 1/2
λ	.163	.02314	.0001259	.121	.1618	.2118
μ	6.259	.9034	.004947	4.721	6.181	8.264

BC 7.1

```
model;
{
lamda~dgamma(.001,.001)
for( i in 1:50){
T1[i]~dexp(lamda)}
mu<-1/lamda
}
list(
T1 = c(5.968,6.741,9.346,6.269,6.117,
3.056,5.674,1.377,1.864,1.956,
0.1391,14.28,22.06,3.203,6.415,
5.078,5.958,0.9036,7.865,5.154,
1.078,5.025,18.92,8.998,24.05,
2.433,0.7362,9.205,0.9738,3.878,
0.9797,1.961,6.133,5.866,2.523,
14.51,3.125,4.142,7.126,2.256,
20.31,17.88,5.138,2.076,1.866,
9.726,0.5665,0.6489,2.325,2.697)))
list(lamda=.16)
```

The parameter of interest is μ, the average holding time for adenine, which has a posterior mean of 6.259 with a 95% credible interval of (4.721,8.264). Note the credible interval contains the value 6, which was used to generate the observations in the list statement of BC 7.1.

It appears that the distributions are symmetric about their posterior means and that the simulation errors are reasonably small. In summary based on the posterior median, the estimate of the mean holding time is 6.181. Clearly, the type of analysis can be repeated for the other three holding times. There is nothing new to be learned because the mean holding time μ is the same for all four holding times. The student will be asked to estimate the holding times for the other three DNA bases as an exercise at the end of Chapter 7.

Now consider another aspect of Bayesian inference for the holding time for the DNA base adenine. Remember that the value $\lambda = 1/6(\mu = 6)$ is used to generate the adenine holding times listed in the list statement of BC 7.1. It is of paramount interest to test the hypothesis that $\lambda = 1/6(\mu = 6)$ is a plausible value of the mean holding time.

Thus, using the Bayesian approach, consider a test of the null hypothesis

$$H_0 : \lambda = 1/6 \quad \text{versus} \quad H_1 : \lambda \neq 1/6 \tag{7.39}$$

The approach presented by Lee [5, pp. 126–128] is employed to test a simple null hypothesis versus the two-sided alternative (7.39).

Recall that the posterior probability of the null hypothesis is given by

$$p_0 = \left[\pi_0 f\left(t \mid \lambda = 1/6\right)\right] / \left[\pi_0 f(t \mid \lambda = 1/6) + \pi_1 \int_0^\infty \rho_1(\lambda) f(t \mid \lambda) d\lambda\right], \quad (7.40)$$

where $\pi_0 = P(\lambda = 1/6)$ is the prior probability of the null hypothesis and $\pi_1 = 1 - \pi_0$ is the prior probability of the alternative hypothesis. Also, the probability density of the n holding times is

$$f\left(t \mid \lambda\right) = \lambda^n e^{-\lambda \sum_{i=1}^{i=n} t_i}, \quad (7.41)$$

where $t = (t_1, t_2, .., t_n)$ is the n by 1 vector of holding times.

Also, it is obvious that

$$f\left(t \mid \lambda = 1/6\right) = \left(1/6\right)^n e^{-(1/6)\sum_{i=1}^{i=n} t_i}. \quad (7.42)$$

In addition, $\rho_1(\lambda)$ is the prior density of λ under the alternative hypothesis $\lambda \neq 1/6$. How does one choose $\rho_1(\lambda)$? It seems reasonable to choose the improper prior density, thus, let

$$\rho_1(\lambda) = 1/\lambda, \lambda > 0. \quad (7.43)$$

Since $\sum_{i=1}^{i=50} t_i = 306.32$, there is sufficient information to compute the posterior probability of the null hypothesis given by (7.40).

The expression (7.40) for the posterior probability of the null hypothesis is formulated as

$$p_0 = \left(1/\left(1 + ra\right)\right) \quad (7.44)$$

where

$$ra = [\pi_1 \int_0^\infty \rho_1(\lambda) f(t \mid \lambda) d\lambda] / [\pi_0 f(t \mid \lambda = 1/6)]. \quad (7.45)$$

Thus, the posterior probability of the null hypothesis is expressed in terms of the ratio ra. Note as the ratio ra approaches zero p_0 approaches 1.

If one lets $\pi_0 = \pi_1 = 1/2$, one can show that

$$ra = \left[\Gamma\left(50\right) 6^{50} e^{51.05444}\right] / \left[\left(306.32\right)^{50}\right] = .7356 \quad (7.46)$$

I took the natural log of *ra* and used the log gamma function, then finally used the natural exponential function to arrive at the value .7356, the posterior probability of the null hypothesis. Thus, based on the 50 exponential holding times for adenine of DNA evolution, and the prior information, one would conclude that $\lambda = 1/6$, that the null hypothesis is plausible. Recall the value $\lambda = 1/6$ was used to generate the 50 holding times included in the list statement of BC 7.1.

The next objective is to determine the predictive density for the holding times of the DNA base adenine. Let $t(n + 1)$ be the future observation for the holding time for adenine.

Note that the predictive density for $t(n + 1)$ is

$$f\left(t(n+1)|\, data\right) = \int_{0}^{\infty} f\left(t(n+1)|\, \lambda\right) f\left(data|\, \lambda\right) \zeta\left(\lambda\right) d\lambda \qquad (7.47)$$

where

$$f\left(t(n+1)|\, \lambda\right) = \lambda e^{-\lambda t(n+1)}, t(n+1) > 0 \qquad (7.48)$$

$$f\left(data|\, \lambda\right) = \lambda^{n} e^{-\lambda \sum_{i=1}^{i=n} t_i}, 0 < t_1 < t_2 < \ldots < t_n \qquad (7.49)$$

where t_i is the *i*-th holding time, and $\zeta(\lambda)$ is the prior density for λ

Choosing the improper prior density

$$\zeta\left(\lambda\right) = 1/\lambda, \quad \lambda > 0, \qquad (7.50)$$

One may show that the predictive density (7.47) reduces to

$$f\left(t(n+1)|\, data\right) = \Gamma\left(n+1\right) / \left[t(n+1) + \sum_{i=1}^{i=n} t_i \right]^{n+1}, t(n+1) > 0$$

The predictive density for $t(n + 1)$ is completely determined when the data $n = 50$ and $\sum_{i=1}^{i=n} t_i = 306.32$ are substituted into (7.50). WinBUGS provides a way to compute future values from the predictive density (7.51). Refer to BC 7.1 and add the command

Z[i]~dexp(lamda) and execute BC 7.1 the usual way for the example when I did the posterior analysis with 55,000 observations for the simulation and a burn in of 5,000, the first five predicted holding times (Table 7.2).

Thus, the mean of the predictive distribution for the first future holding time for adenine is 6.186 time units and a 95% predictive interval of (.1463,23.26). I used a gamma prior (.001,.001) for λ in the WinBUGS program BC 7.1, but

TABLE 7.2

Posterior Predictive Analysis

Future	Mean	SD	Error	2 ½	Median	97 1/2
t(51)	6.186	6.29	.03337	.1463	4.21	23.26
t(52)	6.254	6.393	.03186	.1532	4.236	23.52
t(53)	6.226	6.343	.03236	.1541	4.292	23.36
t(54)	6.209	6.314	.03075	.148	4.264	23.48
t(55)	6.18	6.312	.029	.1498	4.24	23.34

the formula for the predictive density (7.51) was the improper prior (7.50), however there will be very little difference in the predicted future values. Note the uncertainty in the prediction implied by the long width of the prediction intervals.

We next consider a variation of the Jukes-Cantor model called the Kimura [6] model with infinitesimal rates given by the matrix

$$Q = \begin{bmatrix} -(r+2s), & r, & s, & s \\ r, & -(r+2s), & s, & s \\ s, & s, & -(r+2s), & r \\ s, & s, & r, & -(r+2s) \end{bmatrix} \tag{7.51}$$

Thus, the evolution remains in the base nucleotide adenine for a time with an exponential parameter $r+2s$. This model distinguishes between the substitutions $a \leftrightarrow g$(from purine to purine) or (from pyrimidine to pyrimidine, and transversions (from purine to pyrimidine or vice versa). Recall chapter five Section 5.7, where these two evolutionary models (Jukes-Cantor, and the Kimura) were analyzed in discrete time. Thus, referring to (7.51) the r rate is the exponential time the process remains in adenine until guanine is substituted. The rate s is the exponential parameter for the holding time in adenine until cytosine is substituted for adenine, and the same rate s is the exponential parameter for the holding time of adenine, until adenine is substituted by thymine.

Note, that corresponding to the infinitesimal rate matrix Q (7.51) the probability transition matrix

$$\begin{aligned} P_{ij}(t) &= \left(1 + e^{-4st} - 2e^{-(r+s)t}\right)/4, (i,j) \in \{ag, ga, ct, tc, \\ &= \left(1 - 2e^{-4t}\right)/4, (i,j) \in \{ac, at, gc, gt, ca, cg, ta, tg\}, \\ &= 1 + e^{-4st} + 2e^{-2(r+s)t})/4, (i,j) \in \{aa, gg, cc, tt\}. \end{aligned} \tag{7.52}$$

See Dobrow [1, p. 282] for additional information about the derivation of (7.52).

The three phases of Bayesian inference will be presented for the Kimura model of molecular evolution. To that end, one must generate holding times for the two rates r and s, and let $r = 1/2$ and $s = 1/8$, thus, the holding time for adenine until the substitution by guanine has an average of 2 time units, while the holding time for adenine until the substitution by cytosine is 8 time units.

I generated data for the holding times T_{12} and T_{13} of adenine until substituted by guanine and cytosine, respectively The list statement of BC 7.2 contains the15 holding times, where the exponential parameter for T_{12} is $\lambda_{12} = 1/2$ and for T_{13}, $\lambda_{13} = 1/8$. BC 7.2 is executed with 35,000 observations for the simulation and 5,000 for the burn in.

BC 7.2

```
model;
{
#lamda13 is the exponential parameter s
lamda13~dgamma(.001,.001)
for ( i in 1:15){

T13[i]~dexp(lamda13)}
# m13 is the average holding time for adenine before it is
substituted by #cytosine
mu13<-1/lamda13

# lamda12 is the exponential parameter r
lamda12~dgamma(.001,.001)
for ( i in 1:15){

T12[i]~dexp(lamda12)}
# mu12 is the average holding time for adenine before it is
substituted by #guanine
mu12<-1/lamda12
# d23 is the difference in the two holding times for adenine
d23<-mu12-mu13
}

list(T13 = c(
11.98,12.58,7.757,24.86,5.816,
8.416,2.104,18.0,3.069,7.62,
0.01324,27.58,3.004,6.996,1.003),
T12 = c(
2.996,3.145,1.939,6.215,1.454,
2.104,0.5259,4.5,0.7673,1.905,
0.003311,6.896,0.751,1.749,0.2509))

list(lamda13=.125,lamda12=.5)
```

The posterior analysis for the two holding times is reported in Table 7.3.

TABLE 7.3

Posterior Analysis for the Kimura Model

Parameter	Mean	SD	Error	2 1/2	Median	97 1/2
d_{23}	−7.556	2.858	.01387	−14.29	−7.14	−3.164
λ_{12}	.427	.1109	.000541	.2394	.4163	.6694
λ_{13}	.1064	.0274	.000127	.05981	.1039	.1668
μ_{12}	2.51	.6957	.003384	1.494	2.402	4.178
μ_{13}	10.07	2.776	.0133	5.996	9.62	16.72

Using the posterior mean of 2.51 time units as the estimate of the average adenine holding time until adenine is substituted by guanine, and 10.07 time units as the estimate of the adenine holding time until substituted by cytosine, leads to a difference between the two estimates as −7.556 time units, which in turn implies the that two are indeed different (because the 95% credible interval of (−14.29, −3.164) does not include zero). This is an informal inference about the difference in two estimates, and it appears that the Kimura model is indeed appropriate and is to be preferred to the Jukes-Cantor model.

However, a more formal Bayesian test of hypothesis of

$$H : \lambda_{12} = \lambda_{13} \quad \text{versus} \quad A : \lambda_{12} \neq \lambda_{13} \tag{7.53}$$

will be presented.

Consider the posterior probability of the null hypothesis

$$p_0 = 1 / (1 + ratio) \tag{7.54}$$

where
  ratio = N/D

$$N = \pi_1 \int_0^\infty \int_0^\infty \rho_1(\lambda_{12}, \lambda_{13}) f(T_{12} | \lambda_{12}) f(T_{13} | \lambda_{13}) d\lambda_{12} d\lambda_{13}, \tag{7.55}$$

$$D = \pi_0 \int_0^\infty \rho_0(\lambda) f(T_{12}, | T_{13}, | \lambda_{12} = \lambda_{13} = \lambda) d\lambda, \tag{7.56}$$

$$\rho_1(\lambda_{12}, \lambda_{13}) = 1 / \lambda_{12}\lambda_{13}, \lambda_{12} > 0, \lambda_{13} > 0$$
$$\rho_0(\lambda) = 1 / \lambda, \lambda > 0 \tag{7.57}$$

In addition

$$f\left(T_{12},|\,T_{13},|\,\lambda_{12}=\lambda_{13}=\lambda\right)=\lambda^{n_1+n_2}\exp-\lambda\left(\sum_{i=1}^{i=n_1}T_{12}(i)+\sum_{i=1}^{i=n_2}T_{13}(i)\right),\quad (7.58)$$

$$f\left(T_{12}|\,\lambda_{12}\right)=\lambda_{12}^{n_{12}}\exp[-\lambda_{12}\left(\sum_{i=1}^{i=n_1}T_{12}(i)\right),\qquad (7.59)$$

and

$$f\left(T_{13}|\,\lambda_{13}\right)=\lambda_{13}^{n_{13}}\exp-\lambda_{13}\left(\sum_{i=1}^{i=n_2}T_{13}(i)\right).\qquad (7.60)$$

Note that $n_1 = n_2 = 15$, $\sum_{i=1}^{i=15}T_{12}(i)=35.2014$, and $\sum_{i-1}^{i=15}T_{13}(i)=140.7934$.

From the above information and assuming $\pi_0 = \pi_1$, it can be shown that the ratio $= 403$, thus, from (7.54) the posterior probability that the null hypothesis is true is $p_0 = .016$.

It is plausible that the null hypothesis is not true and that $\lambda_{12} \neq \lambda_{13}$.

Of course, this is not surprising because the $T_{12}(i)$ data are generated using the exponential distribution with parameter $\lambda_{12} = .5$, and the $T_{13}(i)$ data are generated using the exponential distribution with parameter $\lambda_{13} = .125$. The overall conclusion is that the average holding time for adenine until substituted with guanine is different (much smaller) than the holding time for adenine until substituted with cytosine.

Another generalization of DNA molecular evolution is described by Felsenstein and Churchill [7] with infinitesimal rate matrix

$$Q=\begin{pmatrix}-\alpha(1-p_a),\alpha p_g,\alpha p_c,\alpha p_t\\ \alpha p_a,-\alpha(1-p_g),\alpha p_c,\alpha p_t\\ \alpha p_a,\alpha p_g,-\alpha(1-p_c),\alpha p_t\\ \alpha p_a,\alpha p_g,\alpha p_c,-\alpha(1-p_t)\end{pmatrix}\qquad (7.61)$$

where the total holding time for adenine has an exponential distribution with parameter $\alpha p_g + \alpha p_c + \alpha p_t = \alpha(1-p_a)$, or mean $= 1/\alpha(1-p_a)$, until substituted with guanine, or cytosine, or thymine. It can be shown that the stationary distribution of this chain is $\pi = (p_a, p_g, p_c, p_t)$, where $p_a + p_g + p_c + p_t = 1$. Using Q

and π, thus determining that $P(t) = \exp(tQ)$, provides the probability transition matrix as

$$P_{ij}(t) = \left(1 - e^{-\alpha t}\right)p_j, i \neq j$$
$$= e^{-\alpha t} + \left(1 - e^{-\alpha t}\right)p_j, i = j$$

(7.62)

with $i, j = a, g, c, t$. Note these probabilities do not depend on the initial state i and that the effect of the scalar is to contract or expand the holding time parameter $= \alpha(1 - p_a)$ for adenine; therefore, it is of interest to investigate the value of α. This will be achieved in the special case $\pi = (.292, .207, .207, .292)$, the stationary distribution for humans. The first part of the Bayesian analysis is to estimate α using observations for the holding time of adenine. Of course, the holding time of any base could have been used to estimate α. I will assume that $\alpha = 1$, thus, the exponential parameter for the holding time of adenine is $(1 - p_a) = (1-.292) = .708$, which corresponds to an average holding time of 1.4124 time units. Fifteen observations will be generated from an exponential distribution with parameter .708, then based on these observations, a Bayesian analysis will be executed in order to estimate α. The Bayesian analysis is executed with 35,000 observations for the simulation and 5,000 for the burn in.

The results of the analysis are reported in Table 7.4. The prior distribution for λ is a noninformative gamma distribution, and the 15 data values included in the first list statement are generated with an exponential distribution with parameter .708.

BC 7.3

```
model;
{
#lamda has a gamma prior distribution with parameters .001 and
.001.
lamda~dgamma(.001,.001)
for ( i in 1:15){
# the HTa vector are the 15 holding times for adenine
HTa[i]~dexp(lamda)
}
# mu is the average holding time for adenine
mu<-1/lamda
# alpha is the main parameter of interest
alpha<-lamda/.708
}
list(
HTa = c(
2.116,2.221,1.37,4.389,1.027,
```

TABLE 7.4

Posterior Analysis for Felsenstein and Churchill [7] Model

Parameter	Mean	SD	Error	2 1/2	Median	97 1/2
α	.8528	.2202	.001089	.4789	.8325	1.337
λ	.6038	.1559	.000770	.339	.5894	.9464
μ	1.774	.4892	.002441	1.057	1.697	2.95

```
1.486,0.3714,3.178,0.5419,1.345,
0.002338,4.87,0.5304,1.235,0.1772))
# this is the starting value for lamda
list(lamda=.7)
```

Note that λ is the parameter for the exponential holding time for adenine, α is the main parameter of interest and is scale factor for the holding time, while μ is the average waiting time for adenine.

The main parameter of interest is α and is estimated as .8325 with the posterior median and a 95% credible interval of (.4789,1.337) which implies that it is plausible and reasonable to believe that $\alpha = 1$. Perhaps a more formal test of the null hypothesis

$$H : \alpha = 1 \quad \text{versus} \quad A : \alpha \neq 1. \tag{7.63}$$

is in order. Note the posterior density of α appears in Figure 7.1.

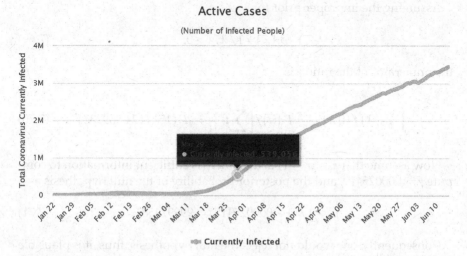

Active Cases

(Number of Infected People)

FIGURE 7.1

Number of infected versus time.

Note that the testing problem in terms of λ is

$$H : \lambda = .708 \quad \text{versus} \quad \lambda \neq .708. \tag{7.64}$$

The explanation of Lee [5, p. 126–127] is adopted for the Bayesian approach to testing a point null hypothesis. The posterior probability of the null hypothesis is given by

$$p_0 = 1/(1+\gamma) \tag{7.65}$$

where

$$\gamma = \pi_1 \int_0^\infty p_1(\lambda) f(t|\lambda) d\lambda / \pi_0 f(t|\lambda = .708). \tag{7.66}$$

In addition

$$f(t|\lambda = .708) = f(t|\lambda = .708) = (.708)^n \exp\left(-.708\left(\sum_{i=1}^{i=n} t_i\right)\right) \tag{7.67}$$

where the vector t is the $n = 15$ holding times in the list statement and

$$\sum_{i=1}^{i=n} t_i = 24.869239. \tag{7.68}$$

Assuming the improper prior for λ

$$p_1(\lambda) = 1/\lambda, \lambda > 0, \tag{7.69}$$

the numerator of the ratio γ is

$$\int_0^\infty p_1(\lambda) f(t|\lambda) d\lambda = \Gamma(n) / \left(\sum_{i=1}^n t_i\right)^n = \Gamma(15)/(24.869238)^{15}. \tag{7.70}$$

Now assume that $\pi_0 = \pi_1 = 1/2$, then there is sufficient information to compute $\gamma = .000025419$, and the posterior probability of the null hypothesis as

$$p_0 = 1/(1+.000025419) = .999974581. \tag{7.71}$$

Consequently, one would not reject the null hypothesis, thus, it is plausible to believe that $\alpha = 1$ and that the holding time for adenine has parameter $(1 - .292) = .708$, or an average holding time of 1.4124 time units.

Our last example for DNA evolution is a generalization of the Felsenstein-Churchill model to the Hasegawa, Kishino, and Yano [8] version for molecular evolution, with infinitesimal rate matrix

$$
Q = \begin{pmatrix}
-(\alpha p_g + \beta p_r), \alpha p_g, \beta p_c, \beta p_t \\
\alpha p_a, -(\alpha p_a + \beta p_r), \beta p_c, \beta p_t \\
\beta p_a, \beta p_g, -(\alpha p_t + \beta p_s), \alpha p_t \\
\beta p_a, \beta p_g, \alpha p_c, -(\alpha p_c + \beta p_s)
\end{pmatrix}.
\tag{7.72}
$$

where

$$
p_r = p_c + p_t, p_s = p_a + p_g,
$$

and

$$
p_a + p_g + p_c + p_t = 1.
$$

The parameters α and β are unknown positive parameters and the stationary distribution of the process is $\pi = (p_a, p_g, p_c, p_t)$.

This model makes a distinction between transitions and transversions, which distinguishes between the substitutions $a \leftrightarrow g$ (from purine to purine) or from pyrimidine to pyrimidine, and transversions, from purine to pyrimidine or vice versa, that is, the substitutions $c \leftrightarrow t$.

At the time this approach was based on a new statistical method for estimating divergence dates of species from DNA sequence data by a molecular clock. This method takes into account effectively the information contained in a set of DNA sequence data.

The molecular clock of mitochondrial DNA (mtDNA) was calibrated by setting the date of divergence between primates and ungulates at the Cretaceous-Tertiary boundary (65 million years ago), when the extinction of dinosaurs occurred.

Our investigation will center on the conjecture that $\alpha = \beta$, that the Hasegawa, Kishino, and Yano model (7.72) reduces to the Felsenstein-Churchill evolutionary process (7.61), that is, that the evolutionary process does not distinguish transversions from transitions. Thus, let the null hypothesis be

$$
H : \alpha = \beta \quad \text{versus the alternative } A : \alpha \neq \beta.
\tag{7.73}
$$

Then the null hypothesis supports the Felsenstein-Churchill process, and in order to illustrate Bayesian inferences, holding time data will be generated that favor the alternative hypothesis, the Hasegawa, Kishino, Yano model. Suppose $\alpha = 2$, $\beta = 8$ and the stationary distribution for humans, namely $p_a = .292$, $p_g = .207$, $p_c = .207$, and $p_t = .292$ is employed to fix the values of the first row of Q (2.72). Consider the holding time for adenine until substituted by quinine which is denoted by αp_g, and the holding time for thymine until substituted by adenine denoted by βp_a. I used $\alpha = 2$ and $\beta = 8$ to generate the holding times for adenine (until substituted by guanine) and thymine (until substituted by adenine), respectively, and these values appear in the list statement of BC 7.4.

There is sufficient information to execute the Bayesian analysis with 35,000 observations for the simulation and 5,000 for the burn in.

BC 7.4

```
model;
{
lamdaa~dgamma(.001,.001)
lamdat~dgamma(.001,.001)
for( i in 1:12){
# holding time for adenine
HTa[i]~dexp(lamdaa)
# holding time for adenine
HTt[i]~dexp(lamdat)}
# average holding time for thymine
# average holding time for adenine
mua<-1/lamdaa
# average holding time for thymine
mut<-1/lamdat
alpha<-lamdaa/pg
beta<-lamdat/pt
dat<-alpha-beta
# DNA nucleotide DNA bases for humans
pa<-.292
pg<-.207
pr<-.499
pt<-.292
}
list(
HTa = c(
2.831,0.4571,5.36,0.583,0.02068,
2.604,2.556,0.8819,2.356,1.371,
0.9336,1.711,1.012,0.324,0.2455),
HTt = c(
0.08592,0.01524,0.07607,0.5035,0.01662,
0.3833,1.271,0.714,1.07,0.04821,
0.2838,0.03206,1.259,0.7526,0.1634))
list(lamdaa=.414,lamdat=2.92)
```

The prior distribution for the exponential parameters λ_a and λ_t are non-informative gamma (.001,.001) distributions, the conjugate prior to the

TABLE 7.5

Posterior Analysis for the Hasegawa, Kishino, and Yano Model

Parameter	Mean	SD	Error	2 1/2	Median	97 1/2
α	2.675	.7658	.004055	1.389	2.599	4.379
β	9.135	2.642	.01419	4.736	8.858	15.04
d_{at}	−6.46	2.748	.01492	−12.51	−6.221	−1.749
λ_a	.5538	.1585	.000839	.2876	.538	.9064
λ_t	2.667	.7714	.004143	1.383	2.587	4.392
μ_a	1.968	.6191	.003331	1.103	1.859	3.477
μ_t	.4104	.1298	.000687	.2279	.3877	.7273

exponential distribution, thus, most of the information for the Bayesian analysis is based on the holding time observation HTa and HTt listed in BC 7.4 (Table 7.5).

Some of the posterior distributions are skewed; thus, the Bayesian estimates will be based on the posterior median. For example, consider α with an estimate of 2.559, which in turn should be compared with $\alpha = 2$, the value used to generate the data in the list statement of BC 7.4.

Also note that the posterior median of λ_a is .538 which is an exponential parameter for the holding time of adenine (before being substituted by guanine) and should be compared to $\lambda_a = .414$, the value used to generate the exponentially distributed holding times. The key parameter d_{at} is the difference between alpha and beta and its posterior median of −6.221 with a 95% credible interval of (−12.51,−1.747), which implies that $\alpha \neq \beta$.

It is left for the student to develop a formal Bayesian test of $\alpha = \beta$. For the Bayesian method of testing hypotheses, see Lee [5, p. 126–127]. Also, as in the previous example of molecular evolution (the Jukes-Cantor model), it is easy to derive the predictive density of a future adenine (or thymine) holding time, and this will be left as an exercise for the student.

7.6.2 Birth and Death Processes

The discrete time version of birth and death processes are presented in Chapter 5, Section 5.2, and the continuous time analog will be described in this section. Such processes are time reversible Markov chains that are quite valuable in a variety of scientific disciplines.

Let the present state of the chain be i, then the process can gain one unit corresponding to a birth or decrease one unit corresponding to a death, where $X(t), t > 0$ is the size of the population at time t. Since this is a continuous time process, the chain is defined in terms of the infinitesimal rate matrix

$$Q = \begin{pmatrix} -\lambda_0, \lambda_0, 0, 0, \ldots\ldots\ldots\ldots \\ \mu_1, -(\lambda_1 + \mu_1), \lambda_1, \ldots\ldots\ldots \\ 0, \mu_2, -(\lambda_2 + \mu_2), \lambda_2, \ldots\ldots \\ 0, 0, \mu_3, -(\lambda_3 + \mu_3), \lambda_3, \ldots \\ \ldots \\ \cdot\cdot \\ \cdot\cdot \end{pmatrix} \tag{7.74}$$

corresponding to the state space $S = \{0, 1, 2, \ldots \ldots\}$. The state 0 is an absorbing barrier, that is, once the population size reaches 0 it dies out. Thus, if the population size is 1, the holding time distribution of state 1 until the next death is exponential parameter μ_1, while on the other hand the holding time distribution of state 1 until a birth has an exponential distribution with parameter λ_1. Note the birth rates λ_i and death rates μ_i depend on the present size of the population.

Since the process is time reversible, one can derive the stationary distribution via the local balance equations

$$\pi_i \lambda_i = \pi_{i+1} \mu_{i+1}, \quad i = 0, 1, 2, \ldots \tag{7.75}$$

which implies that

$$\pi_1 = \pi_0 \lambda_0 / \mu_1,$$

and

$$\pi_2 = \pi_1 \lambda_1 / \mu_2 = \pi_0 \lambda_0 \lambda_1 / \mu_1 \mu_2$$

Thus, the pattern is

$$\pi_k = \pi_0 \lambda_0 \lambda_1 \ldots \lambda_{k-1} / \mu_1 \mu_2 \ldots \mu_k$$
$$= \pi_0 \prod_{i=1}^{i=k} \lambda_{i-1} / \mu_i, k = 0, 1, 2, \ldots \tag{7.76}$$

Since the stationary distribution is a probability distribution

$$1 = \sum_{k=0}^{k=\infty} \pi_k = \pi_0 \sum_{k=0}^{k=\infty} \prod_{i=0}^{i=k} \lambda_{i-1} / \mu_i, k = 0, 1, 2 \ldots \tag{7.77}$$

However, it is necessary to impose the constraint

$$\sum_{k=0}^{k=\infty}\prod_{i=0}^{i=k}\lambda_{i-1}/\mu_i < \infty, i = 1,2..$$

so that (2.77) converges, then the unique stationary distribution is determined as

$$\pi_k = \pi_0 \prod_{i=1}^{i=k}\lambda_{i-1}/\mu_i, k = 0,1,2,.. \text{ where}$$

$$\pi_0 = \left(\sum_{k=0}^{k=\infty}\prod_{i=1}^{i=k}\lambda_{i-1}/\mu_i\right)^{-1}. \tag{7.78}$$

In the infinite case, notice all states are transient except the absorbing state 0.

Now consider a finite state space with infinitesimal rate matrix and state space $S = \{0,1,2,3,4\}$

$$Q = \begin{pmatrix} -\lambda_0, \lambda_0, 0.0, 0.0, 0.00 \\ \mu_1, -(\mu_1 + \lambda_1), \lambda_1, 0, 0 \\ 0, \mu_2, -(\mu_2 + \lambda_2), \lambda_2, 0 \\ 0, 0, \mu_3, -(\mu_3 + \lambda_3), \lambda_3 \\ 0.0, 0.0, 0.0, \mu_4, -\mu_4 \end{pmatrix} \tag{7.79}$$

For the purpose of illustration, suppose $\mu_1 = 2$, $\lambda_1 = 1$, $\mu_2 = 3$, $\lambda_2 = 2, \mu_3 = 4$, and $\lambda_3 = 3$.

Using these values, I generated 20 holding times for six exponential holding times: From state 1 to 0 with parameter 2, from state 1 to 2 with parameter 1, from state 2 to 1 with parameter 3, from state 2 to 2 with parameter 2, from state 3 to 2 with parameter 4 and state 3 to 4 with parameter 3. These 6 holding tines are reported in the list statement of BC 7.5. Note that the birth rate for a population of size i is $\lambda_i/(\mu_i + \lambda_i)$ and the corresponding death rate is $\mu_i/(\mu_i + \lambda_i)$, $i = 1,2,3$. The following Bayesian analysis is executed with 45,000 observations for the simulation and 5,000 for the burn in.

BC 7.5

```
model;
{
mul~dgamma(.001,.001)
lamda1~dgamma(.001,.001)
mu2~dgamma(.001,.001)
lamda2~dgamma(.001,.001)
mu3~dgamma(.001,.001)
```

```
lamda3~dgamma(.001,.001)

for ( i in 1:20){
# is the vector of holding times when the process is in state
1 until the process switches to state 0
HT10[i]~dexp(mu1)
HT12[i]~dexp(lamda1)
HT21[i]~dexp(mu2)
HT23[i]~dexp(lamda2)
HT32[i]~dexp(mu3)
HT34[i]~dexp(lamda3)}
#p10 is the death rate when the population size is 1
p10<-mu1/(mu1+lamda1)
# p12 is the birth rate when the population is size 1
p12<-lamda1/(mu1+lamda1)
# p21 is the death rate when the population is size 2
p21<-mu2/(mu2+lamda2)
#p23 is the birth rate when the population is size 2
p23<-lamda2/(mu2+lamda2)
# p32 is the death rate when the population is size 3
p32<-mu3/(mu3+lamda3)
#p34 is the birth rate when the population is size 3
p34<-lamda3/(mu3+lamda3)
# the following is the average holding time for the process in
state 1 until it switches to state 0
nu1<-1/mu1
#the following is the average holding time for the process in
state 1 until it switches to state 2
vu1<-1/lamda1
nu2<-1/mu2
vu2<-1/lamda2
nu3<-1/mu3
vu3<-1/lamda3
}
list(
HT10 = c(
0.4236,0.0738,0.01755,0.2506,0.1679,
0.1345,0.1335,0.2103,0.5676,0.1256,
1.25,0.08106,0.08959,0.789,0.966,
0.4133,0.01223,0.08178,0.7944,0.2417),
HT12 = c(
0.6452,0.3766,0.4237,0.8919,0.1333,
0.2981,0.4902,0.1167,0.2695,0.7278,
0.2951,3.941,1.342,0.4537,0.9498,
1.354,0.5427,0.5481,0.1861,0.8717),
HT21 = c(
0.3853,0.0437,0.05582,0.1248,0.2109,
0.2065,0.5253,0.9537,0.07334,0.01717,
0.1436,0.2864,0.7099,0.04587,0.4547,
0.2007,0.438,0.5084,0.3366,0.4267),
```

```
HT23 = c(
0.2497,0.1747,0.09605,0.08779,0.1217,
0.1621,0.1332,0.255,2.358,1.472,
0.2527,0.6953,1.937,0.191,1.772,
0.2749,0.03768,0.1866,0.41,1.134),
HT32 = c(
0.007235,0.07714,0.02351,0.3239,0.1192,
0.2329,0.3503,0.1093,0.1339,0.5003,
0.2394,0.336,0.08296,0.229,0.06038,
0.07797,0.125,0.035,0.2428,0.4869),
HT34 = c(
1.067,0.2683,0.6207,0.1697,0.1857,
0.1188,0.2984,0.03796,0.2262,0.4814,
0.5348,0.4655,0.3812,0.1125,0.00313,
0.9027,0.0557,0.4312,0.4711,0.1909))
list(mu1=2,mu2=3,mu3=4,lamda1= 1,lamda2=2,lamda3=3)
```

The Bayesian analysis employs the exponential distribution with parameter μ_i, as the likelihood function for μ_i, and uses the non-informative prior gamma (.001,.001) for the μ_i, while for the birth rate parameter λ_i, its likelihood has an exponential distribution with parameter λ_i and prior gamma (.001,001). Refer to **BC 7.5** for the statements corresponding to the likelihood function and prior of the λ_i and μ_i, $i = 1, 2, 3$ (Table 7.6).

TABLE 7.6

Posterior Analysis for Birth and Death Process

Parameter	Mean	SD	Error	2 ½	Median	97 1/2
λ_1	1.345	.3015	.001345	.8237	1.322	2
λ_2	1.666	.3725	.001656	1.016	1.637	2.475
λ_3	2.852	.6333	.002825	1.749	2.806	4.222
μ_1	2.927	.6571	.002994	1.787	2.877	4.347
μ_2	3.25	.7288	.003365	1.988	3.196	4.825
μ_3	5.268	1.174	.005562	3.225	5.176	7.089
η_1	.3598	.08517	.0003899	.23	.3476	.5595
η_2	.3239	.0763	.0003522	.2072	.3129	.50321
η_3	.1997	.04686	.000214	.1281	.1932	.31
p_{10}	.6812	.06828	.000299	.5362	.6852	.8032
p_{12}	.3188	.06828	.000299	.1968	.31248	.4638
p_{21}	.6575	.07082	.000335	.5092	.6612	.7852
p_{23}	.3425	.07082	.000335	.2148	.3388	.4908
p_{32}	.6454	.07145	.000327	.498	.6488	.7756
p_{34}	.3546	.07145	.000327	.2244	.3512	.502
ν_1	.7827	.1847	.000854	.5001	.7567	1.214
ν_2	.6317	.1487	.000664	.4041	.6109	.9846
ν_3	.3689	.08655	.000398	.2369	.3564	.5718

The Bayesian analysis is for the three birthrates λ_i, $i = 1, 2, 3$ and death rates μ_i, $i = 1, 2, 3$. The corresponding average holding times for the deaths are given by the η_i, $i = 1, 2, 3$ and by the ν_i, $i = 1, 2, 3$ for the births.

The transition probabilities are denoted by p_{10}, p_{12}, p_{21}, p_{23}, p_{32}, and p_{34}, and 20 exponential holding times for the death and births are generated, thus the transition probabilities are based on 20 transition to the neighboring states.

Consider the transition probability p_{12} from a population of one to a population of size 2 (because of a birth), then the corresponding posterior mean is .3188 with 95% credible interval (.1968,.4638). On the other hand, the posterior mean of p_{10} is .6812 with 95% credible interval (.5362,.8034) implying that the chances are higher for the population to become extinct than to increase by 1.

The next inference to be considered is the estimation of the average time to extinction for the process

$$Q = \begin{pmatrix} -\lambda_0, \lambda_0, 0.0, 0.0, 0.00 \\ \mu_1, -(\mu_1 + \lambda_1), \lambda_1, 0, 0 \\ 0, \mu_2, -(\mu_2 + \lambda_2), \lambda_2, 0 \\ 0, 0, \mu_3, -(\mu_3 + \lambda_3), \lambda_3 \\ 0.0, 0.0, 0.0, \mu_4, -\mu_4 \end{pmatrix} \tag{7.80}$$

where $\mu_1 = 2$, $\lambda_1 = 1$, $\mu_2 = 3$, $\lambda_2 = 2$, $\mu_3 = 4$, $\lambda_3 = 3$, and $\mu_4 = 4$. In the list statement of BC 7.6 appears the 20 observations for the data labeled HT4, the holding times with exponential parameter $\mu_4 = 4$.

The other holding times were used in BC 7.5. Our main goal is the estimation of the average time to extinction using the patter (2.79), and the following formula given that parameter.

Consider a birth and death process with state space $\{0,1,2,\ldots,k\}$ with one absorbing state 0, where the remaining are transient states and let V be the $(k-1)$ by $(k-1)$ matrix of transient states, and let $F = -V^{-1}$, then the average time to absorption from state i, $i = 1,2,\ldots k$ is

$$a_i = \sum_{i=1}^{i=k} F_{ij}, \tag{7.81}$$

where F_{ij} is the ij-th element of F. See Dobrow [1, pp. 288–289] for a proof.

BC 7.6. is the WinBugs code for estimating the average time to extinction for the birth and death process with matrix Q (2.79). Non-informative gamma (.001,.001) distributions were used as priors for the parameters: the death rates μ_i, $i = 1, 2, 3, 4$ and birth rates λ_i, $i = 1, 2, 3$. The Bayesian analysis is executed with 57,000 observations and 1,000 for the burn in (Table 7.7).

TABLE 7.7

Posterior Analysis for Extinction

Parameter	Mean	SD	Error	2 ½	Median	97 1/2
a_1	.4248	.4461	.001472	.2738	.399	.6533
a_2	.5676	1.36	.004491	.3172	.493	1.028
a_3	.6699	5.77	.01083	.2741	.4882	1.638
a_4	1.063	5.77	.01919	.3704	.7253	2.844

BC 7.6

```
model;
{

#prior distributions for the parameters

lamda1~dgamma(.001,.001)
mu1~dgamma(.001,.001)
lamda2~dgamma(.001,.001)
mu2~dgamma(.001,.001)
lamda3~dgamma(.001,.001)
mu3~dgamma(.001,.001)
mu4~dgamma(.001,.001)
for ( i in 1:20){
# the seven holding times for (2.79)
HT10[i]~dexp(mu1)
HT12[i]~dexp(lamda1)
HT21[i]~dexp(mu2)
HT23[i]~dexp(lamda2)
HT32[i]~dexp(mu3)
HT34[i]~dexp(lamda3)
HT4[i]~dexp(mu4)}
# the -V matrix
v[1,1]<-mu1+lamda1
v[1,2]<-(-lamda1)
v[1,3]<-0
v[1,4]<-0
v[2,1]<-(-mu2)
v[2]<-mu2+lamda2
v[2, 3]<- (-lamda2)
v[2, 4]<-0
v[3,1]<-0
v[2, 3]<-(-mu3)
v[3]<-mu3+lamda3
v[3, 4]<-(-lamda3)
v[4,1]<-0
v[2, 4]<-0
```

```
v[3, 4]<-(-mu4)
v[4]<-mu4
# F is the inverse of -V.
F[1:4,1:4]<-inverse(v[1:4,1:4])
}
list(
HT10 = c(
0.4236,0.0738,0.01755,0.2506,0.1679,
0.1345,0.1335,0.2103,0.5676,0.1256,
1.25,0.08106,0.08959,0.789,0.966,
0.4133,0.01223,0.08178,0.7944,0.2417),
HT12 = c(
0.6452,0.3766,0.4237,0.8919,0.1333,
0.2981,0.4902,0.1167,0.2695,0.7278,
0.2951,3.941,1.342,0.4537,0.9498,
1.354,0.5427,0.5481,0.1861,0.8717),
HT21 = c(
0.3853,0.0437,0.05582,0.1248,0.2109,
0.2065,0.5253,0.9537,0.07334,0.01717,
0.1436,0.2864,0.7099,0.04587,0.4547,
0.2007,0.438,0.5084,0.3366,0.4267),
HT23 = c(
0.2497,0.1747,0.09605,0.08779,0.1217,
0.1621,0.1332,0.255,2.358,1.472,
0.2527,0.6953,1.937,0.191,1.772,
0.2749,0.03768,0.1866,0.41,1.134),
HT32 = c(
0.007235,0.07714,0.02351,0.3239,0.1192,
0.2329,0.3503,0.1093,0.1339,0.5003,
0.2394,0.336,0.08296,0.229,0.06038,
0.07797,0.125,0.035,0.2428,0.4869),
HT34 = c(
1.067,0.2683,0.6207,0.1697,0.1857,
0.1188,0.2984,0.03796,0.2262,0.4814,
0.5348,0.4655,0.3812,0.1125,0.00313,
0.9027,0.0557,0.4312,0.4711,0.1909),
HT4 = c(
0.7442,0.4533,0.07353,0.03283,0.1242,
1.001,0.1311,1.057,0.09183,0.226,
0.3407,0.1795,0.01064,0.003547,0.3841,
0.6416,0.06772,0.06674,0.2898,0.1095)))
list(mu1=2,mu2=3,mu3=4,mu4=4,lamda1= 1,lamda2=2,lamda3=3)
```

The posterior distributions are skewed thus the posterior medians should be used as point estimators. For example, when the process is in state 4, the posterior median is .7252 time units, but if the process is in state 1, the posterior median time to extinction is .399 time units. This seems to appear to be reasonable because closer states to the absorbing state 0 have smaller posterior medians.

7.6.3 A Random Walk

The random walk is a birth and death process with constant birth rate $\lambda_i = \lambda$ and death rate $\mu_i = \mu$, that is, the birth and death rates do not depend on the population size. From what is known about the general birth and death process, see (7.79), the stationary distribution is

$$\pi_k = \pi_0 \prod_{i=1}^{i=k} (\lambda / \mu) = \pi_0 (\lambda / \mu)^k, k = 0,1,.. \tag{7.82}$$

where $\lambda < \mu$ and

$$\pi_0 = \left(\sum_{k=0}^{k=\infty} (\lambda / \mu)^k \right)^{-1} = 1 - \lambda / \mu. \tag{7.83}$$

Thus, the stationary distribution is geometric, namely

$$\pi_k = (1 - \lambda / \mu)(\lambda / \mu), k = 0,1,2,.. \tag{7.84}$$

Bayesian inferences will focus on estimating the rates μ and λ, and testing the hypothesis that $\lambda < \mu$. Recall that for this process, the infinitesimal rate matrix is

$$Q = \begin{pmatrix} -\lambda, \lambda, 0, 0, \dots\dots\dots\dots \\ \mu, -(\mu + \lambda), \lambda, 0, 0, \dots\dots \\ 0, \mu, -(\mu + \lambda), \lambda, 0, \dots\dots \\ 0, 0, \mu, -(\mu + \lambda), \lambda, 0, \dots \\ \cdot \\ \cdot \end{pmatrix}. \tag{7.85}$$

Observations for the holding times with exponential parameters λ and μ will be generated; then based on those observations, Bayesian inferences will be presented. Suppose that $\lambda = 2 < \mu = 5$. The likelihood functions for λ and μ are determined by the exponential density and the 17 holding time observations denoted by HT2, for λ and HT5 for μ. Non-informative gamma (.001,.001) distributions are assumed for the two unknown parameters. The objective of the Bayesian analysis is to estimate the stationary distribution of the random walk and to estimate

$\Pr(\lambda > \mu \mid data)$, thus testing the hypothesis $H : \lambda > \mu$.

The following WinBUGS code BC 7.7 is executed with 35,000 observations for the simulation, and a burn in of 5,000 (Table 7.8).

TABLE 7.8

Posterior Analysis for Random Walk

Parameter	Mean	SD	Error	2 1/2	Median	97 1/2
diff	−5.66	1.985	.01111	−9.939	−5.506	−2.185
λ	2.19	.526	.003034	1.286	2.148	3.332
m_2	.4846	.1241	.000729	.3002	.4656	.7778
m_5	.1345	.03501	.000207	.08321	.1304	.219
μ	7.85	1.915	.01085	4.567	7.671	12.01
π_1	.1974	.03646	.000126	.1209	.2013	.2495
π_2	.06812	.03107	.000106	.01713	.05645	.1354
π_3	.02151	.01953	.000066	.00242	.01581	.07544
π_4	.008273	.01373	.000046	.000341	.00442	.04181
π_5	.003485	.01363	.000046	.000482	.00124	.02316
$\Pr(\lambda > \mu)$	.0001333	.01155	.000053	0	0	0

BC 7.7

```
model;
{
# the prior distributions for lamda and mu
lamda~dgamma(.001,.001)
mu~dgamma(.001,.001)
for ( i in 1:17){
HT2[i]~dexp(lamda)
HT5[i]~dexp(mu) }
m2<-1/lamda
m5<-1/mu
# the pi[k] are the stationary probabilities
for( k in 0:5){
pi[k]<-(1-lamda/mu)*pow(lamda/mu,k) }
diff<-lamda-mu
#prob is the Pr(λ > μ)
prob<-step(diff)
}
list(
HT2 = c(
1.155,0.1775,1.513,0.1776,0.9627,
0.602,0.05385,0.2169,0.1129,0.3904,
0.7396,0.06482,0.09624,0.1167,0.5177,
0.511,0.3539),
HT5 = c(
0.09529,0.1754,0.4323,0.04315,0.01035,
0.05834,0.05996,0.09225,0.07383,0.1131,
0.1176,0.1822,0.1276,0.2809,0.001542,
0.01506,0.2859))
list( mu=5,lamda=2)
```

The posterior distributions for the parameters of the random walk appear to be symmetric about the posterior mean, and it also appears that $\lambda < \mu$ because the 95% credible interval for the difference $\lambda - \mu$ excludes zero and has a negative posterior mean of -5.66. It should be remembered that the 17 holding times are generated with the values $\lambda = 2 < \mu = 5$. With such a small sample size, it is not surprising that the posterior means for λ and μ are not very close to their hypothetical values.

The hypothesis $\lambda > \mu$ has posterior probability 0, as measured by the posterior median; thus, one would conclude that $\lambda < \mu$, further implying that the stationary distribution is well defined in that the geometric series (7.84) converges!

7.6.4 The Yule Process

The Yule process is a pure birth process where each individual has the same rate λ of a birth; thus, if the population size is i, the rate probability of a birth is λi, $i = 1, 2, 3, ..$ with infinitesimal rate matrix

$$Q = \begin{pmatrix} -\lambda, \lambda, 0, 0, 0, 0, 0, 0, 0, 0...... \\ 0, -2\lambda, 2\lambda, 0, 0, 0, 0, 0........ \\ 0, 0, -3\lambda, 3\lambda, 0, 0, 0, 0, 0..... \\ . \\ 0, 0, 0, 0, 0, -i\lambda, i\lambda, 0, 0, 0,... \\ : \\ . \end{pmatrix} \qquad (7.86)$$

Note for such a process all states are transient and the limiting probability does not exist. It is easily shown that the transition function is

$$P_{ij}(t) = \binom{j-1}{i-1} e^{-i\lambda t} \left(1 - e^{-\lambda t}\right)^{j-1}, i \le j, t > 0 \qquad (7.87)$$

which is the negative binomial distribution. In particular, starting with a population of size 1, the probability the size remains at 1 at time t is given by

$$P_{11}(t) = \exp(-\lambda t). \qquad (7.88)$$

Of concern to the Bayesian is the estimation of λ and of the transition probability (7.87). This is easily accomplished by generating holding times with an exponential distribution with parameter λ.

Using the 20 observations for the holding times with exponential parameter $\lambda = 3$, the Bayesian analysis consists of estimating λ and the probability function (7.88), the probability that the population remains at one individual for times $t = 1,2,...$ The analysis is executed with 35,000 observations for the simulation and a burn in of 5,000.

BC 7.8

```
model;
{
lamda~dgamma(.01,.01)
for ( i in 1:20){
HT[i]~dexp(lamda)}
for ( t in 1:10){
p11[t]<-exp(-lamda*t)}
}
list(
HT = c(
0.9923,0.6045,0.09804,0.04378,0.1655,
1.335,0.1748,1.409,0.1224,0.3013,
0.4542,0.2393,0.01419,0.004729,0.5122,
0.8555,0.09029,0.08898,0.3865,0.146))
list(lamda=3)
```

The results of the Bayesian analysis are reported in Table 7.9. Note that the posterior mean of λ is 2.4876 with a 95% credible interval of (1.525,3.691), and the posterior mean of $P_{11}(1)$ is .096 and that the posterior mean of b $P_{11}(t)$, $t = 2, 3$ is decreasing as it should.

It is straightforward to test hypotheses about λ and to derive the formula for future holding times with exponential parameter λ. The student will be asked to perform these inferences as problems in the end of Chapter 7.

7.6.5 Birth and Death With Immigration

From the least complex, such as the Yule process, to the more complicated, we now study the so-called birth and death process with immigration. Note these processes are highly related to epidemics, in that in an epidemic, there are deaths, and at the same time births too indeed occur.

TABLE 7.9

Posterior Analysis for the Yule Process

Parameter	Mean	SD	Error	2 1/2	Median	97 1/2
λ	2.486	.5562	.003134	1.525	2.441	3.691
$P_{11}(1)$	.096	.05049	.0002882	.02494	.08711	.2176
$P_{11}(2)$	.01177	.01308	.0000755	.0006221	.007589	.04733
$P_{11}(3)$	.001757	.003381	.0000201	.0000155	.000661	.0103

Suppose the immigration with rate ν is included in the simple birth and death process, then the infinitesimal rate matrix is

$$Q = \begin{pmatrix} -\nu,\nu,0,0,0,0,0,0,0,\ldots\ldots\ldots\ldots\ldots\ldots\ldots\ldots \\ \mu,-(\nu+\lambda+\mu),\nu+\lambda,0,0,0,0,\ldots\ldots\ldots\ldots \\ 0,2\mu,-(\nu+2(\lambda+\mu)),\nu+2\lambda,0,0,0,0,\ldots\ldots \\ 0,0,3\mu,-(\nu+3(\lambda+\mu)),\nu+3\lambda,0,0,0\ldots\ldots \\ \vdots \end{pmatrix}$$ (7.89)

where the rates μ, ν, and λ are positive and are the parameters of the relevant holding times, which have an exponential distribution.

Referring to (7.89), it is apparent that if the population is 0 it can increase by one person if one person immigrates to the population. Our goal is to estimate the parameters and to test hypotheses about those parameters. In order to perform a Bayesian analysis, let $\mu = 1/2$, $\nu = 1/3$, and $\lambda = 1$, that is, if the population is size i ($i = 1,2,..$), the average number of immigrants per day is 3, the average number of births is 1, and the average number of deaths is 2 per day. Note the birth and death rates depend on the present population size, but the immigration rate does not. The Bayesian analysis is relatively straightforward and is executed with **BC 7.9** with noninformative prior gamma(.01,.01) distributions and using 35,000 observations for the simulation and a burn in of 5,000.

BC 7.9

```
model;
{
lamda~dgamma(.01,.01)
mu~dgamma(.01,.01)
nu~dgamma(.01,.01)
for( i in 1:16){
HTmu[i]~dexp(mu)
HTvu[i]~dexp(nu)
HTlamda[i]~dexp(lamda)}
mua<-1/mu
nua<-1/nu
lamdaa<-1/lamda
}
list(
HTlamda = c(
1.159,1.833,0.2687,0.1907,0.2907,
0.2291,0.6853,0.5028,0.6184,2.253,
0.3,3.233,0.9386,0.9576,1.274,
0.2392),
```

```
HTmu = c(
0.1633,0.3263,0.7803,0.5374,0.9227,
0.2175,0.6166,0.9843,7.635,0.8423,
0.2366,0.7924,3.172,0.6005,0.4124,
0.08125),
HTvu = c(
2.049,1.409,3.333,4.758,5.905,
0.03409,6.001,1.666,0.281,1.086,
3.418,1.319,2.271,0.4253,6.108,
5.066))
list(lamda=1,vu=.333,mu=.5)
```

The Bayesian analysis for the immigration model is portrayed in Table 7.10.

The main parameter of interest is the immigration rate and the average number of immigrants per day.

With regard to this rate, the posterior mean is .3544 with a 95% credible interval (.2003,.5478), while for the average, the posterior median is 2.884 with posterior standard deviation .7985. Note the asymmetry in the posterior distribution of $E(\nu)$ which is easily seen with its posterior density. Also note that the 95% credible interval for λ includes the value 1, the 95% credible interval for μ includes ½ and that for ν contains 1/3. What does this imply about the generated holding times HTmu, HTnu, and HTlamda?

TABLE 7.10

Posterior Distributions for Birth and Death with Immigration

Parameter	Mean	SD	Error	2 1/2	Median	97 1/2
λ	1.07	.2679	.001294	.6131	1.047	1,661
$E(\lambda)$	.9971	.2663	.001282	.6002	.9551	1.631
μ	.8717	.2181	.001046	.4999	.8513	1.35
$E(\mu)$	1.223	.3249	.001632	.7408	1.175	2.001
ν	.3544	.08832	.000458	.2033	.3468	.5478
$E(\nu)$	3.008	.7985	.004228	1.825	2.884	4.919

7.6.6 SI Epidemic Models

This section introduces the continuous time version of epidemic models and is a generalization of the discrete version of stochastic epidemic model of Sections 5.4.2 and 5.4.3 of Chapter 5. Recall the dynamics of SI and SIS models where the number of susceptible people at time t is denoted by $S(t)$ and the number of infected individuals given by $I(t)$. Infected individuals are also infectious that is there is no latent period and the total population size $N = I(t) + S(t)$ remains constant over the period of observation. This SI model has been used to explain such diseases as the common cold and influenza where the epidemic is best described by the system of differential equations

$$dS(t)/dt = -(\beta/N)S(t)I(t)$$
and $\qquad\qquad\qquad\qquad\qquad\qquad\qquad\qquad$ (7.90)
$$dI(t)/dt = (\beta/N)S(t)I(t)$$

where $S(0) + I(0) = N$ and β is the transmission rate , the number of contacts per unit time that result in an infection of a susceptible individual. Allen [3, pp. 302–308] presents a more detailed account of the SI and SIS models and is an excellent reference of the general area of stochastic epidemics.

For the stochastic version the infinitesimal generator matrix for the number of infected individuals with state space $\{0,1,2,...,N\}$ is given as

$$Q = \begin{pmatrix} -\beta(N-1)/N, \beta(N-1)/N, 0, 0, 0, ... \\ 0, -2\beta(N-2)/N, 2\beta(N-2)/N, 0, 0, 0, ... \\ 0, 0, -3\beta(N-3)/N, 3\beta(N-3)/N, 0, 0, ... \\ . \\ . \\ . \\ 0, 0, 0, 0, ...-\beta(N-1)/N, \beta(N-1)/N \\ 0, 0, 0, 0, ...0, 0 \end{pmatrix} . \quad (7.91)$$

The only unknown parameter is the transmission rate β, the number of contacts per unit time of infected individuals with susceptible people resulting in an infection.

The holding time for state 1 (with one infected individual) is $2\beta(N-2)/N$, How should β be estimated ? Remember that $\gamma = 2\beta(N-2)/N$ is the parameter for the holding time for one infected individual (until the number of infected increase to 2 infected individuals) and that holding time has an exponential distribution. Suppose that $\beta = 3$ and $N = 6$, then $\gamma = 4$, thus, I will generate 16 holding times with parameter $\gamma = 4$ and use those to estimate γ and consequently $\beta = 3\gamma/4$. The main parameters of interest are β, the contact rate, γ the parameter of the exponential distribution for the holding time of one infected individual, and $E(HT1)$ the average holding time for one infected individual. Bayesian inferences are based on BC 7.10 which is executed with 35,000 observations for the simulation and a burn in of 5,000 (Table 7.11):

TABLE 7.11

Posterior Analysis for the SI Epidemic Model

Parameter	Mean	SD	Error	2 1/2	Median	97 1/2
β	3.204	.8015	.004305	1.839	3.131	4.966
γ	4.272	1.069	.00574	2.452	4.174	6.621
E(HT1)	.2496	.06625	.000362	.151	.2396	.4078

BC 7.10

```
model;
{
# gamma is the parameter for the exponential distribution of
the holding time for one infected
# gamma has a noninformative gamma distribution
gamma~dgamma(.001,.001)
for ( i in 1:16){
HT1[i]~dexp(gamma)}
beta<-3*gamma/4
EFT1<-1/gamma
}
# the following times were generated with an exponential
distribution with parameter 4
list(
HT1 = c(
0.3804,0.03817,0.1017,0.3212,0.2032,
0.4066,0.3085,0.4867,0.2681,0.07279,
0.1096,0.04133,0.5914,0.2417,0.1273,
0.04811))
list(gamma=4)
```

The values of the parameters used to generate the holding times in the list statement of BC 7.11 are $N = 6$, $\gamma = 4$, and $\beta = 3$, and these values should be compared to the corresponding posterior means appearing in Table 7.10, the posterior analysis for the epidemic model. For example, the posterior mean of γ is 4.272 with a 95% credible interval of (2.452,6.621), implying informally that the generated holding times were indeed distributed as an exponential with parameter $\gamma = 4$. Note the average holding time for one infected individual is .2496 days as estimated by the posterior mean.

7.6.7 Stochastic SIS Epidemic Model

A generalization of the SI model is the SIS where individuals who are infected can recover but do not develop immunity and can immediately become infected again, which is graphically represented as

$S \to I \to S$. This is a birth and death process with $\mu_i = (\gamma + b)i$ and $\lambda_i = \max\{0, (\beta/N)i(N - i)\}$, where i is the size of the population.

Let $S(t)$ and $I(t)$ be the number of susceptible and infected individuals at time t then the number of new susceptible individuals at the next instant equals the people that did not become infected $[1 - \beta I(t)/N]$, plus those that recovered $\gamma I(t)$, plus newborns among the infected class $bI(t)$.

Corresponding to the number of infected $\{I(t), t > 0\}$, the infinitesimal rate matrix is

$$Q = \begin{pmatrix} -(\beta/N)N, (\beta/N)N, 0, 0, \dots \dots \dots \dots \dots \dots \dots \dots \dots \dots \dots \dots \\ (b+\gamma), -\big[(\beta/N)(N-1)+(b+\gamma)\big], (\beta/N)(N-1), 0, 0, 0, \dots \\ 0, 2(b+\gamma), -\big[2(\beta/N)(N-2)+2(b+\gamma)\big], 2(\beta/N)(N-2), 0, 0, \dots \\ \vdots \end{pmatrix}$$

Consider the example presented by Allen [3, pp. 308–309] with $\beta = 2$, $N = 100$, and $\gamma + b = 1$. Our goal is to estimate β, $(b + \gamma)$, and $R_0 = \beta - (b + \gamma)$. Note that for one infected individual the holding time (until a new infection) is $(\beta/N)(N-1) + (b+\gamma) = 2.98$, and the holding time for a population with two infected people is $(2\beta/N)(N-2) + 2(b+\gamma) = 5.92$.

Using the values $\lambda_1 = 2.98$ and $\lambda_2 = 5.92$ for the parameters of the exponential distribution for the holding times for one and two infected individuals, 17 observations are generated for both and labeled as HT1 and HT2, respectively. These holding times are in the list statement of BC 7.11 which is the Bayesian analysis executed with 45,000 observations for the simulation and 5,000 for the burn in.

BC 7.11

```
model;
{
lamda1~dgamma(.001,.001)
lamda2~dgamma(.001,.001)
for( i in 1:18){
HT1[i]~dexp(lamda1)
HT2[i]~dexp(lamda2)}
beta<-(lamda1-1)/.99
delta<-(lamda2-1.96*beta)/2
 R<-beta-delta
S<-step(R)
p10<-delta/(delta+beta*.99)
}
list(
HT1 = c(
0.3496,0.9303,0.6686,0.7489,0.1625,
0.2897,0.06194,0.3293,0.1065,0.04272,
0.07717,0.2257,0.3087,0.004282,0.0615,
0.5061,0.1497,0.3919),
HT2 = c(
0.3002,0.01733,0.3756,0.02314,0.2873,
0.1072,0.2551,0.474,0.1629,0.1206,
0.4864,0.1873,0.01003,0.01907,0.3545,
0.2151,0.03929,0.007648)))
list(lamda1=2.98,lamda2=5.92)
```

TABLE 7.12

Posterior Analysis for a SIS Epidemic

Parameter	Mean	SD	Error	2 ½	Median	97 1/2
$R = \beta - \delta$	2.035	1.681	.00784	−.9977	1.935	5.607
Pr $(R > 0)$	.8947	.3069	.001435	0	1	1
β	2.346	.789	.003505	.9849	2.284	4.057
$\delta = b + \gamma$	.3112	.9907	.004777	−1.696	.3269	2.224
λ_1	3.323	.7811	.00347	1.975	3.261	5.017
λ_2	5.221	1.237	.005924	3.091	5.111	7.93
p_{10}	.06774	.392	.002323	−.8665	.1262	.6561

The posterior analysis is reported in Table 7.12. One can see the effect of the data, the holding time on the estimation of the parameters. For example, the value of $b + \gamma$ used to generate the holding times is 1, but the posterior mean of this parameter is .3112 with a 95% credible interval (−1.696,2.224) does indeed include 1. Also, the value of β was set to 2 for generating the holding times; however, its posterior mean is 2.346 with a 95% credible interval (.0035,2.284) but does include the value 2.

Consider

$$p_{10} = (b+\gamma)/\left[.99\beta + (b+\gamma)\right], \tag{7.92}$$

the probability the epidemic will change from one to zero infected people. It is seen that its posterior mean is .06774 and its posterior median is .1262, implying skewness in this posterior distribution.

7.7 The SIR Model

How many people are now infected with the coronavirus, SARS CoV-2, and how many will be infected tomorrow? This is the question asked by Patrick Bell, Director of research at the Human Rights Data Analysis Group. See pages 12-13 of the June 2020, Volume 12, Issue 3 of *Significance*. These are difficult questions to answer, because we do not know just who is infected, which people are interacting with others, and we do not know if the people around an infected person become infected or not. The basic ideas on how to estimate how many people are likely to become sick will be described.

In the US as of April 9, there is a severe shortage of tests for SARS-CoV-2, the virus that causes people to become sick with covid-19. Thus, even individuals in the hospital displaying obvious symptoms are rarely tested. In addition, it is now apparent that people infected with the disease display little or no symptoms. The combination of these factors implies that only a small fraction of SARS-CoV-2 cases are confirmed by a positive test. In reality, the confirmed cases count gives us the message more about the availability and extent of tests than the prevalence of infection. Thus, the true number of SARS-CoV-2 positive cases is higher than the reported counts.

The total size of the infected population determines how many people will need critical care, and how many will eventually die. It is important for those dealing in health-planning, economic policy, and public communication to be able to determine the population prevalence if SARS-CoV-2. The foundation of epidemiological modeling is the SIR model, which allows one to estimate the daily progression of three subpopulations: S, the number of susceptible people, I, the number of infected and, R the number removed. See the previous section for the Bayesian analysis of how to examine such an epidemic.

For any one day, the population is partitioned into people still susceptible to the virus, the people infected with the virus, and the people who have been removed. This relationship is depicted as

$$N = S_t + I_t + R_t \qquad (7.93)$$

Where t denotes day t.

The number of deaths on each day is specified by D_t and is usually determined without too much error. There is still some error in this term because deaths due to the virus a sometimes mistaken as death due to other causes.

What does one mean by susceptible? It means those who have the opportunity to become infected. It is important to note that the number susceptible on day t is equal to the number susceptible on day t-1, minus the number η_t who are infected for the first time at day t , which is given by the formula

$$S_t = S_{t-1} - \eta_t \qquad (7.94)$$

As long as people can only become infected once, the number of infected continue to decrease.

It is important to know that the people who recover and are no longer sick each day is a fraction δ of all the people infected up to and including yesterday, minus all the people who succumbed up to and including yesterday denoted by $\delta(I_{t-1} - D_{t-1})$ where δ is a fraction between 0 and 1 and denotes how many people are recovering.

Now we turn our attention to the number of infected I_t, where

$$I_t = I_{t-1} + \eta_t - D_{t-1} - \delta\left(I_{t-1} - D_{t-1}\right) \qquad (7.95)$$

that is the number of people infected today is equal to the number infected yesterday, plus the number newly infected today, minus the people who died yesterday, minus the number who recovered yesterday. Note this number increases as new infections occur and decrease as people recover or die.

How about the number removed? The number removed on day t is equal to the number removed yesterday, plus the number who died yesterday, plus those that recovered yesterday, which gives one the formula

$$R_t = R_{t-1} + D_{t-1} + \delta\left(I_{t-1} - D_{t-1}\right). \tag{7.96}$$

What about those who are newly infected? The appropriate formula is

$$\eta_t = S_{t-1}\beta I_{t-1} / N \tag{7.97}$$

where β is an index of infectiousness and is related to the term R_0 found in epidemiology which signifies the average number of people that each person newly infects.

Another important concept is the infected fatality rate. Consider the fraction of the infected who will eventually die must equal the total deaths (adding over all days) divided by the total number infected, given by

$$\rho = \left[\sum_{i=0}^{i=t} D_i / \left(I_t + R_t\right)\right]. \tag{7.98}$$

A careful interpretation of this rate is in order. The rate may change as the health care system becomes overloaded, or if new treatments prove successful. Of course, it varies with age and with co-morbidities such as diabetes, hypertension, etc.

This is all very relevant to the coronavirus pandemic, and the reader is referred to the daily briefings of the CDC.

We now summarize the ideas and concepts introduced in the current Section 7.7. The SIR values can be estimated by knowing the relationship among them and from information from clinical trials. The New York Times for an interactive online tool (nyti.ms/3cFqpNf) and gives the user a chance to see the immediate effects of changing the parameters of the model. It is understood that Covid-19 is a generic epidemic which has its own values as parameters. Of course, policy and human behavior influence the value of the parameters in the model. We have seen this before in Section 7.6.6, where the main parameters if the SIR epidemic model are expressed with the infinitesimal generator matrix Q. There are different models to express different aspects of the behavior of the coronavirus pandemic.

The figures below give the relevant information for calculating the unknown parameters λ, β, and ρ of the SIR model for the coronavirus pandemic.

The first is the number of infections recorded from January 22 to June 10, 2020 (Figures 7.2 and 7.3)

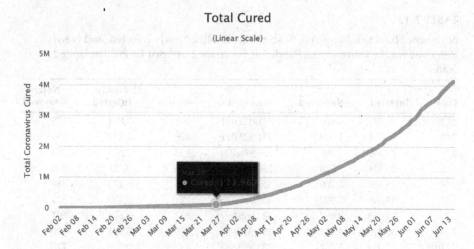

FIGURE 7.2
Number recovered versus time.

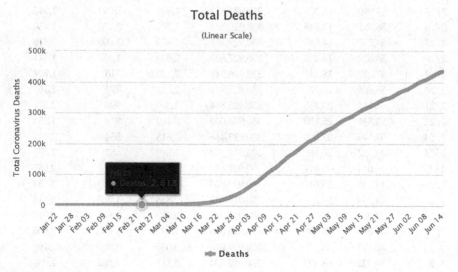

FIGURE 7.3
Number of deaths versus time.

   The table below displays the number of infected cases, the number removed, the susceptible, the deaths, the newly infected, and the newly recovered. The number of removed is the number of deaths plus the number of recovered cases. This assumes that once recovered the person cannot be re-infected (Table 7.13).

TABLE 7.13

Number of Infected, Removed, Susceptible, Deaths, Newly Infected, and Newly Removed for the Coronavirus Pandemic February 2 to April 12, 2020 in United States

Date	Infected	Removed	Susceptible	Deaths	Newly Infected	Newly Removed
2/2	16,523	866	331,022,651	362	2,838	176
2/3	19,561	1,069	331,022,021	426	3,239	139
2/4	23,146	1,399	330,998,106	492	3,915	264
2/5	26,528	1,738	330,894,385	565	3,721	266
2/6	29,239	2,200	330,971,212	638	3,173	389
2/7	32,069	2,807	330,967,775	724	3,437	521
2/8	34,055	3,497	330,965,099	813	2,676	601
2/9	36,320	4,233	330,962,098	910	3,001	639
2/10	38,038	5,061	330,959,552	1,018	2,546	720
2/11	39,216	5,918	330,957,517	1,115	2,035	760
2/12	52,039	7,248	330,944,694	1,261	14,153	1,184
2/13	56,247	8,191	330,936,682	1,383	5,151	821
2/14	57,378	9,722	330,934,066	1,526	2,662	1,385
2/15	57,990	11,207	330,931,823	1,669	2,097	1,342
2/16	58,581	12,748	330,929,395	1,775	2,132	1,435
2/17	58,747	14,585	330,929,315	1,873	2,003	1,739
2/18	58,622	16,426	330,927,603	2,009	1,852	1,841
2/19	57,217	18,483	330,926,941	2,126	516	1,804
2/20	55,906	20,771	330,925,974	2,247	977	2,167
2/21	54,418	23,255	330,925,884	2,360	996	2,371
2/22	53,541	25,110	330,924,000	2,460	978	1,755
2/23	51,596	27,609	330,923,446	2,618	554	2,341
2/24	49,922	30,165	330,922,563	2,699	882	2,475
2/25	48,014	32,814	330,921,823	2,763	741	2,585
2/26	46,215	35,611	330,920,825	2,806	992	2,754
2/27	43,739	39,378	330,919,543	2,858	1,288	3,715
2/28	42,262	42,353	330,918,036	2,923	1,507	2,910
2/29	41,298	45,307	330,916,046	2,977	1,990	2,900
3/1	40,413	48,172	330,914,066	3,050	1,980	2,792
3/2	39,222	51,225	330,912,204	3,117	1,862	2,986
3/3	38,872	54,146	330,909,633	3,202	2,571	2,836
3/4	38,515	56,809	330,907,327	3,285	2,306	2,580
3/5	39,426	58,992	330,904,233	3,387	3,094	2,081
3/6	40,957	61,102	330,900,5932	3,493	3,641	2,004
3/7	42,347	63,770	330,896,534	3,598	4,058	2,563
3/8	43,909	66,104	330,892,638	3,826	3,896	2,106
3/9	46,369	68,079	330,890,178	4,023	4,435	1,778

(Continued)

Table 7.13 (Continued)

Date	Infected	Removed	Susceptible	Deaths	Newly Infected	Newly Removed
3/10	48,101	70,918	330,883,632	4,297	4,571	2,565
3/11	53,401	72,934	330,876,315	4,627	7,316	1,686
3/12	59,284	75,340	330,868,027	4,980	8,259	2,053
3/13	67,525	78,002	330,859,786	5,427	10,933	2,215
3/14	74,746	81,766	330,846,139	5,841	10,985	3,350
3/15	85,558	83,985	330,823,108	6,532	13,031	1,528
3/16	95,661	86,806	330,820,184	7,189	12,927	2,176
3/17	107,622	90,620	330,804,409	8,000	15,776	2,995
3/18	124,659	94,324	330,783,668	8.983	20,737	2,717
3/19	146,920	98,242	330,757,489	10,077	26,179	2,824
3/20	172,841	103,033	330,726,777	11,457	30,712	4,411
3/21	196,767	108,599	330,697,285	13,101	29,492	3,922
3/22	224,474	113,369	330,664,808	14,739	32,477	3,132
3/23	260,724	118,745	330,659,432	16,671	41,626	3,444
3/24	295,309	128,054	330,579,288	19,157	43,894	6,823
3/25	336,105	135,995	330,530,551	21,747	48,737	5,351
3/26	384,545	148,610	330,469,496	24,643	61,105	9,719
3/27	436,801	161,259	330,404,591	28,163	64,855	9,129
3/28	491,115	173,825	330,337,711	31,835	66,880	8,894
3/29	539,506	186,528	330,277,067	35,179	60,644	9,359
3/30	585,242	204,770	330,212,639	39,341	64,428	14,080
3/31	642,008	222,224	330,138,419	44,056	74,217	12,739
4/1	698,225	243,462	330,060,964	49,246	77,458	16,048
4/2	754,357	267,783	329,980,511	55,519	80,453	18,048
4/3	816,404	290,169	329,896,078	61,484	84,433	16,421
4/4	874,249	314,116	329,814,286	67,553	81,792	17,878
4/5	923,258	336,029	329,743,464	72,560	70,920	16,904
4/6	975,691	356,887	329,670,073	78,171	73,287	15,243
4/7	1,022,894	388,287	329,591,470	86,068	78,608	23,508
4/8	1,071,419	424,605	329,506,627	92,808	84,839	29,574
4/9	1,124,589	456,916	329,421,146	100,479	85,486	24,645
4/10	1,189,922	484,089	329,328,940	107,835	92,206	19,817
4/11	1,236,610	516,757	329,249,284	114,048	79,656	26,455
4/12	1,282,063	543,016	329,177,572	119,617	71,712	20,690

The entries in the table can be downloaded from https://www.worldme-ters.info/coronavirus/worldwide-graphs/.

The histogram of the number of recovered individuals of coronavirus patients is presented in Figure 7.4.

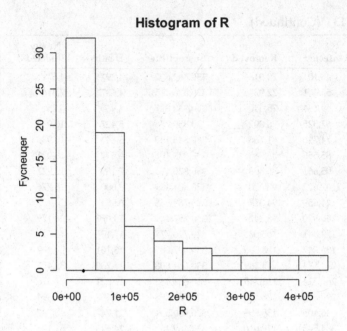

FIGURE 7.4
Histogram of the number of recovered individuals.

It appears safe to assume that the number of recovered coronavirus patients follows an exponential distribution. The same can be verified for the number of infected and number of deaths. Thus, in the Bayesian analysis of BC 7.12, the number of infected, number of recovered, and number of deaths are specified as exponentially distributed random variables. Of interest is the dependence of the deaths on time given by

$$D[i] = \theta \exp(\phi i), i = 2,\dots,71. \tag{7.99}$$

Remember that the number of susceptible individuals is the population size of the United States minus the number of infected minus the number of removed. The information in the above table is needed to estimate δ of Equation (9.95), β of equation (7.97), and ρ of equation (7.98). Estimation of δ and β will be conducted with WinBUGS. The code is given by BC 7.12, and the analysis executed with 75,000 observations for the simulation with 5,000 initial values.

BC 7.12

```
model;
{
for( i in 2:71){INF[i]~dexp(lamda1[i])
lamda1[i]<-1/(INF[i-1]+nu[i]-D[i-1]-delta*(INF[i-1]-D[i-1]))

R[i]~dexp(lamda2[i])
lamda2[i]<-1/(R[i-1]+D[i-1]+delta*(INF[i-1]-D[i-1]))

nu[i]~dexp(lamda3[i])
lamda3[i]<- 1/(beta*S[i-1]*INF[i-1]/331002651)

D[i]~dexp(lamda4[i])
lamda4[i]<-1/(theta*exp(phi*i))

}

beta~dbeta(4,5)
delta~dbeta(4,5)
theta~dbeta(4,5)
phi~dbeta(4,5)

}
list(R = c(504,643,907,1173,1563,2083,2684,3323,4043,4803,5987,
6808,8196,9538,10973,12712,14553,16357,18524,20895,22650,24991,
27466,30051,32805,36520,39430,42330,45122,48108,50944,53524,
55605,57609,60172,62278,64056,66621,68307,70360,72575,75,925,7
7453,79629,82624,85341,88165,91576,95498,98630,102074,108897,
114248,123967,133096,141990,151349,165429,178168,194216,
212264,228685,246563,263469,278716,302218,331797,356437,
376254,402709,423300),

D = c(362,426,392,565,638,724,813,910,1018,1115,1261,1383,1526
,
1669,1775,1873,2009,2126,2247,2360,2460,2618,2699,2763,2808,
2858,2923,2977,3050,3117,3202,3285,3387,3493,3598,3826,4023,
4297,4627,4980,5427,5841,6532,7180,8000,8983,10077,11457,
13101,14739,16671,19157,21747,24493,28163,31835,35179,39341,
44056,49246,55519,61484,67553,72560,78171,86068,92808,
100479,107835,114048,119617),
INF = c(563,786,1238,1910,2669,4415,5823,7519,13921,16523,19561,
23146,26528,29239,32069,34055,36320,38038,39216,52039,56247,
57378,57990,58581,58747,58622,57217,55906,54418,53541,51596,
49922,48014,46215,43730,42262,41298,40413,39222,38872,38515,
39426,40957,42347,43909,46369,48101,53401,59284,67525,74746,
85558,95661,107622,124659,146920,172841,196767,224474,
260724,295309,336105,384545,436801,491115,539056,585242,
642008,698225,754357,816404,874249,923258,974691,1022894,
1071419,1124589,1189622,1236610,1282063),
```

TABLE 7.14

Posterior Analysis for Coronavirus

Parameter	Mean	SD	Error	2 1/2	Median	97 1/2
β	1	.000013	.0000000869	.999	1	1
δ	.1387	.04714	.0000028	.0563	.1356	.2382
ϕ	.464	.007994	.00000197	.4494	.4637	.48
θ	.9902	.004322	.000000635	.9801	.9909	.9967

```
nu= c(260,265,472,698,785,1781,1477,1755,2010,2603,2838,3239,
3915,3721,3173,3437,2676,3001,2546,2035,14153,5151,2662,2097,
2132,2003,1852,516,977,996,978,554,882,741,992,1288,1507,
1990,1980,1862,2571,2306,3094,3641,4058,3896,4435,4571,7316,
8259,10933,10985,13031,12927,15776,20737,26179,30712,29492,
32477,41626,43894,48737,61105,64855,66880,60644,64428,74217,
77458,80453,84433,81792,70920,73287,78608,84839,85486,
92206,79656,71712),

S= c(331022,331002,330998,330894,330971212,330967775,
330965099,330962098,330959552,330957517,330744694,
330,936682,330934066,330931823,330929395,330929319,
330927603,330926951,330925974,330925884,330924000,
330923446,330922563,330921834,330920825,330919543,
339918036,330915046,330914066,330912204,330909633,
330907327,330904233,330900592,330896534,330892638,
330890178,330883632,330876316,330868027,330859786,
330846139,330833108,330820184,330804409,330783668,
330757489,330726777,330697285,330664808,330659432,
330579288,330530551,330469496,330404591,339337711,
330277067,330212639,330138419,330060964,329980511,
329896078,329814286,329743364,328670073,329591470,
329506627,329421146,329328940,329249284,329177572))

list( delta=10,beta=10)
```

The results of the Bayesian analysis appear in Table 7.14.

The student will be asked to interpret the estimates of the parameters given in Table 7.14, and how they relate to the coronavirus epidemic. With regard to estimating θ and ϕ, the evolution of deaths over time given by (7.99), one sees that the rate of increase is estimated as .464 deaths per day.

Also, the student will be asked to estimate the infected fatality rate $\rho = \left[\sum_{i=0}^{i=t} D_i\right] / (I_t + R_t)$ of (7.98) by adding the appropriate WinBUGS code BC 7.12.

7.8 Summary and Conclusions

The chapter begins with laying the theoretical foundation for the study of continuous time Markov chains (CTMC). First, the Markov property is defined which is the most important concept for such processes. Next to be described are the ideas of time homogeneity and the probability transition function. One of the most important concepts for CTMC is the infinitesimal transition rate matrix which leads to the transition probabilities of the imbedded chain. Next to be introduced is the Kolmogorov forward and backward system of differential equations involving the transition rate matrix Q and the derivatives of the transition probability function. The solution to this system is the transition probability function $P(t)$. It is demonstrated how one may use R and the exponential function $\exp(tQ)$ to compute the transition probability function. Next it is shown how to compute the stationary distribution (if it exists) by solving a system of equation involving the transition rates of the infinitesimal rate matrix Q.

With Section 7.4, CTMC with an absorbing state is considered and it is demonstrated with a liver disease process and using R how to determine the average time to absorption from a transient state of the chain. Also explained are the concepts of time reversibility and global stability, which depends on the stationary distribution of the chain.

Section 7.6 introduces several biologic examples including three versions of DNA evolution. The first to be considered is the simplest model of DNA evolution called the Jukes-Cantor model. One of the holding time parameters is estimated using BC 7.1 and the posterior reported in Table 7.1. Also presented is a test of hypothesis involving the holding time parameter and a derivation of the predictive density of a future holding time. The Kimura model is a generalization of the Jukes-Cantor model and allows one to distinguish between tranversions and transitions of DNA substitutions. A Bayesian test of hypothesis investigates if the Kimura model reduces to the Juke-Cantor model, which is followed by an examination of the Felsenstein-Churchill model, which generalizes the Kimura model. A Bayesian analysis is conducted that estimates the alpha parameter of the generalization. Bugs code 7.3 is executed to estimate alpha and the posterior analysis reported in Table 7.7. Lastly considered is the DNA evolution model referred to as the Hasegawa, Kishino, and Yano model, and a Bayesian test that the model reduces to the Felsenstein-Churchill model is performed.

Section 7.6.2 is the first regarding the important class of CTMC, namely birth and death processes. Its stationary distribution corresponding to the infinitesimal rate matric Q given by (7.74) is explained, and this is followed by an example with five states determined by the Q matrix (7.80). The Bayesian analysis depends on holding times generated with an exponential distribution with known parameters. Using 45,000 observations for the simulation and a burn in of 5,000, BC 7.5 is executed with the prior information defined as a non-informative gamma distribution for the holding time parameter. Posterior analysis results are reported in Table 7.5 and consist of the characteristics of the posterior distribution of the four average extinction times.

A special case of the birth and death process is the random walk with instantaneous rate matrix Q given by (7.85) from which the stationary distribution is derived. The process depends on two infinitesimal rates: (1) the one move to the right (corresponding birth rate), and (2) one move to the left (corresponding to the death rate). With known values assigned to these two rates, the corresponding holding times with exponential distributions are generated and appeared in the list statement of BC 7.6 with the posterior analysis reported in Table 7.6.

Another special birth and death process is the Yule process which is a birth process (no deaths are possible). This implies that all states are transient and that the stationary distribution does not exist. As with the previous examples, a particular value is assigned to the birth rate which allows one to generate exponentially distributed holding times (for the various states) which are in turn used for the Bayesian analysis reported in Table 7.8.

A generalization of the birth and death process is the birth and death process with immigration, which allows only an increase in the population; however, births and deaths are possible. The Bayesian analysis is executed with BC 7.9 and the results appearing in Table 7.9.

Section 7.6.6., last part of the chapter, introduces stochastic epidemic processes, the so-called SI model, meaning two types of individuals are followed in the epidemic, namely the susceptibles and those that are infected. Assigning known values to the infinitesimal rate matrix allows one to generate exponentially distributed observations for the Bayesian analysis executed with BC 7.10 and results reported in Table 7.11.

A generalization of this epidemic process to the so-called SIS model is the last example of the chapter and the analysis is similar as that for the SI model.

Bayesian inferences for continuous type Markov chains has been an active area of research and the following references should be appealing to the student who wants to contribute to the literature on the subject.

In the area of reliability, see Cano, Moguerza, and Insua [9] and Cano, Moguerza, and Insua [10] while those interested in Markov-modulated Poisson processes should read Fearnhead and Sherlock [11]. Geweke [12] studies mobility indices for CTMC and Scott [13] emphasizes Bayesian inferences applicable to Markov modulated Poisson chains. With regard to DNA evolutionary models, refer to Suchard, Weiss, and Sinsheimer [14]. But for a more comprehensive list of work related to Bayesian techniques with CTMC, see Insua, Ruggeri, and Wiper [2, pp. 103–104]

Lastly, the degree of infectiousness of the coronavirus is investigated, and Chapter 8 will present more information on infectious diseases, including the recent coronavirus worldwide pandemic.

7.9 Exercises

1. Define the Markov property and the transition probability function for a CTMC.

2. a. Define time homogeneity for a CTMC.

   b. Give an example of a CTMC which is time homogenous.

3. Define the memoryless property of a CTMC. What is the distribution of the holding time of a CTMC?

4. What is the association between the infinitesimal transition rates and the transition probabilities of the imbedded chain?

5. From the infinitesimal transition rates (7.8) derive the transition probabilities (7.9).

6. The Kolmogorov forward equations are a system of differential equation involving the derivative $P'(t)$ of the transition probability function. Show the solution to this system is the transition probability function.

7. Using R code 7.1, compute the probability transition function $P(t)$ as $P(t) = \exp(tQ)$, where Q is the matrix of instantaneous transition rates.

8. If it exists, define the limiting distribution of a CTMC.

9. Under what conditions does the unique stationary distribution of a CTMC exist?

10. Based on the infinitesimal rate matrix Q (7.19), find the unique stationary distribution given by (7.14). RC 7.2 should be employed to find the stationary distribution.

11. Use RC 7.3 with the matrix Q specified by (7.24) with state 3 (death) as an absorbing state and starting in state 1 (cirrhosis of the liver), compute the mean time to death.

12. Define time reversibility of a CTMC. Consider the 3-state chain with probability transition matrix P of the imbedded chain:

    a. What is the corresponding Q matrix?

    b. Is the process time reversible? Why? Explain.

13. Based on the Q matrix (7.32) of the Jukes-Cantor DNA evolution model, derive the corresponding probability transition function.

14. Execute BC 7.1 with 45,000 observations for the simulation and a burn in of 5,000 and verify the posterior analysis of Table 7.1.

    a. What is the posterior mean of λ?

    b. What is the posterior mean of μ?

    c. Is this process time reversible? Why?

    d. Which posterior distributions appear as symmetric about the posterior mean?

15. Refer to the Jukes-Cantor model and test the hypothesis $H : \lambda = 1/6$ versus $A : \lambda \neq 1/6$. Show the posterior probability of the null hypothesis is .7356.

Parameter	Mean	sd	Error	2 1/2	Median	97 1/2
beta	1	.000013	.0000000594	.9999	1	1
delta	.1388	.04726	.00000183	.05584	.1357	.2395

16. Derive the predictive density (7.51) of $t(n + 1)$ for the holding time with exponential parameter λ.

17. Refer to the Felsenstein-Churchill model with instantaneous rate matrix Q (7.61).

    a. What is its stationary distribution?

    b. What is its probability transition function matrix $P(t)$?

18. Refer to the Felsenstein-Churchill model for DNA evolution with matrix Q given by (7.61). In order to estimate the parameter α of the matrix Q, execute BC 7.3 with 35,000 observations for the simulation and 5,000 for the burn in. Your results should be similar to those reported in Table 7.4.

    a. What is the posterior median of α?

    b. Is the posterior distribution of α symmetric about its posterior mean?

    c. What is the 95% credible interval for α?

19. Refer to the birth and death process with infinitesimal rate matrix Q given by (7.74) and derive the corresponding stationary distribution (7.78).

20. Refer to the birth and death process with matrix Q given by (7.80) and with states 0,1,2,3, and 4, where $\mu_1 = 2, \lambda_1 = 1, \mu_2 = 3, \lambda_2 = 2, \mu_3 = 4, \lambda_4 = 3$.

    a. With BC 7.5 verify the posterior analysis of Table 7.6.

    b. What are the a_i, $i = 1, 2, 3$ in the posterior analysis?

    c. Assume the process is in state 3. What is the posterior mean of the average time to extinction?

    d. Is the posterior distribution of a_3 symmetric about its posterior mean? Why?

21. For the birth and death process with $\lambda = 2$ and $\mu = 5$, execute BC 7.7 and verify the posterior analysis of Table 7.7.

    a. What is the posterior mean and median of $P(\lambda > \mu)$.

    b. Display the posterior density of $P(\lambda > \mu)$.

    c. What does the posterior mean of $P(\lambda > \mu)$ imply about this birth and death process?

22. For the Yule process with Q matrix given by (7.86), show all states are transient and that the stationary distribution does not exist.

23. For the Yule process with infinitesimal rate matrix (7.86), let the holding time parameter be $\lambda = 2$. The holding time observations are in the list statement of BC 7.9. Execute BC 7.8 and verify the posterior analysis appearing in Table 7.10.

    a. What is the posterior mean of λ?

    b. What prior distribution is used for λ?

    c. Name the posterior distribution of λ.

    d. Does the posterior analysis suggest $\lambda = 2$? Why?

24. For the birth and death process with immigration and Q matrix (7.89), let $\mu = 1$, $\nu = 1/3$, $\lambda = 1$ be the assigned values for the death, immigration, and birth rates, respectively. These values are used to generate the exponentially distributed holding times appearing in the list statement of BC 7.9. Execute BC 7.9 and verify the posterior analysis of Table 7.10.

    a. What is the posterior mean of the immigration rate ν?

    b. What is the posterior median of the average number of immigrants per day?

    c. Do you believe $\lambda = 1$?

    d. Display the posterior density of μ?

    e. Specify the prior distribution for the three rates.

25. Refer to the SI epidemic with Q matrix (7.91) for the number of infections. Execute BC 7.10 and verify Table 7.11.

    a. What is the posterior mean of β?

    b. For this epidemic, what is the interpretation of β?

    c. What is the average holding time for one infected individual. Refer to the parameter labeled E(HT1) in Table 7.11.

    d. What prior distributions did you specify for β?

26. For the SIS epidemic, let $\beta = 2$, $N = 100$, $\lambda_1 = 2.98$, $\lambda_2 = 5.92$, $(b + \gamma) = 1$. Execute BC 7.11 and verify the posterior analysis of Table 7.12.

    a. What is the posterior mean of the holding time for one infected individual?

  b. What is the posterior mean of the holding time for two infected individuals?

  c. What did you use for the prior distribution of β?

  d. Explain the difference between an SI epidemic and an SIS epidemic.

27. Refer to (7.98) the formula for the infected fatality rate ρ. Estimate this parameter by adding the appropriate programming statement to BC 7.12.

References

1. Dobrow, R.P. (2016). *Introduction to Stochastic Processes with R*, John Wiley & Sons Inc., New York.

2. Insua, D.R., Ruggeri, F., and Wiper, M.P. (2012). *Bayesian Analysis of Stochastic Process Models*, John Wiley & Sons Inc., New York.

3. Allen, L.J.S. (2011). *An Introduction to Stochastic Processes with Applications to Biology*, 2nd Edition, Taylor and Francis, Boca Raton, FL.

4. Bartolomeo, P., Trerotoli, P., and Serio, G. (2011). Progression of liver cirrhosis to HCC: an application of hidden Markov model. *BMC Med. Res. Methodol.*, 11(380), 1-8. http://www.biomedcentral.com/1471-2288/11/38.Openaccess.

5. Lee, P.M. (1997). *Bayesian Statistics: An Introduction*, 2nd Edition. John Wiley & Sons Inc., New York.

6. Kimura, M. (1980). A simple method for estimating evolutionary rates of base substitution of comprehensive studies of nucleotide sequences, *J. Mol. Evol.*, 16(20), 111-120.

7. Felsenstein, J. and Churchill, G.A. (1996). A hidden Markov model approach variation among sites in rate of evolution, *Mol. Biol. Evol.*, 13, 93-101.

8. Hasegawa, M., Kishino, H., and Yano, T. (1980). Dating of human ape splitting by a molecular clock of mitochondrial DNA, *J. Mol. Evol.* 22(2), 160-174.

9. Cano, J., Moguerza, J.M., and Insua, R. (2010). Bayesian reliability, availability, and maintainability analysis for hardware systems described through continuous time Markov chains, *Technometrics*, 52, 324-334.

10. Cano, J., Moguerza, J., and Insua, R. (2011). Bayesian analysis for semi Markov processes with application to reliability and maintenance, Technical Report. Madrid, University Rey Juan Carlos.

11. Fearhead, P. and Sherlock, C. (2009). An exact Gibbs sampler for the Markov-modulated Poisson Process, *J. Royal Stat. Soc.*, B68, 767-784.

12. Geweke, J., Marshall, R., and Zarkin, G. (1986). Mobility indices in continuous time Markov chains, *Econometrica*, 54, 1407-1423.

13. Scott, S.L., and Smyth, P. (2003). The Markov modulated Poisson process cascade with application to webb traffic modeling. In *Bayesian Statistics 7*, J.M. Bernardo, M.J. Bayarri, J.O. Berger, A.P. Dawid, D. Heckerman, A.F.M. Smith, and M. West (Eds.), Oxford University Press, Oxford, 1–10.

14. Suchard, M., Weiss, R., and Sinsheimer, J. (2001). Bayesian selection of continuous time Markov chain evolutionary models. *Mol. Evol. Biol.*, 18, 1001-1013.

8

Additional Information about Infectious Diseases

8.1 Introduction

The aim of this chapter is to describe the statistical analysis of observational information of the behavior of infectious diseases. A disease is infectious if the infected host transitions through an infectious period, during which the person is capable of passing the disease to a susceptible individual, either by direct contact or by infecting the surrounding environment in such a way that the person becomes infected. Another way for a person to contract a disease is by an intermediate vector, that is, the disease is carried by the vector which subsequently infects the host. For example, a mosquito which has malaria transmits the disease to another by biting the victim. The infected immediate surroundings might include linen and utensils of a household or the ambient air in the house.

8.2 Contagious Diseases Today

According to Becker [1], in the past, infectious diseases were the scourge of humanity and were the primary causes of mortality and morbidity. Over the past, some of these diseases were tamed, but in the 1930s and 1940s, pneumonia and tuberculosis were successfully treated with antibiotics. But, it should be noted that diseases such as malaria, schistosomiasis, filariasis, hookworm, and trachoma still infect several million people, at the present time. In addition, tens of millions of people are infected with leprosy and onchocerciasis.

Public health problems are prevalent, even among nations that are relatively free from infectious diseases. When the more serious diseases appear under control, the more minor diseases receive more attention with the view of bringing them under control. For example, in Denmark, a survey revealed that 18% of measle cases involved associated maladies such as otitis media, pneumonia, and encephalitis, which implies that measles deserves to be considered a serious disease. See Horowitz et al. [2] for additional information. Thus, it is desirable to have vaccination campaigns directed toward controlling the spread of coronavirus, and other diseases which induce maladies leading to complications. Another type of public health problem is with vaccinations that have a small fraction of people developing a full-blown case of the disease they were vaccinated against. Often, when the disease is eradicated, it is difficult to discern whether damage due to additional vaccinations is more or less than that attributed to the residual spread of the disease. According to Lane et al. [3] such was the case for smallpox during the period 1965–1975 and in some countries at present it is the case for whooping-cough, see Miller and Pollock [4]. In addition, with the increase in air traffic, the global population is in danger of endemic diseases such as coronavirus and other infectious diseases. Finally, cholera, even in those nations essentially free from it, still can reoccur in that country as well as those surrounding the affected country. As another more relevant example, AIDS does indeed illustrate the point.

In summary, infectious diseases continue to confront the public with serious public health challenges. The Bayesian statistical methods described in the book have as its objective the improvement of one's understanding of contagious diseases and their spread through the community, with the sincere desire that such additional knowledge will aid in the control of these maladies.

8.3 A Preview of Data Analysis and Models

Knowledge is expanded by the analysis of data from the repetition of designed experiments. This is not the case when analyzing the data from an epidemic. Note that infectious disease data are usually found by observing epidemics, which makes it difficult to accumulate data with the precision one would desire, that is, often such data lack sufficient detail. When studying the behavior of infections, at most one can observe the times that people show symptoms. It is virtually impossible to know the times at which infections occur, or to know which infected person is responsible for transmitting the disease to a susceptible host.

An epidemiological investigation of such maladies should in general begin with the statement of the objectives of this scientific undertaking. In an ideal world, one would use those objectives to design the appropriate experiment. Since epidemics are not planned, the researcher uses the objectives to determine the scope of the information to be collected. Of course, it is important to determine which observations are required to know the infectious disease and the surrounding environment and insure that the proposed objective is achieved. Thus, it follows that when describing the various means of investigation, one should make it clear, an attempt is executed to answer the questions that must be answered in order to achieve a successful study.

In statistics there is a tendency to make inferences with distribution-free techniques, so that the problems of adopting incorrect models are avoided. Of course, this position can also be a constraint on the analysis, because as will be seen, it is often appropriate to use parametric methods that do indeed achieve one's goal to analyze the data in an efficient way. Indeed, on what is to follow, a Bayesian approach will provide inferences that are very informative in providing succinct information about the behavior of an infectious disease. The advantage of basing statistical analysis based on specific parametric models is that it usually implies to more efficient inferences. In other words, by designing a model that describes how the data were generated, it can assist in compensating for lack of detail that is part of infectious disease data. Of course, it is important to make the sure the model assumptions are supported empirically and by known biological and social truths. Of course, once a model is adopted, those parameters should be able to interpret the underlying biological or social tenants.

Also, of concern is the statistical analysis and the associate stochastic models which takes into account the random nature of the observations. Deterministic models can be initially useful, and the parameters estimated from the data, but usually the precision (variances), are not known. Thus, the deterministic models serve as an approximation to the corresponding version. Indeed, the deterministic version is quite useful in enriching the general theory of epidemics than in applications to real data. One problem with stochastic models is that they tend to lead to equations that can be quite difficult to solve. Fortunately, this problem has been to a large extent negated, because of the sophistication of Bayesian models, that rely on resampling techniques (such as Markov chain Monte Carlo, or MCMC) that determine the posterior distribution of the parameters of the model.

An important aspect of modeling concerns the degree of complexity as part of the model. Of course, a model can be based on assumptions that are not realistic or are too "simple." According to Becker, [1, p. 34] "indeed this property of mathematical formulations coupled with the fact that many concepts, models, methods of analysis, and their interpretations are most clearly described in a mathematical framework helps to explain why in most areas of science mathematics is recognized as a most useful means of communication between research workers." Nevertheless, it is true, that simplifying assumptions are a part of epidemic models that are prevalent in the literature, but of course it would be folly to reject such models merely on the basis of simplicity. It should be noted that simplicity can be a virtue.

It should be asserted that a model is an idealization and would not be viewed as an exact representation describing the evolution of an infectious disease. There are statistical techniques that can test just how well a model fits the data. It is indeed true, that if a simple model does provide an adequate fit to some data, then it is often the case that it could prove to be more useful than a detailed complex model that also fits the data in an adequate manner. See Box [5] for a general discussion on models and adequacy of fit. Indeed, it is standard procedure of statistical analysis to compare data sets by comparing the models that adequately describe them.

8.4 The Epidemic Threshold Theorem

Most likely, the most important conclusions deduced from an investigation of epidemic models are a result of the epidemic threshold theorem.

The theorem quantifies the probability distribution for the final size of the epidemic in a close large population in terms of the critical parameter μ and other aspects of the infection process. At the early stage of the infection, μ may be defined as the average number of susceptible individuals infected by one infected person while that person is infected. This parameter takes on various values for different diseases and different types of specialized populations or communities, so that it is important to estimate it for every epidemic. It would be interesting to compare the estimated value of μ for the coronavirus with its estimate for ordinary influenza at the present time (May 2020). One of the useful statistical techniques is to determine the number of observations necessary to estimate μ to a given degree of accuracy. In view of the scarcity of data in epidemics, it is difficult to estimate the epidemic threshold μ, to the desired degree of accuracy.

Is the present interpretation of threshold parameter μ based on simplified assumptions? It is true that certain details of the theorem will change as these assumptions are relaxed, it can be shown that the value of the estimated μ is very robust under a relaxation of these assumptions. The interpretation of μ is as follows: (1) the probability of a minor outbreak in large populations is unity when $\mu < 1$; (2) when $\mu > 1$, the probability of a major epidemic is positive. The details of this assertion will be presented later in this chapter. Suppose a fraction α of the population is immunized against the disease, then the threshold parameter is reduced to $\mu* = (1 - \alpha)\mu$. If $\alpha > 1 - 1/\mu$, then $\mu* < 1$ and the partially immunized population satisfies the condition under which a minor epidemic occurs with probability one. This implies that the threshold theorem indicates what fraction of the community must be immunized for a serious outbreak to be prevented. Of course, one must have a reliable estimate of μ and this will be examined at various sections of the book. It would be of value to know the value of μ for the coronavirus.

The evidence which supports the claim that the estimate of the threshold parameter is not sensitive to the simplifying assumptions of epidemic formulations is implied by the association between a minor epidemic occuring in a large population and the extinction of a branching process. This association can be traced to Bartlett [6] and to latter derivations by Whittle [7] and Becker [8]. Once this association is found credible, the results concerning multi-type branching process may be used. Also relevant are branching processes in random environments, and branching processes with different households in order to make the safe conjecture that the epidemic threshold parameter μ applies under general conditions for large populations. It can be demonstrated under these general assumptions that the corresponding epidemic threshold parameter is still feasible to establish the fraction of susceptible individuals that must be immunized to prevent major epidemics.

8.5 Basic Characteristics of the Infectious Process

The infectious disease is transmitted to a susceptible host, to be referred to as a susceptible, when the individual contracts a sufficient quantity of causative organism. When a susceptible acquires a quantity of infectious material, sufficient to induce an infection, it is said the host has made an infectious contact. The first infectious contact a susceptible makes results in an infection and further infectious contacts are assumed to have no further effect on the individual, unless they occur again when they become susceptible. See Becker [1, p. 10] for additional details. Following the infected person through time, this person passes through a period called the latent period, during which the infection is confined to the individual, without the transmission of any kind of infectious material. The latent period is terminated when the individual ceases to be to be infectious and either becomes infectious again or becomes removed for some reason (death or leaves the population under study). A removal is an individual that plays no part in the spread of the malady. An individual becomes a removal by being isolated or by death or becoming immune again. The states of isolation and immunity may be temporary or be permanent. Each infected individual is often called a case.

8.6 Chain Binomial Representations

Our first excursion into the analysis of infectious diseases is with the chain binomial model, using data for the spread of infection within a household. We consider a group of households that are homogeneous with regard to the spread of the disease. Furthermore, the households are partitioned into classes, within which the malady is assumed to expand in a common way. This implies that outbreaks with the affected household evolve independently of one another. This constrain will be relaxed to consider a more general way the disease spreads within households.

8.7 The Size of the Outbreak is Compared

According to Becker [1, p. 11], Consider n households which are affected by a certain disease. For the analysis of data from such households, it is convenient to assume that the households are homogeneous with respect to the spread of the disease. It is not wise to adopt such an assumption blindly and we begin our discussion with a test of this assumption. Suppose then that a classification of n households suggests itself which is such that households within the same class are thought to be similar, while prior epidemiological evidence suggests there might be differences between classes. For example, households might be classified according to the degree of crowding or according to the number of susceptible people in the household. The aim is to test whether the sizes of outbreaks differ significantly between such classes."

The presentation is clarified by assuming that the households are of all the same size, containing prior to being affected, s susceptible individuals. Consider the distribution for the size of outbreaks first under the assumption that all households are similar. Let θ_j represent the probability that j of the s susceptible people in a household become cases by the end of the outbreak, and let N_j be the number of households with exactly j cases, j = 1,2,...,s. Under this constraint, N_j has a binomial distribution with probability mass function

$$P\left(N_j = x\right) = \binom{n}{x} \theta_j^x \left(1-\theta_j\right)^{n-x}, x = 0,1,...,n \qquad (8.1)$$

Therefore, the joint probability mass function of the vector $(N_1, N_2, ..., N_s)$ is

$$P\left(N_1 = x_1, N_2 = x_2,...,N_s = x_s\right) = \left[n! / x_1! x_2!,...,x_s!\right] \theta_1^{x_1} \theta_2^{x_2} ... \theta_s^{x_s} \qquad (8.2)$$

where $\sum_{j=1}^{j=s} x_j = n$ and $\sum_{j=1}^{j=s} \theta_j = 1$.

Under the alternative hypothesis, there are k different classes, or types of households. By now assume that there are n_i households of type I among the affected households. Of the n_i households of type I, suppose there are N_{ij}

households with a total number of cases equal to j, then for each type there is a separate multinomial distribution for $(N_{i1}, N_{i2}, ..., N_{is})$ with joint probability mass function

$$P(N_{i1} = x_{i1}, N_{i2} = x_{i2}, ..., N_{is} = x_{is}) = [n_{i.}! / x_{i1}! x_{i2}!, ..., x_{is}!] \theta_{i1}^{x_{i1}} \theta_{i2}^{x_{i2}} ... \theta_{is}^{x_{is}} \quad (8.3)$$

where θ_{ij} is the probability that an affected household of type i will have a total of j cases.

Note that the data are classified as the n households according to both type of household and the number of cases. This can be summarized by a contingency table such as that shown in Table 8.1.

It should be noted that the first row can be considered a realization from a multinomial distribution where the total of n_1 households are allocated to the s cells with probability vector $(\theta_{11}, \theta_{12}, ..., \theta_{1s})$. The multinomial mass function for the counts in the first row is

$$P(N_{11} = n_{11}, N_{12} = n_{12}, ..., N_{1s} = n_{1s}) = [n_{1.}! / n_{11}! n_{12}! ... n_{1s}!] \theta_{11}^{n_{11}} \theta_{12}^{n_{12}} ... \theta_{1s}^{n_{1s}} \quad (8.4)$$

If one uses the improper prior density for $(\theta_{11}\theta_{12}, ..., \theta_{1s})$ denoted by

$$g(\theta_{11}\theta_{12}, ..., \theta_{1s}) \propto 1 / \theta_{11}\theta_{12}, ..., \theta_{1s}, \quad (8.5)$$

where $\theta_{11} > 0$, $\theta_{12} > 0$, ..., $\theta_{1s} > 0$ and $\sum_{j=1}^{j=s} \theta_{1j} = 1$, it can be shown that the resulting posterior density is

$$h(\theta_{11}, |, \theta_{12}, |, ..., |, \theta_{1s}, |, n_{11}, |, n_{12}, |, ..., |, n_{1s}) \propto \prod_{j=1}^{j=s} \theta_{1j}^{n_{1j}-1}. \quad (8.6)$$

TABLE 8.1

Frequency Data Classified by Type and Size of Outbreak

Type	1	2	...	s	Total
1	n_{11}	n_{12}		n_{1s}	$n_{1.}$
2	n_{21}	n_{22}		n_{2s}	$n_{2.}$
.					
.					
k	n_{k1}	n_{k2}		n_{ks}	$n_{k.}$
Total	$n_{.1}$	$n_{.2}$		$n_{.s}$	n

This is the density of a Dirichlet distribution with parameter vector $(n_{11}, n_{12}, \ldots, n_{1s})$. See DeGroot [9, p. 50] for additional information about the multinomial and Dirichlet distributions. Knowing this, it is easy to make inferences about the theta parameters.

8.8 The Evolution of an Epidemic: Epidemic Chains

What is an epidemic chain? It is describing the behavior of the epidemic as it spreads through a household. To do this, the idea of a generation is introduced. Now suppose a contagious disease enters the community, the first generation of cases is made up of those infected by coming into contact with introductory cases. Those individuals becoming infected by contact with the first generation of cases consist of the second generation of contact. The introductory group is referred to as the zero generation. An epidemic chain for an affected household is a counting of the number of individuals in each generation, including the initial generation. For instance, $1 \to 1 \to 2$ denotes a chain consisting of one introductory case, one first-generation case, two second-generation cases, and zero third-generation cases. For more generality, $i_0 \to i_1 \to \ldots \to i_r$ this chain has i_t infectious people at generation t, t = 0,1,2,...,r. There is the possibility that the information that is available is not sufficient in detail, for the classification of outbreaks into separate epidemic chains. See Becker [1, p. 14] for more information about this topic. On the other hand, it remains crucial to describe epidemic chain models as they lead to outbreak size distributions in terms of parameters that have clear meanings as to the description of the outbreak.

8.9 A Chain Binomial Model

To express the probability of each possible chain, it is necessary to make some assumptions about the nature of the epidemic's spread. Assume that susceptible individuals make infectious contacts independently of each other and that each remaining susceptible has the same probability of making an infectious contact with the infectives of each generation. Let q_i, i = 1,2,... signify the probability that a given susceptible escapes infection when exposed to i infectious individuals of a specific generation. At this stage assume that q_i does not vary from generation to generation. Denote S_t as the number of susceptible individuals of the household exposed to the I_t infectives of generation t = 0,1,2,..... The chain binomial model is represented by the binomial probability mass function

$$P\left(I_{t+1} = x | , S_t = s | , I_t = i\right) = \binom{s}{x} p_i^x q_i^{s-x}, x = 0, 1, 2, ..., s \qquad (8.7)$$

where $p_i = 1 - q_i$. This implies that the probability of a given epidemic chain is the product of probability terms from different binomial distributions. Is this a realistic model? To be realistic, one needs to know, for each generation, how many infectives, and how many susceptible people there are. This implies that there is sufficient machinery for the epidemiologist to actually acquire this information. Thus, two further assumptions are proposed in order that one actually knows the number of susceptible individuals and the number of infected: (1) assume there are no subclinical infections (i.e. all infectives can be recognized), (2) after each infection period the number of infectives become removals, by becoming immune for the remaining duration of the outbreak. This in turn implies that the number of people who become a susceptible at the end of each generation is given by

$$S_{t+1} = S_t - I_{t+1} \qquad (8.8)$$

for t = 0,1,2,... with beginning values $I_0 = i_0$ and $S_0 = s_0$

To make this more understandable, consider some example of chain probabilities, where a household consists of four susceptible individuals and one initial infective, denoted by $i_0 = 1$ and $s_0 = 4$. For this situation, consider the model representation that gives the probability of the epidemic chain $1 \to 1 \to 2$ as

$$\begin{aligned} P(1 \to 1 \to 2) &= P\left(I_3 = 0 | S_2 = 1, I_2 = 2\right) \\ &= P\left(I_1 = 1 | , S_0 = 4 | , I_0 = 1\right) P\left(I_2 = 2 | , S_1 = 3 | , I_1 = 1\right) \\ &= 4p_1 q_1^3 \ldots 3p_1^2 q_1.q_2 \\ &= 12p_1^3 q_1^4 q_2 \end{aligned} \qquad (8.9)$$

More generally, the probability of the complete epidemic chain $i_0 \to i_1 \to . \ldots \to i_r$ is

$$P\left(i_0 \to i_1 \to .... \to i_r\right) = \left[s_0! / i_0! i_1! .... i_r! s_r!\right] \prod_{t=0}^{t=r} p_{i_t}^{i_{t+1}} q_{i_t}^{s_{t+1}}, \qquad (8.10)$$

where $i_{r+1} = 0$ and $s_{r+1} = s_r$.

The epidemic chain probabilities for households of sizes 3, 4, and 5 are listed in Table 8.2 corresponding to chains with one introductory case,

TABLE 8.2

Chain Binomial Probabilities -One Introductory Case Household Size

Chain				5	4	3
1				q_1^4	q_1^3	q_1^2
$1 \to 1$				$4q_1^6 p_1$	$3q_1^4 p_1$	$2q_1^2 p_1$
$1 \to 1$	$\to 1$			$12q_1^7 p_1^2$	$6q_1^4 p_1^2$	$2q_1 p_1^2$
$1 \to 2$				$6q_1^2 p_1^2 q_2^2$	$3q_1 p_1^2 q_2$	p_1^2
$1 \to 1$	$\to 1$	$\to 1$		$24q_1^7 p_1^3$	$6q_1^3 p_1^3$	
$1 \to 1$	$1 \to 2$			$12q_1^4 p_1^3 q_2$	$3q_1^2 p_1^3$	
$1 \to 3$				$4q_1 p_1^3 q_3$	p_1^3	
$1 \to 1$	$\to 1$	$\to 1$	$\to 1$	$24q_1^6 p_1^4$		
$1 \to 1$	$\to 1$	$\to 2$		$12q_1^5 p_1^4$		
$1 \to 1$	$\to 2$	$\to 1$		$12q_1^4 p_1^3 p_2$		
$1 \to 1$	$\to 3$			$4q_1^3 p_1^4$		
$1 \to 2$	$\to 1$	$\to 1$		$12q_1^2 p_1^3 q_2 p_2$		
$1 \to 2$	$\to 2$			$6q_1^2 p_1^2 p_2^2$		
$1 \to 3$	$\to 1$			$4q_1 p_1^3 p_3$		
$1 \to 4$				p_1^4		

Source: Based on Table 2.2 of Becker [1, p. 16].

while in Table 8.3 when there are two introductory cases. Note these probabilities are actually conditional probabilities, given the number of introductory cases.

TABLE 8.3

Household Counts for Size of Outbreaks of Common Cold

	Number of Cases			
	1	2	3	4
Overcrowded	112	35	17	11
Crowded	155	41	24	15
Uncrowded	156	55	19	10
Total	423	131	60	36

8.10 What is the Size of an Epidemic?

Infectious disease data are observational, rather than data from a designed experiment. This can result in the difficulty of soliciting reliable and detailed information. Possibly the readily available data for contagious maladies are taken about the size of outbreaks in households. With the aid of serological tools for diagnosis, such data are usually quite reliable. It goes without saying that it is essential to use the appropriate tools to analyze the data, which will be for this book, the Bayesian approach to inference.

Recall that the probability that the size of an epidemic equals j is denoted by θ_j, where $\sum_{j=1}^{j=s} \theta_j = 1$. With the chain binomial model, the number of parameters can be reduced, where the θ_j can be expressed in terms of $q_1, q_2, \dots, q_{s-2}$. It is assumed that the data are detailed enough to specify the number of initial cases and the initial number of susceptible people. The explanation is set in households of size four where initially there is one case and three susceptible individuals. The distribution is easily determined by accumulating the appropriate chain probabilities for the sixth column of Table 8.2. Therefore,

$$\theta_1 = pr[1] = q_1^3,$$

$$\theta_2 = pr[1 \to 1] = 3q_1^4 p_1, \tag{8.11}$$

and

$$\theta_3 = pr[1 \to 1 \to 1] + pr[1 \to 2] = 3q_1 p_1^2 \left(2q_1^3 + q_2 \right),$$

where $\theta_4 = 1 - \theta_1 - \theta_2 - \theta_3$.

Consider n households containing $s_0 = 3$ susceptible individuals and one $i_0 = 1$ initially infected person. Also, let n_j be the number of households with j cases, then the likelihood is given by

$$l(\theta_1, |, \theta_2, |, \theta_3, |, \theta_4, |, n_1, |, n_2, |, n_3, |, n_4) \propto \theta_1^{n_1} \theta_2^{n_2} \theta_3^{n_3} \theta_4^{n_4}, \tag{8.12}$$

where $\sum_{j=1}^{j=4} \theta_j = 1$.

Now assume the improper prior density

$$h(\theta_1,\theta_2,\theta_3,\theta_4) = 1 / \prod_{j=1}^{j=4} \theta_j, \qquad (8.13)$$

Then the posterior density is

$$l(\theta_1,\theta_2,\theta_3,\theta_4 \mid n_1,n_2,n_3,n_4) \propto \theta_1^{n_1-1}\theta_2^{n_2-1}\theta_3^{n_3-1}\theta_4^{n_4-1}, \qquad (8.14)$$

which is the density of a Dirichlet distribution with parameter vector (n_1,n_2,n_3,n_4). Also, note that $n = \sum_{j=1}^{j=4} n_j$ and that the expectation or average of θ_j is

$$E(\theta_j \mid n_1,n_2,n_3,n_4) = n_j / n \qquad (8.15)$$

For additional information about the Dirichlet, see DeGroot [9, pp. 49–51].

As an example, suppose there are n = 175 overcrowded households where, $n_1 = 112$, $n_2 = 35$, $n_3 = 17$, $n_4 = 11$, that is, there are 112 households with one case, 35 with two cases, 17 with three cases, and four with 11 cases, then using the improper prior (8.13), the posterior distribution of $(\theta_1,\theta_2,\theta_3,\theta_4)$ is Dirichlet with density

$$l(\theta_1,\theta_2,\theta_3,\theta_4 \mid n_1 = 112,\ n_2 = 35,\ n_3 = 17,\ n_4 = 11) \propto$$
$$\propto \theta_1^{112-1}\theta_2^{35-1}\theta_3^{17-1}\theta_4^{11-1} \qquad (8.16)$$

namely a Dirichlet distribution with parameter vector (112,35,17,11). The above data appear in the first row of Table 8.3.

Does the extent of crowding affect the number of cases? In the second row the number of households with one case is 155, with 2, 41, with 3, 24, and the number of households with 4 is 15.

Corresponding to the second row of table and associated with crowded households, and assuming the improper prior density is comparable to (8.13), the posterior density of the Dirichlet distribution with parameter vector (155,41,24,15) is

$$\pi(\phi_1,\phi_2,\phi_3,\phi_4 \mid m_1 = 155,\ m_2 = 41,\ m_3 = 24,\ m_4 = 15) \propto$$
$$\propto \phi_1^{155-1}\phi_2^{41-1}\phi_3^{24-1}\phi_4^{15-1}, \qquad (8.17)$$

where $\sum_{j=1}^{j=4} \phi_j = 1$.

Consider a test of the null hypothesis

H: $\theta_i = \phi_i$, $i = 1, 2, 3, 4$. versus the alternative hypothesis A: $\theta_i \neq \phi_i$ for at least one i, i = 1,2,3,4. The null hypothesis states that the proportion of households with one case is the same for the undercrowded and crowded households, that the proportion of households with two cases is the same for under-crowded and crowded households, etc. The Bayesian test procedure is based on [10, pp. 124–127].

Consider the following quantities

$$p(n,m) = \pi_0 \int p(n, | m, | \theta = \phi = \gamma) d\gamma$$
$$+ \pi_1 \int \rho_1(\theta, \phi) p(n, |, m, |, \theta, |, \phi) d\theta d\phi \qquad (8.18)$$

where

$$p(n, |, m, |, \theta, |, \phi) = [n! m! / n_1! n_2! n_3! n_4! m_1! m_2! m_3! m_4!] \int \prod_{i=1}^{i=4} \theta_i^{n_i} \phi_i^{m_i}, (8.19)$$

and

$$p(n, | m, | \theta = \phi = \gamma) = [n! m! / n_1! n_2! n_3! n_4! m_1! m_2! m_3! m_4!] \prod_{i=1}^{i=4} \gamma_i^{n_i + m_i}, \qquad (8.20)$$

Furthermore, suppose that $\rho_1(\theta, \phi)$ is the prior density of (θ, ϕ) under the alternative hypothesis. Consider the improper prior density for (θ, ϕ) to be

$$\rho_1(\theta, \phi) = 1 / \prod_{i=1}^{i=4} \theta_i \phi_i \qquad (8.21)$$

According to Lee, the posterior probability of the null hypothesis is

$$p_0 = \pi_0 \int p(n, | m, | \theta = \phi = \gamma) d\gamma / \left[\begin{array}{c} \pi_0 \int p(n, | m, | \theta = \phi = \gamma) d\gamma \\ + \pi_1 \int \rho_1(\theta, \phi) p(n, |, m, |, \theta, |, \phi) d\theta d\phi \end{array} \right] (8.22)$$

where π_0 is the prior probability of the null hypothesis and $\pi_0 + \pi_1 = 1$.

Recall that $n_1 = 112$, $n_2 = 35$, $n_3 = 17$, $n_4 = 11$, $m_1 = 155$, $m_2 = 41$, $m_3 = 23$, $m_4 = 15$. Then it can be shown that

$$p_0 = 1/2/ = [1/2 + 0] = 1, \qquad (8.23)$$

assuming $\pi_0 = 1/2 = \pi_1$.

Thus, one is confident in believing that the evidence in favor of the null hypothesis is overwhelming. Also, note that the calculation of the posterior probability of the null hypothesis is quite involved and time consuming.

Note, if one calculates the proportion of households in each of the four categories, for overcrowded households, the proportions are .64,.20,.097, and .062, while for the crowded households, the corresponding proportions are .65,.17,.102, and .0638. Of course, there is strong evidence that the null hypothesis is true, the same result confirmed by the Bayesian posterior probability of the null hypothesis. (8.23).

8.11 Chain Data for the Common Cold

There are obstacles with the classification of cases of common cold into generations, because the latent time for the common cold may be shorter than the infectious period. However, this did not deter Heasman and Reid [11] to have used the known properties of common cold to classify outbreaks in household of size 5 into various possible chains. The chain frequencies for 664 households with one introductory case are represented in Table 8.4. The three-parameter chain model is fitted to this information.

The likelihood function corresponding to the chain frequency data is

$$l\left(q_1, \mid q_2, \mid q_3, \mid data\right) \propto q_1^{3000} p_1^{397} q_2^{70} p_2^{18} q_3^3 \tag{8.24}$$

where q_1 is the probability a person escapes infection when exposed to 1 infected person, whereas q_2 is the probability a person is not infected when exposed to 2 infected people. Quick estimates of these parameters lead to $q_{\tilde{1}} = .86$ and $q_{\tilde{2}} = .11$, etc. then these are substituted into the expressions for the expected frequencies to obtain the fitted frequencies given in Table 8.4. Continuing with the Bayesian analysis based on the likelihood (8.24), let the improper prior density for the parameters be

$$\xi\left(q_1, q_2, q_3, p_1, p_2\right) = 1 / q_1 q_2 q_3 p_1 p_2 \tag{8.25}$$

then the posterior density is,

$$h\left(q_1, \mid q_2, \mid q_3, \mid data\right) \propto q_1^{3000-1} p_1^{397-1} q_2^{70-1} p_2^{18-1} q_3^{3-1} \tag{8.26}$$

which is recognized as the density of a Dirichlet distribution with parameter vector (3000,397,70,18,3).

TABLE 8.4

Observed and Expected Chain Counts for Outbreaks of the Common Cold in Households of Size Five and One Initial Case Chain Fitted

	Expected 7 Parameters	Observed	7 Parameter	3 Parameter	Reed-Frost
1	nq_{11}^4	423	421.0	403.9	405.2
$1 \rightarrow 1$	$4nq_{11}^3 p_{11} q_{21}^3$	131	130.4	147.3	147.1
$1 \rightarrow 1 \quad 1 \rightarrow 1$	$12nq_{11}^3 p_{11} q_{21}^2 p_{21} q_{31}^3$	36	40.0	45.6	45.3
$1 \rightarrow 2$	$6nq_{11}^3 p_{11}^2 q_{22}^2$	24	23.2	26.9	25.6
$1 \rightarrow 1 \quad 1 \rightarrow 1 \quad 1 \rightarrow 1$	$24nq_{11}^3 p_{11} q_{21}^2 p_{21} q_{31} p_{31} q_{41}$	14	15.4	10.7	10.5
$1 \rightarrow 1 \quad 1 \rightarrow 2$	$12nq_{11}^3 p_{11} q_{21} p_{21}^2 q_{32}$	8	7.9	6.2	6.0
$1 \rightarrow 2 \quad 2 \rightarrow 1$	$12nq_{11}^3 p_{11}^2 q_{22} p_{22} q_{31}$	11	9.6	12.2	12.7
$1 \rightarrow 3$	$4nq_{11} p_{11}^3 q_{23}$	3	3.0	3.7	2.5
$1 \rightarrow 1 \quad 1 \rightarrow 1 \quad 1 \rightarrow 1 \quad 1 \rightarrow 1$	$24nq_{11}^3 p_{11} q_{21}^3 p_{21} q_{31} p_{31} p_{41}$	4	4.4	1.4	1.4
$1 \rightarrow 1 \quad 1 \rightarrow 1 \quad 1 \rightarrow 2$	$12nq_{11}^3 p_{11} q_{21}^2 p_{21} p_{31}^2$	2	2.5	0.8	0.8
$1 \rightarrow 1 \quad 1 \rightarrow 2 \quad 2 \rightarrow 1$	$12nq_{11}^3 p_{11} q_{21} p_{21}^2 p_{32}$	2	2.0	1.6	1.7
$1 \rightarrow 1 \quad 1 \rightarrow 3$	$4nq_{11}^3 p_{11} q_{21} p_{21}^3$	2	0.5	0.3	0.3
$1 \rightarrow 2 \quad 2 \rightarrow 1 \quad 1 \rightarrow 1$	$12nq_{11}^2 p_{11}^2 q_{22} p_{22} p_{31}$	3	2.4	1.6	1.7
$1 \rightarrow 2 \quad 2 \rightarrow 2$	$6nq_{11}^2 p_{11}^2 p_{22}^2$	1	1.5	1.8	2.0
$1 \rightarrow 3 \quad 3 \rightarrow 1$	$4nq_{11} p_{11}^3 p_{22}^2$	0	0.0	0.0	1.1
$1 \rightarrow 4$	np_{11}^4	0	0.1	0.1	0.1
Total	N	664	663.9	664.1	664.0

Source: Table 2.7 from Becker [1, p. 31].

Also, the marginal posterior distribution of $q_1 \sim beta(3000, 488)$, with mean $E(q_1 \mid data) = 3000/3488) = .86009$.

8.12 Generalized Linear Models for the Analysis of Binomial Chain Information

The binomial distribution in chain binomial epidemic models arise as a consequence of the underlying constraints that each exposure which arises during the course of the epidemic chain is an independent Bernoulli trial, with an outcome either an infection or an escape from an infection. During the process of classifying the outbreaks into various epidemic chains, a person is actually making a decision as to whether each exposure results in an infection. This implies that whatever reliable epidemic chain data are observable one can in fact record the result of each of the exposures that arose during the course of the outbreak. To be more specific, it is possible to perform a logistic regression analysis that allows the escape probability (not to be infected) to depend on epidemiological considerations such as age, sex, generation, and health properties of both susceptible and infectives to whom one is exposed. In addition, epidemic chain data are not available that include detail on the characteristics of individuals. The method is illustrated with reference to the factors: "generation" and number of infected people that are exposed. Consider an example of epidemic chain data based on a sample of n affected households. Suppose that over all n outbreaks, generation i is formed as a result of a total of m_{ij} exposures to j infectives, and that for x_{ij} of these exposures the susceptible people escape infection. Thus, x_{ij} is an observation from a binomial distribution with m_{ij} trials and success probability q_{ij}. We now employ generalized linear models in order to capture a more detailed description of the infection process. We will make use of WinBUGS to execute the Bayesian analysis using generalized linear models (such as logistic linear regression) to estimate the unknown parameters of the model. In this way, the relationship between the escape probability q_{ij} and the number of infectives j is easily programmed with WinBUGS and other statistical software such as SAS or Stan, which is another Bayesian package that employs MCMC methods. For binomial data, a linear logistic regression model is often used, namely

$$\ln\left[q_{ij} / \left(1 - q_{ij}\right) \right] = \alpha_i + \beta_i j \qquad (8.27)$$

which is referred to as a generalized linear model,

$$\ln\left[q_{ij} / \left(1 - q_{ij}\right) \right] = \ln\left[\mu_{ij} / \left(m_{ij} - \mu_{ij}\right) \right] \qquad (8.28)$$

and is seen as a function of the mean μ_{ij}, linear in the parameters.

It is seen that the generation is a factor in the model (8.27), and the number of infectives exposed to is introduced as a continuous variable with regression coefficient depending on the generation. In the setting of a binomial epidemic expression, there is a choice of employing the log-linear model in lieu of the linear logistic model (8.27). More emphatically, there is a preferred choice for

$$\ln\left(m_{ij} q_{ij} \right) = \ln\left(m_{ij} \right) + \alpha_i + \beta_i j \qquad (8.29)$$

over the expression (8.27). See Becker [1, p. 38] for more detail concerning this topic. Note that model (8.28) includes the Greenwood and Reed-Frost chain binomial models as special cases. This is seen by letting $\beta_i = 0$, $i = 1, 2,$ ... which in turn implies that $q_{ij} = q_i$, the Greenwood formulation. It is also seen that when $\alpha_i = 0$, $i = 1, 2, ...,$ that $q_{ij} = q_i^j$, which is seen as the Reed-Frost model. If the linear logistic model is used for the analysis, this model and the log-linear model (8.29) usually result in a similar inference. The latter has the advantage that its parameters have epidemiologic interpretations, and one also sees that $\ln(m_{ij})$ of (8.29) can be observed directly.

8.13 Models for the Common Cold

See Table 8.4, which displays the common cold epidemic chain information, then one sees that the binomial distribution can express quite adequately different exposures, thus providing complete descriptions of the epidemic chain data, but the binomial parameters will vary with different types of exposure. The log linear model (8.29) is now employed to determine the extent to which the number of parameters in the model can be reduced. Refer to Table 8.5.

Model (1) of Table 8.5 is the standard Greenwood model determined from (8.29) by letting $\alpha_1 = \alpha_2 = \alpha_3 = \alpha_4 = \alpha$ and $\beta_i = 0$, $i = 1, 2, 3, 4$. This gives the model

$$\ln\left(m_{ij}q_{ij}\right) = \ln\left(m_{ij}\right) + \alpha \tag{8.30}$$

Thus, in particular, based on the information of Table 8.5, the seven equations leading to estimates of alpha are:

TABLE 8.5

Observed Counts for Different Exposures to the Common Cold. Fitted Counts Corresponding to various Log-Linear Models Fitted Counts

Generation i	# Infectives j	# Exposures m_{ij}	Observed Counts x_{ij}	Expected Counts	Model (1)	Model (2)	Model (3)	Model (4)	Model (5)
1	1	2656	2370	$m_{11}q_{11}$	2340	2347.5	2370	2370	2370
2	1	597	515	$m_{21}q_{21}$	526	527.6	510.7	519.3	514.5
2	2	78	62	$m_{22}q_{22}$	68.7	60.9	66.7	59	63.2
2	3	3	3	$m_{23}q_{23}$	2.6	2.1	2.6	2	2.3
3	1	126	101	$m_{31}q_{31}$	111	111.4	101	102.5	101.6
3	2	10	8	$m_{32}q_{32}$	8.8	7.8	8	6.6	7.4
4	1	18	14	$m_{41}q_{41}$	15.9	15.9	14	14	14

$$\ln(2370/2656) = \alpha = -.11393,$$
$$\ln(515/587) = \alpha = -.14775$$
$$\ln(62/78) = \alpha - .22957, \qquad (8.31)$$
$$\ln(3/3) = \alpha = 0,$$
$$\ln(101/126) = \alpha = -.22116,$$
$$\ln(8/10) = \alpha - .22314,$$

and

$$\ln(14/18) = \alpha = -.25131.$$

When one solves for α, one finds that the estimate for α is $\tilde{\alpha} = -.16955$.

We now estimate the q_{ij} using Bayesian methods. Consider the likelihood function for q_{11}

$$l\left(q_{11} \mid , m_{11} = 2656 \mid , x_{ij} = 2370\right) \propto q_{11}^{2370}\left(1 - q_{11}\right)^{286}, 0 < q_{11} < 1 \qquad (8.32)$$

Now suppose the prior information is vague, then it is reasonable to employ the improper density

$$\zeta\left(q_{11}\right) \propto q_{11}^{-1}\left(1 - q_{11}\right)^{-1},$$

Thus, the posterior distribution of q_{11} has density

$$l\left(q_{11} \mid n_{11} = 2656, m_{11} = 2370\right) \propto q_{11}^{2370-1}\left(1 - q_{11}\right)^{286-1}, 0 < q_{11} < 1, \qquad (8.33)$$

which is that of a Beta distribution with parameter vector (2370,286). A plausible estimate of q_{11} is the posterior mean

$$E\left(q_{11} \mid , m_{11} = 2656 \mid , x_{ij} = 2370\right) = 2370 / 2656 = .8923. \qquad (8.34)$$

What is the interpretation of this result? Recall that q_{11} is the probability of not being infected for an individual of generation 1 exposed to 1 infective. Recall the model assumed to apply is the Greenwood model.

We now consider model (2), the Reed-Frost model, by letting the alpha be zero and $\beta_i = \beta$, $i = 1, 2, 3, 4$ in model (8.29), which results in

$$\ln\left(m_{ij}q_{ij}\right) = \ln\left(m_{ij}\right) + \beta_i j. \qquad (8.35)$$

It follows that

$$\ln(515) = \ln(597) + \beta \Rightarrow \beta = -.14775,$$
$$\ln(62) = \ln(78) + \beta \Rightarrow \beta = -.11478,$$
$$\ln(3) = \ln(3) + 3\beta \Rightarrow \beta = 0,$$
$$\ln(101) = \ln(126) + \beta \Rightarrow \beta = -.22116, \qquad (8.36)$$
$$\ln(8) = \ln(10) + 2\beta \Rightarrow \beta = -.11187$$
$$\ln(14) = \ln(18) + \beta \Rightarrow \beta = -.06432$$

Averaging these 7 values of beta gives as an estimate $\tilde{\beta} = -.11054$ and as an estimate of the escape probability $\tilde{q} = \exp(-.11054) = .89535$.

Next is model (3) defined as

$$\ln(m_{ij}) = \ln(m_{ij}) + \alpha_i, i = 1,2,3,4, j = 1,2,3 \qquad (8.37)$$

It follows from the information is Table 8.5 that in particular

$$\tilde{\alpha}_1 = -.11393,$$
$$\tilde{\alpha}_2 = -.12575, \qquad (8.38)$$
$$\tilde{\alpha}_3 = -.22215,$$

and

$$\tilde{\alpha}_4 = -.25131.$$

The corresponding probabilities of not being infected are:

$$\tilde{q}_1 = \exp(\tilde{\alpha}_1) = .89232,$$
$$\tilde{q}_2 = \exp(\tilde{\alpha}_2) = .88183, \qquad (8.39)$$
$$\tilde{q}_3 = \exp(\tilde{\alpha}_3) = .80079,$$

and

$$\tilde{q}_4 = \exp(\tilde{\alpha}_4) = .77775$$

respectively.

If one adopts a uniform prior for α, what is the posterior density of $q = e^\alpha, -1 < \alpha < 0$. This is left as an exercise for the student.

It is seen that the chain binomial model provides a useful basis for analysis even when the data consist of affected households with different number of people across households. These models assume their least complex form when all individuals are equally susceptible and infectious individuals reach equal stages of infectiousness and remain infectious for the same amount of time. Of course, this is somewhat unrealistic, and the more realistic scenario will be taken up later in the chapter. Also, it was discovered that chain binomial models are still applicable when some heterogeneity exists between individuals. This implies that infected and susceptible individuals can be partitioned into groups, and within each group the individuals can be considered homogenous. This further implies that the value of the binomial parameter to be associated with the type of cross-infection. When this is not the case, that'is not possible, that is, to partition individuals into homogenous groups, the chain binomial model is not appropriate. When this is the case, the analysis is executed by employing covariates to describe the heterogeneity. Technically, these are no longer chain binomial models.

8.14 Random Infectiousness Models

Consider a household in which the individuals are uniformly mixed, and assume the susceptible individuals are equally susceptible. It is also assumed that infectives differ in their infectiveness by assigning to each infected individual an infectiousness function chosen independently and at random from a set of infectiousness functions. Assign s_0 as the number of susceptible individuals in a household of size $s_0 + 1$, including one introductory case. Assume that each susceptible escapes infection by the introductory infective with probability ϕ, then given ϕ, the probability distribution of the number of first-generation cases X is binomial with mass function

$$\Pr\left(X = x \mid \phi\right) = \binom{s_0}{x}\left(1-\phi\right)^x \phi^{s_0-x}, x = 0,1,\ldots,s_0. \tag{8.40}$$

Now continue on to the second generation, then the conditional distribution of the number Y of second-generation individuals given X=x in the first generation is binomial with mass function

$$P_r\left(Y = y \mid \phi_{(x)}, X = x\right) = \binom{s_0 - x}{y}\left(1-\phi_{(x)}\right)^y \phi_{(x)}^{s_0-x-y}, y = 0,1,\ldots,s_0 - x \tag{8.41}$$

where $\phi_{(x)}$ is the probability that a susceptible escapes infection when exposed to x infectives for the duration of the infectious period. Note that $\phi_{(x)}$ is considered a random variable.

Example 8.1

A less complex model is the result of determining the way that $\phi_{(x)}$ depends on x. If the Reed-Frost model is adopted, $\phi_{(x)}$ is the product of x independent random variables such as ϕ. Under this scenario, the computation of the chain probabilities is described. Suppose the household is made up of four susceptible individuals and one introductory infective, so that $s_0 = 4$, and for this household let the epidemic chain be $1 \rightarrow 1 \rightarrow 2$. Let $\phi_1, \phi_2, \phi_3, \phi_4$ signify the probabilities that a given susceptible escapes infection by each of the four infected individuals. Therefore, the conditional probability of this chain, $1 \rightarrow 1 \rightarrow 2$, given $\phi_1, \phi_2, \phi_3, \phi_4$, is computed in a similar way as the chain binomial model and thus is

$$\Pr(1 \rightarrow 1 \rightarrow 2 \mid \phi_1, \phi_2\phi_3, \phi_4)$$
$$= \binom{4}{3}\phi_1^3(1-\phi_1)\binom{3}{1}\phi_2(1-\phi_2)^2\binom{1}{1}\phi_3\phi_4(1-\phi_3\phi_4)^0 \qquad (8.42)$$

It is seen that the event $1 \rightarrow 1 \rightarrow 2$ is the product of independent binomial distributions: The first is binomial with parameters n = 4 and p = ϕ_1, the second is binomial with parameters n = 3 and p = ϕ_2, and the third is binomial with parameters n = 1 and p = ϕ_3 and the last is binomial with parameters n = 1 and p = ϕ_4.

Assuming a uniform prior for ϕ_1, the posterior distribution of ϕ_1 is beta with parameters $\alpha = 4$ and $\beta = 2$, thus the posterior mean of ϕ_1 is $\alpha/\alpha + \beta = 2/3$, and the posterior variance is $\alpha\beta/(\alpha + \beta)^2(\alpha + \beta + 1) = .031746$.

Example 8.2

Now consider a household with one introductory case and four susceptible individuals, with chain probability

$$P(1 \rightarrow 1 \rightarrow 1 \mid \phi_1, \phi_2, \phi_3, \phi_4)$$
$$= \binom{4}{3}\phi_1^3(1-\phi_1)\binom{3}{1}\phi_2(1-\phi_2)^2\binom{2}{1}\phi_3(1-\phi_3)\binom{1}{1}\phi_4(1-\phi_4)^0 \qquad (8.43)$$

Assuming a uniform prior for the parameter vector $(\phi_1, \phi_2, \phi_3, \phi_4)$, what is the posterior distribution of these parameters? Following the logic of Example 8.1, the posterior distribution of each of the ϕ_1, ϕ_2, ϕ_3, and ϕ_4 are beta. The details will be left with the reader to fill in.

Following the logic above in the previous example, the posterior distribution of ϕ_3 is beta with parameters $\alpha = \beta = 2$, thus the posterior mean of ϕ_3 is $\alpha/(\alpha + \beta) = 2/(2 + 2) = 1/2$ and its posterior variance is $\alpha\beta/(\alpha + \beta)^2(\alpha + \beta + 1) = .05$

Example 8.3 Simulation of Beta

The following example is a simulation of the beta distribution with parameters $\alpha = \beta = .5$. The R code used for the simulation is:

```
U <- runif(1e4) alpha <- 0.5 beta <- 0.5 b_rand <- qbeta(U, alpha, beta)
hist(b_rand, col = "skyblue", main = "Inverse U")
```

Of course, to obtain the unconditional version of (8.42), one averages (8.42) with respect to the joint marginal distribution of $(\phi_1, \phi_2 \phi_3, \phi_4)$ to obtain

$$\Pr(1 \to 1 \to 2) = E\left[4\phi_1^3 \left(1-\phi_1\right) 3\phi_2 \left(1-\phi_2\right)^2 \phi_3\phi_4 \right]$$
$$= 12\mu_1^2 \left(\mu_3 - \mu_4\right)\left(\mu_1 - 2\mu_2 + \mu_3\right) \qquad (8.44)$$

where $\mu_i = E(\phi_i)$, $i = 1,2,3,4$.

To simplify the following, let $\theta_i = \mu_{i-1} - \mu_i$ and $\beta_i = \mu_{i-1}^2 - \mu_i^2$, and consider the following table of chain probabilities for the random infection model with one introductory case for households of size 5,4, and 3.

For more information about this subject, see Becker [1, pp. 48–67]. It will be left to the student to verify Table 8.6. See Figure 8.1 for a plot of the simulated values,

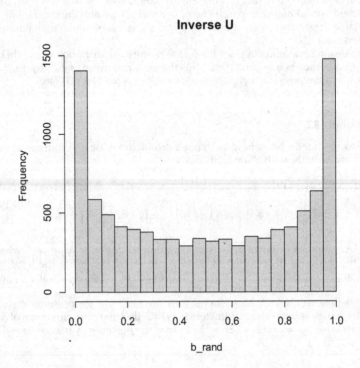

FIGURE 8.1

TABLE 8.6

Chain Probabilities for the Infectious Model with One Introductory Case

Chain	Household Size		
	5	4	3
1	μ_4	μ_3	μ_2
$1 \rightarrow 1$	$4\mu_3\theta_4$	$3\mu_2\theta_3$	$2\mu_1\theta_2$
$1 \rightarrow 1 \rightarrow 1$	$12\mu_2\theta_3\theta_4$	$6\mu_1\theta_2\theta_3$	$2\theta_1\theta_2$
$1 \rightarrow 2$	$6\mu_2^2(\theta_3-\theta_4)$	$3\mu_1^2(\theta_2-\theta_3)$	$(\theta_1-\theta_2)$
$1 \rightarrow 1 \rightarrow 1 \rightarrow 1$	$24\mu_1\theta_2\theta_3\theta_4$	$6\theta_1\theta_2\theta_3$	
$1 \rightarrow 1 \rightarrow 2$	$12\mu_1^2(\theta_2-\theta_3)\theta_4$	$3(\theta_1-\theta_2)\theta_3$	
$1 \rightarrow 2 \rightarrow 1$	$12\mu_1\beta_2(\theta_3-\theta_4)$	$3\beta_1(\theta_2-\theta_3)$	
$1 \rightarrow 3$	$4\mu_1^3(\theta_2-2\theta_3+\theta_4)$	$\theta_1-2\theta_2-\theta_3$	
$1 \rightarrow 1 \rightarrow 1 \rightarrow 1 \rightarrow 1$	$24\theta_1\theta_2\theta_3\theta_4$		
$1 \rightarrow 1 \rightarrow 1 \rightarrow 2$	$12(\theta_1-\theta_2)\theta_3\theta_4$		
$1 \rightarrow 1 \rightarrow 2 \rightarrow 1$	$12\beta_1(\theta_2-\theta_3)\theta_4$		
$1 \rightarrow 1 \rightarrow 3$	$4(\theta_1-2\theta_2+\theta_3)\theta_4$		
$1 \rightarrow 2 \rightarrow 1 \rightarrow 1$	$12\theta_1\beta_2(\theta_3-\theta_4)$		
$1 \rightarrow 2 \rightarrow 2$	$6(\beta_1-\beta_2)(\theta_3-\theta_4)$		
$1 \rightarrow 3 \rightarrow 1$	$4(1-\mu_1^3)(\theta_2-2\theta_3+\theta_4)$		
$1 \rightarrow 4$	$\theta_1-3\theta_2+3\theta_3-\theta_4$		

8.15 Latent and Infectiousness Periods

Information on the size of an outbreak is obtained even though there is sparse information about the times at which cases show their symptoms.

The categorization of outbreaks into several epidemic chains requires a minimum of knowledge of which the symptoms do appear. But, analyses based on size of outbreak data or chain data provide practically no information on the rate the outbreak is spreading as a function of time. We will utilize the arrival time of disease in order to make inferences about how the contagion evolves through time, namely the duration of the latent and infectious periods experienced by the individual, and in addition the instantaneous rate of the outbreak.

8.16 Observable Infectious Period

We first consider where it is possible to determine the end and beginning of the infectious period for each person observed. For example, a person is considered infected as long as they display a rash (as in measles). On the other hand, it might be known that the individual is infectious from two days before the rash and until four days after the rash has disappeared. Obviously in this situation, a great deal must be known about the contagion in question. Also suppose, this disease is mild so that its onset does not affect substantially the behavior of the household individuals. This would not be the situation for such diseases as measles or tuberculosis. Suppose for each person that is infected, one can observe the interval (U,W), the infectious period of the individual. The variables U and W are measured relative to a time origin, and the duration of the disease is Y=W-U, and thus by observing Y for a number of infected people, one can determine the distribution of Y. Based on observation and the knowledge of this distribution, one could compute the mean and standard deviation of the durations observed. Of course, as a part of the summary statistics for this scenario, a histogram or stem and leaf plot is usually computed. On the other hand, one could compare the infectious periods of individuals in separate groups of infected individuals using more sophisticated methods, and this will be implemented by Bayesian inferential techniques. Whatever is the situation, the fact that the durations are observable allows one to employ a variety of methods for making deductions about the spread of the contagion.

It is more difficult to make inferences about the latent periods, because the exact times at which the infectious contact does occur are not observable. This necessitates the stating of assumptions about the nature of the infectiousness function. One's selection of the infectiousness function will of course be based on the knowledge of the disease as well as having a convenient mathematical (including stochastic) formula that will include unknown parameters that will be estimated with various statistical procedures.

Consider the infectiousness function

$$\Gamma(z) = \beta(z-U)(W-x), U \leq z \leq W \qquad (8.45)$$
$$= 0, otw$$

which has the property as a function increasing to a maximum and decreasing finally to zero.

A somewhat less complex function is

$$\Gamma(z) = \beta, U < z < W \qquad (8.46)$$
$$= 0, otw$$

since it describes an adequate description of the behavior of an infection. Note that U and W are random variables.

8.17 Households of Size Two

Now consider the estimation of the infection rate β for households of size two under the following conditions. It is supposed that the observed outbreaks can be grouped in the chains:

2: two introductory cases

1: one introductory case, no secondary case

1 $\rightarrow$ 1: one introductory case and one secondary case

It is obvious that data from an affected household with two introductory cases contain no information about the rate β because one needs information about what is going on inside of the household. Let (U_1, W_1) and (U_2, W_2) signify the infectious intervals for the two cases of a household with two introductory cases, and assume the two outbreaks occur independently of each other. For such scenarios, it is not unreasonable to postulate the cases are infected at the same time. Therefore, it follows that $U_1 - U_2 = X_1 - X_2$, where X_1 and X_2 are the durations of the two latent periods. It follows that $U_1 - U_2$ is a function of (U_1, W_1, U_2, W_2) and contains information about the latent period. Since $E(U_1 - U_2) = 0$ and $Var(U_1 - U_2) = 2Var(X)$, where X is either X_1 or X_2 which implies that $U_1 - U_2$ is informative primarily about the dispersion of the length of the duration interval. As an example, consider the duration of the latent period has density

$$f_X\left(x\mid,\lambda\mid,\gamma\right) = \lambda \exp{-\lambda\left(x-\gamma\right)}, x > \gamma \qquad (8.47)$$

Thus, $U_1 - U_2$ has a distribution depending only on the parameter λ. A household with two introductory cases and associated observations $(U_1, W_1) = (u_1, w_1)$ and $(U_2, W_2) = (u_2, w_2)$ makes the contribution

$$\int_0^\infty f_X\left(x + u_1 - u_2\right) f_X\left(x\right) dx \qquad (8.48)$$

to the likelihood function. It should be noted that Y is the duration of the infectious period on which there are observations $y_1 = w_1 - u_1$ and $y_2 = w_2 - u_2$. Note that the functions f_X and f_Y represent density functions of X and Y respectively, and the integral is the density of $U_1 - U_2$ evaluated at $u_1 - u_2$. Suppose one examines the situation for households of size two with one introductory case, but no secondary cases. Data in this case are not very useful because the only data available are the infectious periods

(U, V) of the observed case and the observations that the remaining susceptible did indeed escape infection. This information is sparse about the latent period but does contain information about the infection rate parameter β. For example, a household with one introductory case and no secondary producing the observation $(U, W) = (u, w)$ makes the contribution

$$f_Y (w - u) e^{-\beta(w-u)} \tag{8.49}$$

to the likelihood function.

Notice that the exponential term represents the probability that the remaining susceptible escapes infection when exposed to one infected person who is contagious for the duration (w-u) time units.

Next consider affected households of size two having observed the chain $1 \rightarrow 1$, and suppose (U_1, W_1) signifies the infectious interval of the introductory infected individual, let (U_2, W_2) that of the other case. Now, where X_2 is the duration of the latent period for the secondary case and Z represents the time from U_1 until the infection of the secondary case. The conditional density of $U_2 - U_1$ given that the introductory infective has an infectious period of duration y_1 and chain $1 \rightarrow 1$ is observed as, is

$$f_{U_2-U_1} \left(a | , Y_1 = y_1 |, 1 \rightarrow 1 \right) = \int_0^{y_1} \beta e^{-\beta z} f_X (a - z) dz / \left(1 - e^{-\beta y_1} \right). \tag{8.50}$$

It follows that a household with chain $1 \rightarrow 1$ and observed infectious periods (u_1, w_1) and (u_2, w_2) makes a contribution

$$f_Y (y_1) f_Y (y_2) \int_0^{y_1} \beta e^{-\beta z} f_X (u_2 - u_1 - z) dz \tag{8.51}$$

to the likelihood function. That part of the likelihood function appropriate for inferences about β or parameters of the distribution of X is given by

$$\left[\prod_{(2)} \int_0^\infty f_X(x + u_1 - u_2) f_X(x) dx \right] \left[\prod_{(1)} e^{-\beta(w-u)} \right]$$
$$\left[\prod_{(1\rightarrow 1)} \int_0^{w_1 - u_1} \beta e^{-\beta x} f_X(u_2 - u_1 - x) dx \right] \tag{8.52}$$

where $\prod_c$ denotes the product of such terms over households of chain type $c = 1, 2, 1 \rightarrow 1$.

The likelihood function depends on β and the parameters involved with the f_X distribution, thus one is able to provide inferences for these parameters. However, to use this likelihood function, a family of distributions should be expressed. Obviously, this family should be chosen in such a way that that the computation of the likelihood is not too complicated to execute. Becker [1, p. 72] proposes three choices:

1. One possibility for the density is the shifted exponential $f_x(x \mid \lambda, \gamma) = \lambda e^{-\lambda(x-\gamma)}$, $x > \gamma$, which gives

$$\int_0^\infty f_x(x+d)f_X(x)dx = (1/2)\lambda e^{-\lambda|d|)} \tag{8.53}$$

and

$$\int_0^\infty \beta e^{-\beta x} f_x(d-x)dx = \lambda \beta \left\{ y \wedge \left(0 \vee (d-\gamma) \right) \right\} e^{-\lambda(d-\gamma)}, \lambda = \beta \tag{8.54}$$

or

$$\lambda \neq \beta \tag{8.55}$$

which can be substituted into the likelihood function. Note that $a \wedge b$ is the smaller of a and b, while $a \vee b$ denotes the larger of a and b.

2. A second possibility is to assume that X has a uniform distribution over $[\gamma, \gamma + \theta]$, where γ and θ are unknown parameters to be estimated. Employing this choice, one substitutes

$$\int_0^\infty f_X(x+d)f_X(x)dx = (\theta - \|d\|)/\theta^2 \tag{8.56}$$

and

$$\int_0^y \beta e^{-\beta x} f_X(x)dx = \left[e^{\beta\{0 \vee (d-\gamma-\theta)\}} - e^{-\beta\{(\gamma+d) \wedge (d-\gamma)\}} \right]/\theta \tag{8.57}$$

into the expression

3. The third alternative is to assume that X has a normal distribution with mean μ_X and variance σ_X^2. Of course, this is an approximation because X is a positive-valued random variable, whereas a normal variate can

assume negative values, but when the coefficient of variation σ_X/μ_X is say smaller than 0.5, this results in a good approximation. This implies that with this choice, one can approximate terms of the form

$$\int_0^\infty f_X(x+d) f_X(x)\,dx = \left(2\sigma_X\sqrt{\pi}\right)^{-1} \exp\left(-d^2/4\sigma_X^2\right), \qquad (8.58)$$

which is acceptable when σ_X/μ_X is small. The following expression is the likelihood function, namely

$$\int_0^y \beta e^{-\beta x} f_X(d-x)\,dx = \beta e^{-\beta\left(a+(1/2)\beta\sigma^2\right)} \left\{\Phi\left(a/\sigma^x\right) - \Phi\left((a-y\wedge d)/\sigma_X\right)\right\} \quad (8.59)$$

which can be used as a term in the likelihood function. Note, that Φ is the distribution function of the standard normal and that $a = d - \mu_X - \beta\sigma_X^2$.

Thus, there are three choices for the distribution of the latent period of the disease. It is suggested that the normal distribution be used only when the coefficient of variation is small and that both the shifted exponential and the uniform are suitable when the duration of the latent period is small. The uniform distribution is appropriate only if the duration of the latent period is contained in the interval $[\gamma, \gamma + \theta]$. It is important to know that the above is applicable for only households containing two individuals.

8.18 Example of Households of Size Two for a Measles Epidemic

The above equations (8.47) through (8.59) are relevant for estimating the parameters of an epidemic for households of size two. This information involves 264 households containing two children under the age of 15. There were 45 households with a single case and the time duration in days between cases for the 219 households with two cases is presented in Table 8.7. The outbreaks with two cases consist of chains 2 and $1 \to 1$. In the challenge of identifying the chain, one is often helped by tracing contacts. Hence, somewhat arbitrarily, take outbreaks with an observed time interval between the detection of cases less than six to be chains of type 2. In such a manner, there is apart from the 45 chains of type 1, 32 of type 2, and 187 of type $1 \to 1$.

Upon investigating the information, there appears to be a tendency to "round" off the time interval to seven days, and somewhat to a lesser extent

TABLE 8.7

Observed Time Intervals and Frequencies between Detection of Two Cases of Measles

Interval	Frequency	Interval	Frequency
0	5	11	38
1	13	12	26
2	5	13	12
3	4	14	15
4	3	15	6
5	2	16	3
6	4	17	1
7	11	18	3
8	5	19	0
9	25	20	0
10	37	21	1

Source: Table 4.1 from Becker [1, p. 82].

to 14 days, and to 21 days. That is, the overall tendency is to round off the duration to the nearest week (1, 2, or 3). It is possible the local peaks in the observed counts of 7, 14, and 21 days might be occurring at random; however, such peaks are commonly observed phenomena and researchers should be aware of such approximations encroaching into the data.

8.19 Bayesian Analysis of Measles in Households of Size Two

I will analyze the above data in Table 8.7, assuming a multinomial distribution for the frequencies in the 22 cells. Let θ_i, $i = 0, 1, 2, \ldots, 21$, be the probability of cell i, then the joint distribution of the observed frequencies is multinomial with mass function

$$0 < \theta_i < 1, \sum_{i=0}^{i=21} \theta_i = 1 \qquad (8.60)$$

where X = (5,13,5,4,3,2,4,11,5,25,37,38,26,12,15,6,3,1,3,0,0,1).

Assuming a uniform prior for the interval probabilities, the posterior distribution for these cell probabilities has density

Histogram of X

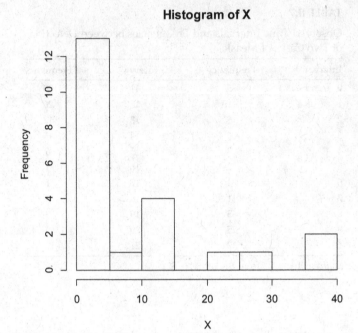

FIGURE 8.2
Histogram of Frequency of Measles Outbreak

$$0 < \theta_i < 1, \sum_{i=0}^{i=21} \theta_i = 1 \qquad (8.61)$$

which is the density function of a Dirichlet distribution with parameter vector Z = (6,14,6,5,4,3,5,12,6,26,38,39,27,13,16,7,4,2,4,1,1,2) . For additional information about the multinomial distribution, see Chapter 5 of DeGroot [9]. It is observed that the marginal distribution of an individual cell probability is Beta. The histogram of the multinomial observed frequencies appears above in Figure 8.2.

The histogram is rather irregular but does resemble, to some extent, an exponential distribution.

8.20 The Exponential Growth of Epidemics

According to Cochran, during the Sean Hannity Show on Fox, President Trump questioned whether New York State would require tens of thousands of ventilators its leaders had estimated would be necessary to deal with the

expected number of coronavirus cases. Then, three days later during a brief-
ing at the White House, Trump wondered out loud why the need for protective masks had increased at one New York Hospital from 10,000-20,000 per
week to 200,000-300,000.

"Where are the masks going?" he asked. "Are they going out the back
door?" He later added "We do have a problem of hoarding. We have some
health care workers, some hospital frankly – individual hospitals and hospital chains – we have then hoarding equipment, including ventilators."
The President's dismissal of the magnitude of these numbers may indicate
a lack of understanding or disregard of exponential growth that plagues a
large portion of the population. Even many who are well educated do not
understand the concept and often use the term "exponential growth" or
"exponentially" as hyperbole instead of a description of a trend in growth
or acceleration. Why should we care about this apparently arcane mathematical principle? Because, under our current circumstances, misunderstanding or disregard of exponential growth and the decisions made
based on the misunderstanding or disregard might have extremely grave
consequences.

Albert Bartlett, who was professor emeritus in nuclear physics at the
University of Colorado at Boulder, emphatically asserted that "The greatest
shortcoming of the human race has quickly brought me (Cochran) in line
with Bartlett's position on the importance of this issue."

To understand the idea of exponential growth, consider Table 8.8, which is
based on the table appearing on page 19 of the Cochran [12] article. In this
table r refers to the growth rate, and the formula for exponential growth of a
variable X at growth rate r at time t is given by

$$X(t) = (1+r)^t \, X(0) \tag{8.62}$$

where $X(0)$ is the initial value at time = 0.

8.21 The Coronavirus

This contribution to the morphology of coronavirus is based on the use
of electron microscopy in a negative contrast investigation of the virus
of transmissible gastroenteritis of swine. Viruses of transmissible gastro-
enteritis are spherical or, in rare cases, pleomorphous particles of typical
coronavirus structure. The viruses investigated by the authors were 132
nm in diameter. The surface projections, consisting of a flattened knob
and conical shaft, are 18 nm in length. Internal bodies, 50+/−2 nm in

TABLE 8.8

Exponential Growth for Three Rates

Day	r = 2	r = 1	r = 0.5
1	.01	.01	.01
2	.03	.02	.02
3	.09	.04	.02
4	.27	.08	.03
5	.81	.16	.05
6	2.43	.32	.08
7	7.29	.64	.11
8	21.87	1.28	.17
9	65.61	2.56	.26
10	196.83	5.12	.38
11	590.49	10.25	.58
12	1771.47	20.48	.86
13	5314.41	40.96	1.30
14	15943.23	81.92	1.95
15	47829.69	163.84	2.92
16	143489.07	327.68	4.38
17	430467.21	655.36	6.57
18	1291401.63	1310.72	9.85
19	3874204.89	2621.44	14.78
20	11622614.67	5242.88	22.17
21	34867844.01	10485.76	33.25
22	104603532.03	20971.52	49.88
23	313810596.09	41943.04	74.82
24	941431788.27	83886.08	112.23
25	2824295364.81	167772.16	168.34
26	8472886094.43	335544.32	252.51
27	25418658283.29	671088.64	378.77
28	76255974549.87	13421777.28	568.15
29	228767924549.61	2684354.56	852.23
30	686303773648.83	5368709.12	1278.34
31	2058911320946.49	10737418.24	1917.51

Source: See Cochran [12, p. 19]

diameter, occur as "filled" or "empty" particles. The thickness of all internal bodies and virus membranes is 8+/−1 nm. Differences were found to exist between virus of transmissible gastro-enteritis and particles similar to coronavirus and isolated from fecal samples. A first comparison had been made for that purpose. Those differences were relating to shape and size of individual particles and to morphological setup of surface projections.

We now use the coronavirus cases to estimate the rate it is expanding via formula (8.62).For the Bayesian analysis, only the first 20 observations of the number of infections (cases) of the time series is used. The main parameter is r, the rate the coronavirus is expanding in an exponential fashion. The analysis assumed an AR(1) process for the time series of the number of coronavirus cases and is executed with 45,000 iterations, and 5,000 initial values.

BC 8.1

```
model;
{
r~dbeta(.1,2)
# r is the rate the cases are increasing
v~dgamma(.1,.1)
theta~dbeta(1,2)
# see formula (8.2)
for(t in 1:20){mu[t]<-pow(1+r,t)}
Y[1,1:20]~dmnorm(mu[],tau[,])
        tau[1:20,1:20]<-inverse(Sigma[,])
            for(i in 1:20){Sigma[i,i]<-v/(1-theta*theta)}
            for(i in 1:20){for(j in i+1:20){Sigma[i,j]<-
v*pow(theta,j)*1/(1-theta*theta)}}
            for(i in 2:20){for(j in 1: i-1){Sigma[i,j]<-
v*pow(theta,i-1)*1/(1-theta*theta)}}
}
list(Y=structure(.Dat
a=c(563,786,1238,1910,2669,4415,5823,7519,13921,16523,19561,
23146,26528,29239,32069,34055,36320,38038,39216,52039),.
Dim=c(1,20)))
list(r=1,theta=. 6, v=4)
```

The Bayesian analysis is executed with 25,000 observations for the simulation and 5,000 initial values.

See Table 8.9 for the associated posterior analysis.

The following WinBUGS code is for the analysis of the mortality rate (based on the formula (8.62)) during the coronavirus epidemic for the first 20 days. The analysis is executed with 45,000 iterations and 5,000 initial values.

TABLE 8.9

Posterior Distribution for Coronavirus Infection Rate

Parameter	Mean	SD	Error	2 1/2	Median	97 1/2
r	.6755	.001534	.00000818	.6724	.6755	.6784
θ	.9999	.00003793	.000000260	.9998	.9999	1

Note that the posterior estimates of these parameters have quite small posterior standard deviations. The theta parameter is that of an AR(1) process.

BC 8.2

```
model;
{
r~dbeta(.1,2)
# r is the mortality rate
v~dgamma(.1,.1)
theta~dbeta(1,2)
for(t in 1:20){mu[t]<-pow(1+r,t)}
Y[1,1:20]~dmnorm(mu[],tau[,])
       tau[1:20,1:20]<-inverse(Sigma[,])
              for(i in 1:20){Sigma[i,i]<-v/(1-theta*theta)}
              for(i in 1:20){for(j in i+1:20){Sigma[i,j]<-
v*pow(theta,j)*1/(1-theta*theta)}}
              for(i in 2:20){for(j in 1: i-1){Sigma[i,j]<-
v*pow(theta,i-1)*1/(1-theta*theta)}}
}
list(
Y=structure(.Dat
a=c(362,426,392,565,638,724,813,910,1018,1115,1261,1383,1526,
1669,1775,1873,2009,2126,2247,2360),.Dim=c(1,20)))
list(r=1,theta=. 6, v=4)
```

See Table 8.10 for the posterior analysis.

The following WinBUGS code is for the Bayesian analysis that estimates the recovery rate of patients during the coronavirus epidemic. Formula (8.62) was used for the rate parameter r. The analysis is executed with 35,000 observations for the simulation and 5,000 initial values.

TABLE 8.10

Mortality Rate during Epidemic First Twenty Days

Parameter	Mean	SD	Error	2 1/2	Median	97 1/2
r	.4308	.005919	.00003187	.4185	.431	.4418
θ	.999	.0006138	.00000482	.9975	.9992	.9998

Based on (8.62), the mortality rate is estimated with the posterior mean as .4308 with an estimated accuracy as measured by the posterior standard deviation, of .005919.

BC 8.3

```
model;
{
r~dbeta(.1,2)
# r is the recovery rate
v~dgamma(.1,.1)
theta~dbeta(1,2)
for(t in 1:20){mu[t]<-pow(1+r,t)}
Y[1,1:20]~dmnorm(mu[],tau[,])
      tau[1:20,1:20]<-inverse(Sigma[,])
            for(i in 1:20){Sigma[i,i]<-v/(1-theta*theta)}
            for(i in 1:20){for(j in i+1:20){Sigma[i,j]<-
v*pow(theta,j)*1/(1-theta*theta)}}
            for(i in 2:20){for(j in 1: i-1){Sigma[i,j]<-
v*pow(theta,i-1)*1/(1-theta*theta)}}
}
list(
Y=structure(.Dat
a=c(504,643,907,1173,1563,2083,2684,3323,4043,4803,5987,6808,8
19695,10973,12712,14553,16357,18524,20895,22650),.
Dim=c(1,20)))
list(r=1,theta=. 6, v=4)
```

TABLE 8.11

Recovery Rate of Coronavirus Patients

Parameter	Mean	SD	Error	2 1/2	Median	97 1/2
r	.02115	.04804	.001272	0	.000237	.1834
θ	1	.0000040	.000000029	1	1	1

Based on (8.62), the recovery rate is estimated with the posterior mean as .02115 with an estimated accuracy, measured by the posterior standard deviation, of .04804.

8.22 Do we Need More Tests for the Virus?

According to Cochran [12, p. 14], we indeed need more tests than we think we need. He continues "In the United States (as of 9 April 2020), President Donald Trump has said that testing for novel coronavirus infection will be limited to people who believe they may be infected." However, if we only test people who believe that they might become infected, one cannot comprehend the extent to which the virus has impacted the population. The only way this could be achieved is if those who accept that they might be infected are emblematic of the population with respect to novel virus infection. What do you believe about this? Does this follow your view?

Of course, the common property of those who believe they might be infected is that they all show common symptoms of the disease typical of the coronavirus. In summary, these people would be disproportionally displaying severe symptoms.

This is not a problem if a person would immediately become infected shows symptoms; however, this is not true. Indeed, some people develop mild cases, do not display attributes, and carry the virus with their knowledge since they do show symptoms. Therefore, efforts to comprehend the virus ability to attack the population should comprise observations of the asymptomatic.

The estimate of the proportion of the population who are infected is given by

$$\tilde{\rho} = (\text{\# of symptomatic infections} + \text{\# asymptomatic infections})/(\,(\text{\# of symptomatic infections} + \text{\# asymptomatic infections} + \text{\# not infected}).$$

This implies what is required is a random sample of the entire population in order to gather information from infected people who are displaying symptoms, infected people who are asymptomatic, and people who are not infected. All have a chance of being included in a true random sample of the population.

On April 23, leaders in Germany and New York State had moved to do random testing to find out the extent of the contagion, but other leaders resisted. This was probably because of ignorance, disregard, or lack of appreciation of statistics – a consequence of the lack of statistical literacy that pervades the general population. On the other hand, it could reflect the concern over the limited availability of tests and the want to devote all of these limited tests to those who display attributes of the disease.

But this had unintended consequences because it inadvertently helped the spread of the virus. If one does not understand the extent of the infection in the general population of its infectiousness, how does society prepare for such an event in an optimal fashion devote its resources to deal with the spread of the disease? For example, what preventive measures are appropriate and necessary? Obviously, masks and social distancing are necessary to limit the spread of the epidemic. Another important question is: how does one minimize the probability that the virus spreads to the point that it overwhelms the health care system? Also, how does one measure the progress of the system to cope with the disease?

Without the evidence, that random sampling would provide, one is essentially operating in an atmosphere of doubt and insecurity. If one is indeed operating in the dark, preventable deaths will occur, and one will continue to take ineffective measure, that do not necessarily result in an overall costly situation.

Much of the world still lacks the ability to test a large number of people, which makes even those leaders who appreciate statistical principles to test random sampling in the general population. Thus, we do indeed need more tests then we think we need. An important statistical question is just how many tests should be done, so that one had an accurate idea of the true extent of the disease?

8.23 Group Testing

Cough, fever, and difficulty breathing are all symptoms of the coronavirus; however, symptoms alone may not qualify someone to be tested for SARS-CoV-2. In the United States, only those individuals who meet strict requirements, for example, hospitalization with no pathogen detected or exposure to an individual with Covid-19, are tested because of the shortage of testing resources. According to Bilder, Iwen, Abdalhamid, Tebbs, and McMahan [13], "shortages like this worldwide, have hampered efforts to understand Covid-19 and to prevent its spread by asymptomatic individual."

In similar situations where resources are minimal, a technique known as group testing is frequently used. Its most fundamental implementation begins with finding specimens from a set number of people and then pooling parts of each specimen into a group for a special test. If the group tests negative, all members of the group are deemed negative. But, on the other hand, if the group tests positive, each member has the remainder of their original specimen tested separately to determine the positive/negative response. This process of forming groups and testing is repeated over all individuals that need to be tested. This technique was originally proposed to screen soldiers for syphilis during World War II and is often referred to as "Dorfman Testing."

When the prevalence of the disease is minimal, say less than 15%, group testing results in an important reduction in the number of tests performed.

Group testing is also used in a large variety of applications, including blood screening for infectious diseases, sexually transmitted diseases, bacterial infection of food, and compound discovery for use in the development of new pharmaceuticals. Group testing was also employed for the investigation for the influenza pandemic (H1N1) of 2009.

There are two significant considerations for applying group testing: (1) pooling specimens leads to each individual specimen being a smaller portion of the whole and (2) a group size needs to be selected. Too large a size results in too many groups that test positive, resulting in a large number of separate tests, while too small a group size results in too many group tests than required. To prevent this from happening, the average number of tests is used to determine the most efficient group size. That is to say, we want the group size that gives the smallest average number of tests if group testing was applied to a continuous stream of specimens coming into the laboratory.

The Nebraska Public Health Laboratory has led this effort among laboratories with respect to applying group testing to detect SARS-CoV-2. According to Bilder, Iwen, Abalhamid, Tebbs, and McMahan [13, p. 15, col. 3], "Their positivity rates were estimated to be 5% from initial testing specimens separately." The most efficient group size for Dorfman testing is 5 with this rate, resulting in 57% fewer tests on average than when testing specimens individually. Validation of group testing showed that pooling five specimens together did not negatively affect the detection of positive specimens with a load viral load. After six days of actual implementation, Dorfman testing resulted in 58% fewer tests than if the same number of people had been tested separately. But from another viewpoint, 137% more individuals were tested employing the same resources as would be required with separate testing.

Figure 8.3 illustrates the expected efficiency of Dorfman testing in general. The reduction in the expected number of tests grows as the disease prevalence decreases, leading to an increase in testing capacity. Especially of interest is the extremely large increase in testing capacity for very low disease prevalence. This would likely occur if the stringent requirements for individuals to be tested were lessened to allow for testing asymptomatic individuals. For example, the increase in expected testing capacity is 411% when disease prevalence is 1%.

There is a reduction in the expected number of tests for group testing algorithms. Group sizes chosen are those that minimize the expected number of tests per individual at a particular disease prevalence and for a specific algorithm. The maximum group size allowed is 40. The right-hand-side y-axis displays the expected increase in the testing capacity (see box, below) relative to the tick marks on the left-hand-side y-axis.

Other group testing algorithms can increase testing capacity even further. This occurs for three-stage hierarchical testing as shown in Figure 8.3. The algorithm is similar to Dorfman testing, but groups that test positive are split into subgroups for further testing. If any subgroup tests positive, each of its members is tested separately. Figure 8.3 also shows that array testing

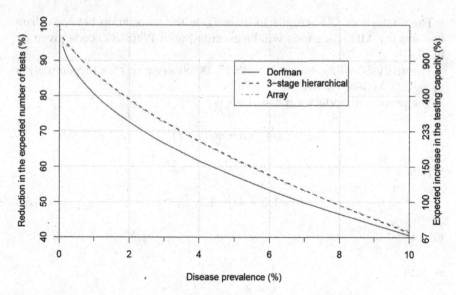

FIGURE 8.3
Reduction in Expected Number of Tests by Disease Prevalence

increases testing capacity further as well. This algorithm involves arranging specimens into a matrix-like structure, where specimens are pooled by rows and by columns to form groups. Those specimens at intersections of positive rows and columns are retested to determine disease outcome. Many other group testing algorithms exist, including those that take advantage of individual-specific probabilities of positivity to increase testing efficiency. Bilder et al. [13] provide introductions to these and other group testing algorithms.

Group testing is one component for solving our world's testing problem. Still, more testing resources are needed. Group testing could also be used to estimate SARS-CoV-2 prevalence. When test accuracy is known, statistics research has shown that prevalence estimators based on group testing data have very similar variability to those obtained through testing each specimen separately. This counterintuitive result means that a smaller number of tests can be used without loss of efficiency for the estimator itself. The research by Cochran was supported by Grant R01 AI121351 from the National Institutes of Health.

8.24 CD4 in HIV Patients

Another example of an infectious disease is now investigated, namely AIDS, which can be transmitted sexually and/or the exchange of bodily fluids.

The analysis of CD4 counts to investigate the association between drug use and the AIDS diagnosis will be executed with WinBUGS code given by BC 8.4.

The analysis will be executed with 45,000 observations for the simulation using 5,000 initial values.

The proposed model for the analysis is

$$CD4_{ij} \sim normal\left(\mu_{ij},\tau\right),$$

Where

$$i = 1, 2, 3, 4, j = 1, 2, \ldots, 80 \tag{8.63}$$

BC 8.4

```
model;
{
for(i in 1:4) {for(j in 1:80){ y[i,j]~dnorm(mu[i,j],tau)
mu[i,j]<-beta0+beta1*i+beta2*Dr[j]+beta3*A[j]}}
beta0~dnorm(0,.001)
beta1~dnorm(0,.001)
beta2~dnorm(0,.001)
beta3~dnorm(0,.001)
tau~dgamma(.001,.001)
}
list(y= structure(.Data=c(4.861,5.074,4.522,4.211,
8.39,7.577,7.644,7.871,
5.02,5.329,4.62,4.284,
1.669,1.934,1.781,.9789,
5.875,5.499,5.475,5.697,
4.855,4.311,4.615,3.573,
5.009,4.943,4.587,3.754,
6.982,6.233,4.797,4.018,
4.507,4.18,3.846,3.433,
3.179,2.876,3.558,4.156,
3.395,4.499,5.115,7.051,
7.029,6.649,7.657,7.572,
7.279,7.47,7.021,6.601,
4.963,4.99,5.022,4.549,
4.999,5.456,3.49,2.291,
```

3.838,3.522,2.55,1.231,
5.811,6.029,7.413,8.735,
3.117,3.07,2.837,2.444,
3.931,3.911,3.955,3.058,
3.768,3.072,3.273,2.595,
5.249,4.761,4.795,4.509,
3.508,3.571,4.061,3.431,
6.885,6.547,7.941,9.102,
6.087,5.795,4.418,2.234,
4.393,4.739,4.312,4.64,
5.163,5.288,5.847,5.797,
4.908,5.608,6.063,7.017,
4.684,4.093,2.583,1.705,
4.248,4.599,3.618,3.036,
4.533,5.061,5.555,6.44,
5.233,5.544,6.21,7.24,
5.397,5.29,5.278,4.885,
4.05,3.847,3.906,3.206,
3.048,4.208,2.528,.9621,
5.712,6.395,6.378,6.743,
4.4,3.713,3.403,3.388,
4.291,4.207,4.395,4.063,
4.798,5.473,6.511,7.89,
7.227,6.513,6.04,4.461,
5.592,5.841,6.062,7.343,
4.097,3.048,3.577,3.908,
5.517,5.622,5.673,5.5,
5.083,4.956,5.567,6.38,
6.318,5.933,4.87,4.488,
3.437,3.829,4.308,4.136,
6.409,6.213,6.042,5.767,
3.302,4.027,4.212,5.31,
3.328,2.649,1.756,.205,
4.528,4.871,4.883,5.355,
6.923,6.082,4.761,3.207,
5.23,5.15,6.229,7.69,
1.59,2.414,3.002,4.31,
2.444,2.27,1.976,1.378,
3.374,3.2,2.865,1.438,

```
3.263,3.829,3.009,2.309,
4.694,3.976,3.088,1.29,
4.7,4.237,4.352,2.965,
7.398,6.621,6.095,5.734,
2.608,2.688,2.154,1.738,
4.696,4.568,4.899,6.678,
4.153,3.854,3.615,3.584,
2.11,2.77,2.895,2.771,
4.709,3.969,4.887,5.687,
6.004,5.135,4.78,3.4,
3.172,4.361,5.458,6.284,
3.322,4.056,5.34,6.698,
4.837,3.382,2.703,2.181,
4.992,5.88,6.148,7.563,
4.327,4.179,5.043,5.036,
5.002,4.215,2.837,1.641,
4.019,4.56,7.055,8.903,
5.499,5.367,5.84,7.49,
5.227,5.182,6.977,5.854,
5.387,5.373,5.328,3.366,
3.481,3.107,2.557,1.874,
5.259,4.82,5.044,4.439,
3.646,4.25,4.984,6.505,
5.41,5.638,5.261,4.965,
4.4,4.322,3.845,2.321,
4.165,4.866,5.25,5.929),.Dim=c(4,80)),
     Dr=c(0,1,1,0,1,0,0,1,0,
          1,0,1,0,1,1,0,0,
          0,1,0,1,1,1,0,0,
          1,0,1,1,0,0,1,1,
          0,1,0,0,1,0,1,0,
          0,0,1,0,1,0,0,1,
          1,1,0,0,0,0,0,1,
          1,0,0,0,0,0,1,1,
          1,1,1,0,1,0,0,1,
          1,1,0,0,1,0,0),
     A=c(1,0,1,1,1,1,1,
          0,1,1,1,0,0,0,
          1,1,0,1,1,1,1,
          0,0,0,1,0,0,1,1,
```

TABLE 8.12

Posterior Analysis of AIDS Study

Parameter	Mean	SD	Error	2 1/2	Median	97 1/2
β_0	5.045	.2678	.005043	4.523	5.042	5.576
β_1	-.097	.07973	.001398	-.2548	-.0969	.05584
β_2	.1083	.1784	.001526	-.2386	.1094	.4567
β_2	-.332	.1849	.001881	-.6954	-.3325	.02629
τ	.4057	.03225	.000162	.3447	.405	.4711

The analysis implies that β_2 might be zero. A formal test of this assertion will be left as an exercise for the reader.

```
0,1,1,1,1,0,1,1,
0,0,0,1,0,0,0,1,0,
1,1,0,0,1,1,1,1,
1,1,1,0,1,1,1,0,
1,1,1,1,1,1,1,
1,1,0,1,1,1,0,1,
0,0,0))
list(beta0=.5,beta1=.5,beta2=.5,beta3=.5,tau=1)
```
The posterior analysis is reported in Table 8.12.

8.25 An Analysis of Smallpox Data

Becker [1, p. 111] analyzes data from a smallpox outbreak in the enclosed community of Abakaliki, near the south eastern part of Nigeria. This information is based on the study of Bailey and Thomas [14]. This information is summarized by 29 time intervals between the detection of cases: 13,7,2,3,0,0, 1,4,5,3,2,0,2,0,5,3,1,4,0,1,1,1,2,0,1,5,0,5,5; where the measurements are in days, and the zeroes indicate cases appearing on the same day. It seems reasonable to assume these measurements follow an exponential distribution with unknown mean λ . W now execute a Bayesian analysis with BC 8.5 using 45000 observations for the simulation and 5,000 initial values.

BC 8.5.

```
model;
{
for (i in 1:29){
```

TABLE 8.13

Posterior Distribution of Average Time Interval of Smallpox Detection

Parameter	Mean	SD	Error	2 1/2	Median	97 1/2
λ	.3816	.07087	.0003172	.2557	.3768	.5332

It is observed that the average time between adjacent detections of smallpox is estimated as .3816, via the posterior mean, while the associated posterior standard deviation is .07078.

```
y[i]~dexp(lamda)}
lamda~dgamma(.01,.01)
}
list(
y=c(13,7,2,3,0,0,1,4,5,3,2,0,2,0,5,3,1,4,0,1,1,1,2,0,1,5,0,5,5
))
list(lamda = 1)
```

The posterior analysis is reported in Table 8.13.

We continue with the analysis of smallpox data using the following information. The number of infectious individuals is I(t), the number of susceptible individuals S(t), and the number of infected is denoted by C(t). This information is displayed in Table 8.14.

TABLE 8.14

The Spread of Smallpox in a Nigerian Village

Time	I(t)	S(t)	C(t)
0	1	119	1
1	1	118	0
2	1	118	0
3	1	118	0
4	1	118	0
5	1	118	0
6	1	118	0
7	1	118	1
8	1	117	0
9	1	117	1
10	1	116	0
11	1	116	0
12	1	116	3
13	1	113	1
14	1	112	0

(Continued)

TABLE 8.14 (Continued)

Time	I(t)	S(t)	C(t)
15	1	112	0
16	1	112	0
17	1	112	1
18	1	111	0
19	1	111	0
20	1	111	0
21	1	111	0
22	1	111	1
23	2	110	0
24	2	110	0
25	2	110	1
26	5	109	0
27	6	109	2
28	5	107	0
29	5	107	2
30	4	105	0
31	5	105	0
32	5	105	0
33	2	105	0
34	1	105	1
35	1	104	0
36	2	104	0
37	2	104	1
38	1	103	1
39	2	102	0
40	2	102	0
41	4	102	0
42	4	102	2
43	5	100	1
44	5	99	1
45	5	98	1
46	5	98	1
47	4	97	2
48	3	95	1
49	3	94	0
50	1	94	0
51	2	94	0
52	3	94	0
53	3	94	2
54	3	92	0
55	2	92	0

(Continued)

TABLE 8.14 (Continued)

Time	I(t)	S(t)	C(t)
56	4	92	0
57	5	92	0
58	5	92	1
59	5	91	0
60	5	91	0
61	7	91	0
62	8	91	0
63	6	91	1
64	5	90	0
65	4	90	0
66	3	90	0
67	5	90	0
68	3	90	0
69	2	90	0
70	2	90	0
71	2	90	0
72	3	90	9
73	3	90	0
74	1	90	0
75	1	90	0
76	1	90	0
77	2	90	0
78	2	90	0
79	1	90	0
80	1	90	0
81	1	90	0
82	1	90	0
83	1	90	0

Source: Table 6.1 of Becker [1, p. 113–114]

Assume the number of infected individuals follows a Poisson distribution with mean $\exp[\mu + \alpha I(t) + \beta S(t)]$, that is to say

$$C(t) \sim Poisson\left\{\exp\left[\mu + \alpha I(t) + \beta S(t)\right]\right\}, t = 1, 2 \ldots \tag{8.64}$$

Using the data of Table 8.15 and the model specified by (8.64), the Bayesian analysis is executed with BC 8.6 with 160,000 observations for the simulation and 5,000 initial values.

BC 8.6

```
model;
{
for (t in 1:83){
C[t]~dpois(lamda[t])
lamda[t]<-exp(mu+alpha*I[t]+beta*S[t])}
mu~dnorm(0,.001)
alpha~dnorm(0,.001)
beta~dnorm(0,.001)
}
list(C=c(0,0,0,0,0,0,0,1,0,1,0,0,3,1,0,0,0,1,0,0,0,0,1,0,0,1,0,
2,0,2,0,0,0,0,1,0,0,1,1,0,0,0,2,1,1,1,0,2,1,0,0,0,0,2,0,0,0,0,
00,0,1,0,0,0,0,1,0,0,0,0,0,0,0,0,0,0,0,0,0,0,0,0,0,0,0,0),
S=c(118,118,118,118,118,118,118,117,117,116,
116,116,112,112,112,112,111,111,111,111,111,110,
110,110,109,109,107,107,105,105,105,105,105,104,
104,104,103,102,102,102,102,100,99,98,97,97,95,
94,94,94,94,94,92,92,92,92,92,91,91,91,91,91,90,90,
90,90,90,90,90,90,90,90,90,90,90,90,90,90,90,90,90,
90,90),
I= c(1,1,1,1,1,1,1,1,1,1,1,1,1,1,1,1,1,1,1,1,1,1,1,2,2,2,5,
6,5,5,4,5,5,2,1,1,2,2,1,2,2,4,4,5,5,5,4,4,3,3,1,2,3,3,
3,2,4,5,5,5,5,7,8,6,5,4,3,5,3,2,2,2,3,3,1,1,1,2,2,1,
1,1,1,1,1))
list(mu=10, alpha=3,beta= -2)
```

The posterior analysis is reported in Table 8.15.

TABLE 8.15

Bayesian Inferences for Smallpox in Nigerian Village

Parameter	Mean	SD	Error	2 1/2	Median	97 1/2
α	.04952	0.2	.009651	−.1847	.04375	.2372
β	−.5425	0.2703	.01363	−.9664	−.5322	−.1676
μ	48.86	24.17	1.218	14.63	48.02	89.33

The posterior distributions appear to be symmetric, and as expected, the number of susceptible individuals has a negative effect on the number of infected individuals.

8.26 Respiratory Disease Data

The respiratory disease data on the island of Tristan da Cunha was collected by British medical officers of the British Medical Research Council in October/November of 1967. The infectious period of each individual is taken to be the group of days on which the individual displayed symptoms. It is assumed the infection occurred one day before symptoms appear. In the study by Becker and Hopper [15], it was deemed reasonable to assume that all natives of the island were initially susceptible.

Under these restrictions, one would be able to trace the number of susceptible individuals and the number of infectious individuals on a daily basis. Becker and Hopper [15] found a significant difference between the within-household infection rate and the between-household infection rate. Also determined was some heterogeneity in the infection rates for different age groups. Based on the results of Becker and Hopper, three age groups were defined as follows: infants from 0-4 years, school children from 5-16, and the rest over 16 years as adults. In Table 8.17, the age groups are designated as 1,2, and 3 respectively. The number of infectious individuals in each age group is recorded.

The data of this epidemic are shown in Table 8.17, where the first column gives the day as measured from the first day on which there is one infectious individual. Column 2 gives the age group, and the third the number of susceptible individuals of that age group who are exposed to IW1 infectious infants, IW2 infectious school children, and IW3 infectious adults within the same household, as well as IB1 infectious infants, IB2 infectious school children, and IB3 infectious adults from other household. It is indeed necessary to explain the notation that IW1 infectious individuals of age group 1 are responsible for within-household infections, whereas IB2 infectious individuals of age group 2 are responsible for between-household infections. Note that the last column of Table 8.17 gives for each row the number of susceptible people who are infected on that day. Of course, these are cases.

We now explain in more detail the entries of Table 8.17 corresponding to the first day. Row one indicates there were 27 susceptible infants in the community who were exposed to just one infectious adult, and that this infected individual was from another household and that none of these infants became infected on that particular day. Rows 2 and 3 indicate that 38 school children and 183 adults were exposed in a similar way and none of them were infected on that day. Rows 4 and 5 indicate that two susceptible school children and four susceptible adults, respectively, are exposed to just one infectious adult, that this infective was a member of their own household and that none of the susceptible individuals became infected on that day. That is to say, there was only one infectious person on day one, this individual was a member of the household containing four other adults, two children, and zero infants. For day 7, there are no entries, because due to the assumptions and the data, there are no infectious individuals, so no cases can occur on that day. By far, Table 8.16 has data that are extremely detailed, not seen up to this point.

TABLE 8.16

The Spread of Respiratory Disease on Tristan da Cunha

Day	Age	S	IW1	IW2	IW3	IB1	IB2	IB3	C
1	1	27	0	0	0	0	0	1	0
1	2	38	0	0	0	0	0	1	0
1	3	183	0	0	0	0	0	1	0
1	2	2	0	0	0	0	0	0	0
1	3	4	0	0	1	0	0	0	0
2	1	27	0	0	0	0	0	1	0
2	2	38	0	0	0	0	0	1	0
2	3	183	0	0	0	0	0	1	0
2	2	2	0	0	1	0	0	0	0
2	3	4	0	0	1	0	0	0	0
3	1	27	0	0	0	0	0	1	0
3	2	38	0	0	0	0	0	1	0
3	3	183	0	0	0	0	0	1	0
3	2	2	0	0	1	0	0	0	0
3	3	4	0	0	1	0	0	0	0
4	1	27	0	0	0	0	0	1	0
4	2	38	0	0	0	0	0	1	0
4	3	183	0	0	0	0	0	1	0
4	2	2	0	0	1	0	0	0	0
4	3	4	0	0	1	0	0	0	0
5	1	27	0	0	0	0	0	1	0
5	2	38	0	0	0	0	0	1	0
5	3	183	0	0	0	0	0	1	0
5	2	2	0	0	1	0	0	0	0
5	3	4	0	0	1	0	0	0	0
6	1	27	0	0	0	0	0	1	0
6	2	38	0	0	0	0	0	1	0

(Continued)

TABLE 8.16 (Continued)

Day	Age	S	IW1	IW2	IW3	IB1	IB2	IB3	C
6	3	183	0	0	0	0	0	1	0
6	2	2	0	0	1	0	0	0	0
6	3	4	0	0	1	0	0	0	0
8	1	25	0	0	0	0	0	1	0
8	2	40	0	0	0	0	0	1	0
8	3	185	0	0	0	0	0	1	0
8	1	2	0	0	1	0	0	0	0
8	3	1	0	0	1	0	0	0	0
9	1	25	0	0	0	0	0	1	2
9	2	39	0	0	0	0	0	1	1
9	3	184	0	0	0	0	0	1	0
9	1	2	0	0	1	0	0	0	0
9	3	1	0	0	1	0	0	0	1
10	1	22	0	0	0	0	1	2	1
10	2	37	0	0	0	0	1	2	1
10	3	178	0	0	0	0	1	2	1
10	1	1	0	0	1	0	0	1	1
10	3	1	0	0	1	0	1	1	0
10	2	1	0	1	0	0	0	2	0
10	3	4	0	1	0	0	0	2	0
10	1	1	0	0	1	0	1	1	0
10	3	2	0	0	1	0	1	1	0
11	1	21	0	0	0	3	2	2	3
11	2	34	0	0	0	3	2	2	0
11	3	167	0	0	0	3	2	2	1
11	3	1	1	0	1	2	2	1	1
11	2	1	0	1	0	3	1	2	0
11	3	4	0	1	0	3	1	2	1
11	2	1	0	1	0	3	1	2	0
11	3	4	0	1	0	3	1	2	1
11	1	1	0	0	1	3	2	1	0
11	3	2	0	0	1	3	2	1	0
11	2	1	0	1	0	3	1	2	0
11	3	3	0	1	0	3	1	2	0
11	2	1	1	0	0	2	2	2	0
11	3	3	1	0	0	2	2	2	0
11	3	4	1	0	0	2	2	2	0
12	1	17	0	0	0	5	3	3	0
12	2	34	0	0	0	5	3	3	0
12	3	162	0	0	0	5	3	3	0
12	2	1	0	1	0	5	2	3	0
12	3	3	0	1	0	5	2	3	0

(Continued)

TABLE 8.16 (Continued)

Day	Age	S	IW1	IW2	IW3	IB1	IB2	IB3	C
12	1	1	0	0	1	5	3	2	0
12	3	2	0	0	1	5	3	2	0
12	2	1	0	1	0	5	2	3	0
12	3	3	0	1	0	5	2	3	0
12	2	1	1	0	0	4	3	3	0
12	3	3	1	0	0	4	3	3	0
12	3	4	1	0	0	4	3	3	0
12	3	1	0	1	0	5	2	3	0
12	1	1	0	0	1	5	3	2	0
12	3	2	0	0	1	5	3	2	0
12	3	1	1	0	0	4	3	3	0
13	1	18	0	0	0	6	2	4	1
13	2	35	0	0	0	6	2	4	0
13	3	169	0	0	0	6	2	4	0
13	2	1	0	1	1	6	1	3	1
13	3	3	0	1	1	6	1	3	0
13	3	1	1	0	0	5	2	4	0
13	1	1	0	0	1	6	2	3	1
13	3	2	0	0	1	6	2	3	0
14	1	17	0	0	0	5	2	4	0
14	2	35	0	0	0	5	2	4	3
14	3	169	0	0	0	5	2	4	3
14	3	3	0	1	1	5	1	3	1
14	2	1	1	0	0	4	2	4	0
14	3	3	1	0	0	4	2	4	0
14	3	1	0	1	0	5	1	4	0
14	3	2	0	0	1	5	2	3	0
14	3	1	2	0	1	3	2	3	0
14	3	2	2	0	0	3	2	4	0
15	1	17	0	0	0	5	3	4	0
15	2	34	0	0	0	5	3	4	0
15	3	164	0	0	0	5	3	4	1
15	3	2	0	2	1	5	1	3	0
15	3	2	1	0	0	4	3	4	0
15	2	1	1	0	0	4	3	4	0
15	3	3	1	0	0	4	3	4	0
15	3	1	0	1	0	5	2	4	0
15	3	2	1	0	1	4	3	3	0
15	3	1	1	0	1	4	3	3	0
15	3	2	1	0	1	4	3	3	0
15	3	1	1	0	1	4	3	3	0
15	3	2	1	0	0	4	3	4	0

(Continued)

TABLE 8.16 (Continued)

Day	Age	S	IW1	IW2	IW3	IB1	IB2	IB3	C
16	1	17	0	0	0	4	4	7	0
16	2	29	0	0	0	4	4	7	1
16	3	150	0	0	0	4	4	7	1
16	3	2	0	2	2	4	2	5	0
16	3	2	1	0	0	3	4	7	0
16	2	1	0	0	1	4	4	6	0
16	3	4	0	0	1	4	4	6	0
16	2	1	1	0	0	3	4	7	0
16	3	4	0	0	1	4	4	6	0
16	2	1	1	0	0	3	4	4	6
16	3	3	1	0	0	3	4	7	0
16	2	1	0	1	0	4	3	7	0
16	3	4	0	1	0	4	3	7	0
16	3	1	0	1	0	4	3	7	0
16	3	2	1	0	0	3	4	7	0
16	3	1	1	0	1	3	4	6	0
16	3	3	0	0	1	4	4	6	0
16	2	3	0	0	1	4	4	6	0
16	3	4	0	0	1	4	4	6	0
17	1	17	0	0	0	3	4	7	0
17	2	28	0	0	0	3	4	7	0
17	3	149	0	0	0	3	4	7	2
17	3	2	0	2	2	3	2	5	0
17	3	2	1	0	0	2	4	7	0
17	2	1	0	0	1	3	4	6	0
17	3	4	0	0	1	3	4	6	0
17	2	1	1	0	0	2	4	7	0
17	3	3	1	0	0	2	4	7	1
17	2	1	0	1	0	3	3	7	0
17	3	4	0	1	0	3	3	7	0
17	2	1	1	0	0	2	4	7	0
17	3	3	1	0	0	2	4	7	1
17	2	1	0	1	0	3	3	7	0
17	3	4	0	1	0	3	3	7	0
17	3	1	0	1	0	3	3	7	0
17	3	1	1	0	1	2	4	6	0
17	3	2	0	0	1	3	4	6	0
17	3	3	0	0	1	3	4	6	0
17	2	3	0	0	1	3	4	6	0
17	3	4	0	0	1	3	4	6	0
18	1	17	0	0	0	3	5	8	0
18	2	28	0	0	0	3	5	8	0

(Continued)

TABLE 8.16 (Continued)

Day	Age	S	IW1	IW2	IW3	IB1	IB2	IB3	C
18	3	142	0	0	0	3	5	8	1
18	3	2	0	0	1	3	5	7	0
18	3	2	0	2	2	3	3	6	0
18	3	2	1	0	0	2	5	8	0
18	2	1	0	0	1	3	5	7	0
18	3	4	0	0	1	3	5	7	0
18	2	1	1	0	0	2	5	8	0
18	3	2	1	0	0	2	5	8	0
18	2	1	0	1	0	3	4	8	0
18	3	4	0	1	0	3	4	8	0
18	3	1	0	1	0	3	4	8	0
18	3	3	0	1	0	3	4	8	0
18	3	1	1	0	1	2	5	7	0
18	3	2	0	0	1	3	5	7	0
18	3	3	0	0	1	3	5	7	1
18	2	3	0	0	1	3	5	7	0
18	3	4	0	0	1	3	5	7	0
19	1	17	0	0	0	3	4	9	0
19	2	30	0	0	0	3	4	9	0
19	3	150	0	0	0	3	4	9	0
19	3	2	0	0	1	3	4	8	0
19	3	2	0	2	2	3	2	7	1
19	3	2	1	0	0	2	4	9	0
19	2	1	1	0	1	2	4	8	0
19	3	2	1	0	1	2	4	8	0
19	3	1	0	1	0	3	3	9	0
19	3	3	0	1	0	3	3	9	0
19	3	1	1	0	1	2	4	8	0
19	3	2	0	0	1	3	4	8	0
19	2	3	0	0	1	3	4	8	0
19	3	4	0	0	1	3	4	8	0
19	3	1	0	0	2	3	4	7	0
20	1	17	0	0	0	3	3	11	0
20	2	30	0	0	0	3	3	11	0
20	3	147	0	0	0	3	3	11	1
20	3	2	0	0	1	3	3	10	0
20	3	1	0	2	2	3	1	9	0
20	3	2	1	0	0	2	3	11	0
20	3	2	0	0	1	3	3	10	0
20	2	1	1	0	1	2	3	10	0
20	3	2	1	0	1	2	3	10	0
20	3	2	0	0	1	3	3	10	0

(Continued)

TABLE 8.16 (Continued)

Day	Age	S	IW1	IW2	IW3	IB1	IB2	IB3	C
20	3	3	0	1	0	3	2	11	0
20	3	1	1	0	1	2	3	10	0
20	3	2	0	0	1	3	3	10	0
20	2	3	0	0	1	3	3	10	0
20	3	4	0	0	1	3	3	10	0
20	3	1	0	0	2	3	3	9	1
21	1	17	0	0	0	0	2	7	0
21	2	33	0	0	0	0	2	7	0
21	3	155	0	0	0	0	2	7	0
21	3	1	0	1	1	0	1	6	0
21	3	2	0	0	1	0	2	6	0
21	2	1	0	0	1	0	2	6	0
21	3	2	0	0	1	0	2	6	0
21	3	2	0	0	1	0	2	6	0
21	3	3	0	1	0	0	1	7	0
21	3	2	0	0	1	0	2	6	0
22	1	17	0	0	0	0	1	5	0
22	2	34	0	0	0	0	1	5	0
22	3	157	0	0	0	0	1	5	0
22	3	2	0	0	1	0	1	4	0
22	3	1	0	0	1	0	1	4	0
22	3	2	0	0	1	0	1	4	0
22	3	2	0	0	1	0	1	4	0
22	3	3	0	1	0	0	0	5	0
23	1	17	0	0	0	0	1	5	0
23	2	34	0	0	0	0	1	5	0
23	3	157	0	0	0	0	1	5	0
23	3	2	0	0	1	0	1	4	0
23	3	1	0	0	1	0	1	4	0
23	3	2	0	0	1	0	13	4	0
23	3	2	0	0	1	0	1	4	0
24	1	17	0	0	0	0	1	3	0
24	2	34	0	0	0	0	1	3	0
24	3	161	0	0	0	0	1	3	0
24	3	2	0	0	1	0	1	2	0
24	3	1	0	0	1	0	1	2	0
24	3	3	0	1	0	0	0	3	0
25	1	17	0	0	0	0	1	2	0
25	2	34	0	0	0	0	1	2	0
25	3	162	0	0	0	0	1	2	0
25	3	2	0	0	1	0	1	1	0
25	3	3	0	1	0	0	0	2	0

(Continued)

TABLE 8.16 (Continued)

Day	Age	S	IW1	IW2	IW3	IB1	IB2	IB3	C
26	1	17	0	0	0	0	0	1	0
26	2	34	0	0	0	0	0	1	0
26	3	165	0	0	0	0	0	1	0
26	3	2	0	0	1	0	0	0	0
27	1	17	0	0	0	0	0	1	0
27	2	34	0	0	0	0	0	1	0
27	3	165	0	0	8	0	0	1	0
27	3	2	0	0	1	0	0	0	0
28	1	17	0	0	0	0	0	1	0
28	2	34	0	0	0	0	0	1	0
28	3	164	0	0	0	0	0	1	1
28	3	2	0	0	1	0	0	0	0
29	1	17	0	0	0	0	0	2	0
29	2	32	0	0	0	0	0	2	0
29	3	160	0	0	0	0	0	2	0
29	3	2	0	0	1	0	0	1	0
29	2	2	0	0	1	0	0	1	0
29	3	3	0	0	1	0	0	1	0
30	1	17	0	0	0	0	0	2	0
30	2	32	0	0	0	0	0	2	0
30	3	160	0	0	0	0	0	2	0
30	2	2	0	0	1	0	0	1	0
30	3	3	0	0	1	0	0	1	0
30	3	2	0	0	1	0	0	1	0
31	1	17	0	0	0	0	0	2	0
31	2	32	0	0	0	0	0	2	0
31	3	160	0	0	0	0	0	2	0
31	2	2	0	0	1	0	0	1	0
31	3	3	0	0	1	0	0	1	0
31	3	2	0	0	1	0	0	1	0
32	1	17	0	0	0	0	0	2	0
32	2	32	0	0	0	0	0	2	0
32	3	160	0	0	0	0	0	2	0
32	2	2	0	0	1	0	0	1	0
32	3	3	0	0	1	0	0	1	0
32	3	2	0	0	1	0	0	1	0
33	1	17	0	0	0	0	0	1	0
33	2	34	0	0	0	0	0	1	0
33	3	163	0	0	0	0	0	1	0
33	3	2	0	0	1	0	0	0	0

Source: Table 6.2 of Becker [1, pp. 121–131]

8.27 Bayesian Analysis of Respiratory Disease Information

We assume that the rows of Table 8.17 are independent and that the number of susceptible individuals have a binomial distribution, that is, in general, S has a binomial distribution with density

$$f(s|\theta) \propto \theta^s (1-\theta)^{n-s}, 0 < s < 1, s = 0,1,2,\ldots,n \tag{8.65}$$

Thus, assuming a uniform prior for θ, gives via Bayes theorem a beta distribution with parameter vector (s+1.n-s+1).

Now consider the first row of Table 8.17, where S has a binomial distribution with parameter vector (27,1), thus assuming a uniform prior, the posterior distribution of θ is beta with parameter vector (28,2).

The WinBUGS code below executes the posterior analysis for the proportion of susceptible individuals of the first row Table 8.17. The list statement contains values generated from a binomial distribution with parameter vector(27,1).

BC 8.7

```
model;
{
for(i in 1:35) { y[i]~dbin(p,28)}
p~dbeta(0.1,1.1)
}
list(
y = c(
27.0,28.0,28.0,28.0,27.0,
28.0,27.0,28.0,28.0,26.0,
27.0,28.0,28.0,28.0,28.0,
28.0,26.0,28.0,26.0,27.0,
27.0,28.0,28.0,28.0,28.0,
27.0,26.0,25.0,26.0,28.0,
28.0,27.0,28.0,27.0,27.0))
```

The WinBUGS code below generates 35 values from the beta (28, 20) posterior distribution of the proportion of susceptible people in the first row of Table 8.1.

TABLE 8.17

Posterior Analysis for the Respiratory Disease Data

Parameter	Mean	SD	Error	2 1/2	Median	97 1/2
A	.9714	.02783	.0002402	.8973	.9789	.9993
B	1.016	.01585	.0001361	1	1.059	1.059

It is seen that the posterior medians for the endpoints are .8973 and 1.059, respectively, which seems reasonable in light of the data.

BC 8.9

```
model;
{
for(i in 1:35) {y[i]~dbeta(28,2)}
p~dbeta(0.1,1.1)
}
```

The values below are the 35 observations generated from the beta(28,2) distribution, the posterior distribution of the proportion p of susceptible individuals in the first row of Table 8.17. This assumes a uniform prior distribution for p.

```
list(
y = c(
0.9551,0.9163,0.9631,0.8759,0.9146,
0.8292,0.9638,0.8644,0.9613,0.9476,
0.9661,0.93,0.9419,0.8815,0.9135,
0.8678,0.8853,0.9263,0.9678,0.9465,
0.9545,0.9337,0.946,0.9482,0.9366,
0.8827,0.8874,0.9191,0.9585,0.9402,
0.9118,0.8462,0.9686,0.9497,0.9734))
```

Of course, it follows that the same above procedure is applicable for the remaining rows of Table 8.16.

We now estimate the values of a and b, the endpoints of the beta distribution of the respiratory values of the first row of Table 8.16.

BC 8.10

```
model;
{
for(i in 1:35) {y[i]~dbeta(a,b)}
a~dunif(0,1)
b~dunif(1,2)
}
list(
y = c(
     0.9551,0.9163,0.9631,0.8759,0.9146,
     0.8292,0.9638,0.8644,0.9613,0.9476,
     0.9661,0.93,0.9419,0.8815,0.9135,
     0.8678,0.8853,0.9263,0.9678,0.9465,
     0.9545,0.9337,0.946,0.9482,0.9366,
     0.8827,0.8874,0.9191,0.9585,0.9402,
     0.9118,0.8462,0.9686,0.9497,0.9734))
list(a=.9,b=1)
```

The posterior analysis is reported in Table 8.17. The Bayesian analysis is executed with 45,000 observations for the simulation and 5,000 initial values.

8.28 Comments and Conclusions

The chapter begins with an explanation of the epidemic threshold theorem and the basic characteristics of an epidemic. The chapter continues the chain binomial representation of an epidemic and how to estimate the size of an epidemic. Does one know the final size of the coronavirus? Some of these ideas are illustrated with the common cold and how it spreads in households of size three, four, and five individuals, assuming that one individual initially is infectious, and the remaining are susceptible. Also introduced are generalized linear models that model the behavior such as its latent and infectiousness periods. Several examples of contagion are explored, including households of size two for measle epidemics, which is analyzed with the Bayesian approach, for households of size two. Epidemics often exhibit explosive exponential growth and the rate of growth is estimated via Bayesian methods, which is implemented with MCMC simulations. Three questions are now asked: (a) do we need more tests? (b) can group testing be done? and (c) how accurate is the test for the coronavirus? A thorough analysis of HIV patients is accomplished using as the main endpoint the CD4 counts of AIDS patients. Two examples of smallpox are explored: one for a small population where the interval between successive infections is estimated using the exponential distribution as the model and Bayesian methods that determine the posterior distribution of the exponential parameter. The other example is for a large population enveloped in a smallpox epidemic. The last example of an epidemic is that of a respiratory ailment in a large population. See Bailey [16] for additional information about epidemics.

8.29 Exercises

1. Describe the implications of the epidemic threshold theorem.

2. Estimate the value of μ of the epidemic threshold theorem for the coronavirus epidemic in the United States over the period from January 1 to August 30 of 2020.

3. Refer to (8.7) and describe the evolution of an epidemic and describe the epidemic chain model for households of size two.

4. Derive the posterior distribution for the size of an epidemic given by (8.14). Note the improper prior density (8.13) was used.

5. Refer to the second row of Table 8.3 and derive the posterior distribution given by equation (8.14).

6. Carefully explain how equation (8.42) defines the epidemic chain $1 \rightarrow 1 \rightarrow 2$.

7. Based on the information of Table 8.7, derive the posterior density of the cell probabilities appearing in that table.

8. Refer to Table 8.8 and explain how equation (8.62) is used to generate the entries in Table 8.8.

9. Using the WinBUGS code BC 8.1, determine the posterior distribution of the rate r at which the coronavirus is expanding in the United States over the period from January 1 to August 30 of 2020.

10. Based on BC 8.2, execute a Bayesian analysis to estimate the mortality rate of the coronavirus. Use 50,000 observations for the simulation with 5,000 initial values. Your results should be similar to Table 8.11.

11. Refer to BC 8.3 and via a Bayesian analysis, estimate the recovery rate from the coronavirus. Use 45,000 observations for the simulation with 5,000 initial values.

12. Briefly summarize section 8.22 which explains group testing. Also, carefully explain how Figure 8.3 was produced.

13. Refer to equation (8.63)), the model for the CD4 counts of AIDS patients. Execute the posterior analysis with BC 8.4 to estimate the unknown parameters of the model (8.63)). Are your results similar to mine, given by Table 8.12?

14. Refer to section 8.26 and the smallpox example, where the focus in on the interval between successive cases of the disease. Using BC 8.5 estimates the average length of the interval. Note this assumes the intervals follow an exponential distribution. Employ 45,000 observations for the simulation with 5,000 initial values. What prior distribution for the parameter of the exponential distribution did you use? Your results should be similar to Table 8.13.

15. Refer to Table 8.14 which provides information about a smallpox epidemic in a small Nigerian town. Based on the Poisson model (8.64), that enumerates the number of infected, use BC 8.6 to estimate the unknown coefficients of the model. Use 160,000 observations for the simulation with 5,000 initial values. Your results should be similar to mine displayed in Table 8.15.

16. Use the first row of Table 8.16 as data and execute BC 8.8 to estimate the parameter θ of the model (8.65). Utilize 45,000 observations for the simulation and 5,000 initial values.

17. Refer to equation (8.16) for the posterior density of θ_i, $i = 1, 2, 3, 4$, and to (8.17) for the posterior distribution of ϕ_i, $i = 1, 2, 3, 4$, test the hypothesis

    $H : \theta_i = \phi_i$, $i = 1, 2, 3, 4$, versus the alternative $A : \theta_i \neq \phi_i$ for at least one I, i = 1,2,3,4. Let $\pi_0 = \pi_1$, where $\pi_0 = \frac{1}{2}$ is the prior probability of the null hypothesis.

    Refer to Lee [10, pp. 126–128] on how to conduct a formal Bayesian test of H versus A.

References

1. Becker, N.G. (1989). *Analysis of Infected Diseases and Hall*. Chapman and Hall. London, UK.
2. Horowitz, O., Grunfeld, K., Lysgaard-Hansen, B., and Kjeldsen, K. (1974). The epidemiology and natural history of measles in Denmark. *Am. J. Epidemiology* 20009100, 136–149.
3. Lane, J.M., Miller, J.D., and Neff, J.M. (1971). Smallpox and smallpox vaccination policy. *Ann. Rev. Medicine* 22, 251–272.
4. Miller, C.L. and Pollock, T.M. (1874). Whooping-cough vaccinations-an assessment. *Lancet* 11, 510–513.
5. Box, G.E.P. (1976). Science and statistics. *J. Am. Stat. Soc.* 71(356), 791–799.

6. Bartlett, M.S. (1949). Some evolutionary stochastic processes. *J. R. Stat. Soc. B.* 11, 211–229.
7. Whittle, P. (1955). The outcome of a stochastic epidemic. -a note on Bailey's paper. *Biometrika*, 42, 116–122.
8. Becker, N.G. (1977). On a general epidemic model. *Theor. Pop. Biol* 11, 23–26.
9. DeGroot, M. (1970). *Optimal Statistical Decisions*. McGraw-Hill Book Company New York, NY.
10. Lee, P.M. (1997). *Bāyesian Statistics, 2nd Edition*. Arnold, A member of the Hodder Headline Group. John Wiley & Sons Inc. New York, NY.
11. Heasman, M.A. and Reid, D.D. (1961). Theory and observation in family epidemics of the common cold. *Brit. J. Prev. Soc. Med.* 15, 12–16.
12. Cochran, J.J. (2020). Why we need more coronavirus tests than we think we need. *Significance* 17(3), 14.
13. Bilder, R.C., Iwen, P.C., Abdalhamild, B., Tebbs, J.M., and McMahan, C.S. (2020). Tests in short supply? Try group testing. *Significance* 17(3), 15.
14. Bailey, N.T.J. and Thomas, A.S. (1971). The estimation of parameters from population data on the general stochastic epidemic. *Theor. Pop. Biol.* 2, 53–70.
15. Becker, N.G. and Hopper, J.L. (1983). Assessing the heterogeneity of disease spread through a community. *Am. J. Epidemiology* 117, 362–374.
16. Bailey, N.T.J. (1975). *The Mathematical Theory of Infectious Diseases and its Applications*. Griffin Publishers. London, UK. Issue 3: 18–20.

Index

Page numbers in *italic* indicate figures. Page numbers in **bold** indicate tables.

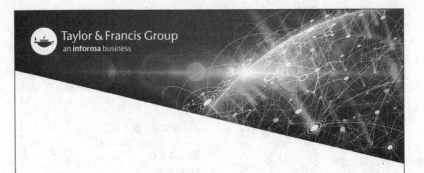

Printed in the United States
By Bookmasters